T0134959

Advances in Non-Invasive Biomedical Signal Sensing and Processing with Machine Learning

Saeed Mian Qaisar
Humaira Nisar • Abdulhamit Subasi
Editors

Advances in Non-Invasive Biomedical Signal Sensing and Processing with Machine Learning

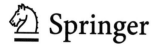 Springer

Editors
Saeed Mian Qaisar
Electrical and Computer Engineering
Department
Effat University
Jeddah, Saudi Arabia

Humaira Nisar
Department of Electronic Engineering
Faculty of Engineering and Green
Technology
Universiti Tunku Abdul Rahman
Kampar, Malaysia

Abdulhamit Subasi
Institute of Biomedicine
Faculty of Medicine
University of Turku
Turku, Finland

ISBN 978-3-031-23241-1   ISBN 978-3-031-23239-8   (eBook)
https://doi.org/10.1007/978-3-031-23239-8

This Springer imprint is published by the registered company Springer Nature Switzerland AG
The registered company address is: Gewerbestrasse 11, 6330 Cham, Switzerland

Foreword

The biomedical signal processing landscape has been enriched by recent advances in machine learning yielding new trends for non-invasive signal estimation, classification, prediction, and manipulation. This is the result of the ever-increasing global demand for affordable healthcare services. The integration of biomedical signal processing and machine learning will have a profound impact on the healthcare scenario around the world. The new technology has the capability to empower humankind to solve the challenges the world is facing towards healthcare by having better, timely, and cost-effective diagnosis and at the same time reaching out to remote parts of the world owing to the non invasive methods of signal sensing and processing.

With the advance in technology, high computation is not a problem. The biomedical signals carry rich and diverse physiological information which can be used to develop new techniques to aid in the prognosis and diagnosis as well as surveillance and treatment of diseases that human beings are suffering from. The field of artificial intelligence (AI) can be found everywhere. A plethora of innovations in AI have occurred as the result of ongoing advances in data acquisition, processing power, cloud computing infra structure, and machine learning. Combining the sheer interest of researchers to pursue research related to biomedical field with the budding potential of machine learning systems, complex problems can be addressed, and this has opened new pathways in healthcare by re-inventing the processes to boost productivity and accuracy as well as maximizing efficacy, decreasing time spent and resources to focus on customized healthcare.

The recent advances in signal sensing and processing and its integration with machine learning are expected to nurture the biomedical research. Hence, the purpose of this work is to highlight the integration of signal sensing and processing with machine learning for high-quality affordable and accessible healthcare to everyone.

President, Universiti Tunku Abdul Rahman   Ir. Prof. Dato' Dr. Ewe Hong Tat
Kampar, Malaysia
18 October 2022

Preface

This book presents the modern technological advancements and revolutions in the biomedical sector. Progress in the contemporary sensing, Internet of Things (IoT), and machine learning algorithms and architectures has introduced new approaches in mobile healthcare. A continuous observation of patients with critical health situation is required. It allows monitoring of their health status during daily-life activities such as during sports, walking and sleeping. Grace of modern IoT framework and wireless biomedical implants, such as smartphones, smartwatches, and belts, it is realizable. Such solutions are currently under development and in testing phases by healthcare and governmental institutions, research laboratories and biomedical companies. The biomedical signals such as electrocardiogram (ECG), electroencephalogram (EEG), electromyography (EMG), phonocardiogram (PCG), chronic obstructive pulmonary (COP) and electrooculography (EoG), photoplethysmography (PPG), positron emission tomography (PET), magnetic resonance imaging (MRI), and computerized tomography (CT) are non-invasively acquired, measured, and processed via the biomedical sensors and gadgets. These signals and images represent the activities and conditions of human cardiovascular, neural, vision and cerebral systems. Multi-channel sensing of these signals and images with an appropriate granularity is required for an effective monitoring and diagnosis. It renders a big volume of data, and its analysis is not feasible manually. Therefore, automated healthcare systems are in the process of evolution. These systems are mainly based on biomedical signals and images acquisition and sensing, preconditioning, features extraction, and classification stages. The contemporary biomedical signal sensing, preconditioning, features extraction, and intelligent machine and deep learning–based classification algorithms are described.

Each chapter starts with the importance, problem statement and motivation. A self-sufficient description is provided. Therefore, each chapter can be read independently by postgraduate students, postdoctoral researchers, engineers and faculty members in the fields of biomedical engineering, health sciences, neural engineering as well as neuropsychology, biomedical image processing, brain computer interaction and automated health diagnosis systems.

In Chap. 1, an overview of non-invasive biomedical signals and images is presented. A comparison between the invasive and non-invasive procedures is also made. The potential applications of non-invasive biomedical signals and images, in the biomedical sector, are also presented.

The procedures for collecting biological signals and extracting features are covered in Chap. 2. It explains the preprocessing and analogue to digital conversion concepts. In addition, a variety of potential feature extraction approaches that are frequently used by researchers for the biomedical signals are also described.

Chapter 3 shows the use of non-invasive EEG readings to spotlight the cerebral activity of depressed individuals. In this framework, the related studies are reviewed. The chapter covers the potential EEG signal collecting protocols, augmentation algorithms, feature extraction methods (both linear and non-linear) and classifier models.

Chapter 4 describes an automated method for the categorization of motor imagery tasks in the context of brain-comp interface. The proposed approach is an effective hybridization of the classification, signal decomposition, feature mining and dimension reduction. The wavelet decomposition is used for sub-bands extraction. A variety of time-frequency features are mined from sub-bands, and dimension reduction is attained with the butterfly optimization. The categorization is carried out by using the machine learning algorithms. It is mentioned that the outcomes of classifier could be used to assist the disabled people by controlling the assistive devices.

In Chap. 5, the authors discuss the development and present state of electrocardiography-based heart failure screening. In the framework of the 4th generation of ECG analysis, the clinical practices of utilizing remote ECG recording devices, data processing and transformation are covered. The use of contemporary machine learning techniques has been highlighted for an automated cardiac system anomaly identification.

The authors describe a comparative analysis of two machine learning–based classifiers for the hand gestures identification in Chap. 6. The intended surface EMG (sEMG) signals are analysed by wavelet decomposition for feature mining. Afterwards, the extracted feature set is processed by the support vector machine and k-nearest neighbour classifiers. Different measures are used for the performance comparison which include F1 score, accuracy, precision and Kappa index.

Chapter 7 gives an overview of machine learning and deep learning techniques for classifying the EEG signals in clinical applications. Additionally, two case studies for the identification of epilepsy and schizophrenia are covered. These studies employ a blended deep learning and machine learning classification architecture.

An overview of machine learning and signal processing techniques for the EoG signals classification in clinical applications is presented in Chap. 8. The principles and practices in the EoG signal acquisition, noise removal, compression, feature extraction and classification are covered. It is described that how the EoG signals can be used for an automatic identification of eye movements.

Chapter 9 describes a segmentation and classification approach for the PCG signals. This method uses the peak spectrogram for an effective segmentation of the

PCG signals. Subsequently, features of the generated peak spectrograms are extracted. Onward, this feature set is processed by the support vector machine and convolutional neural network for an automated anomaly detection in the functionality of the cardiovascular system.

The authors have presented an approach for the atopic eczema skin lesions segmentation using deep neural networks in Chap. 10. A fully automated method is suggested to segment eczema skin lesions. A five-stage U-Net is trained to perform segmentation. The effect of colour space normalization and adaptive light compensation are also examined. The performance is evaluated using multiple measures. This method can be used by dermatologists for an augmented diagnosis of Eczema.

Chapter 11 describes an approach for automated detection of sleep arousals by processing the multi-physiological signals with ensemble learning algorithms. The dataset used in this study is related to polysomnography measurements. Various features are extracted from each instance in the time and frequency domains. The Wilcoxon rank-sum test and genetic optimization algorithm are used to find a set of features with the most discriminative information. A technique for data augmentation is used to tackle the unbalanced classes problem. The feature set is onward processed by the ensemble learning algorithms for detection of sleep arousals.

The author has discussed the progress of deep learning–based solutions, designed to control the biofeedback process in Chap. 12. The incorporation of deep learning models can fill the actual vacuum of precision in current neurofeedback devices. The objective of this research axis is to substitute the current devices and neurofeedback procedures with a robust set of deep learning approaches. It can reduce variability and deliver biofeedback process according to the natural brain waves relations and principles and practice.

Chapter 13 describes an approach for the estimations of emotional synchronization indices for brain regions using the EEG signal analysis. To investigate the synchronization between various brain regions, a hybrid technique combining empirical mode decomposition with wavelet transform is employed. The linear and non-linear features are computed to capture various dynamical properties from emotion-based multi-channel EEG signals. Then, in order to increase the classification accuracy of various emotional states, feature selection is carried out using a statistical analysis. The selected features are classified using the k-nearest neighbours algorithm for the estimations of emotional synchronization indices.

The authors have presented an approach for the recognition of dementia patients' working memory in Chap. 14. The proposed method uses the automatic independent component analysis and wavelet method for EEG signals denoising and analysis. In the next stage, nonlinear entropy features are extracted. A statistical examination of the individual performance is conducted using analysis of variance to determine the degree of EEG complexity across brain regions. Onward, the nonlinear local tangent space alignment based dimensionality reduction is performed. Finally, the selected feature set is processed by the machine learning algorithms for recognition of dementia patients' working memory.

To the best of the editors' knowledge, this book is a comprehensive compilation on advances in non-invasive biomedical signal sensing and processing with machine and deep learning. We believe that theories, algorithms, realizations, applications, approaches and challenges which are presented in this book will have their impact and contribution in the design and development of modern and effective healthcare systems.

Jeddah, Saudi Arabia   Saeed Mian Qaisar
Kampar, Malaysia   Humaira Nisar
Turku, Finland   Abdulhamit Subasi

Acknowledgements

We would like to thank all the contributors for their support in developing this book. We would like to acknowledge all the reviewers for providing time and professional support to this book through their valuable and constructive reviews.

We also acknowledge the support of the Electrical and Computer Engineering Department at Effat University, Jeddah, Saudi Arabia; Department of Electronic Engineering in the Faculty of Engineering and Green Technology at Universiti Tunku Abdul Rahman, Kampar, Malaysia; and the Institute of Biomedicine in the Faculty of Medicine at the University of Turku, Turku, Finland.

Finally, we express our appreciation for Springer Nature who gave us the opportunity for editing this book. We would like to acknowledge Springer Nature and their staff for providing professional support during all phases of the book development.

Jeddah, Saudi Arabia   Saeed Mian Qaisar

Kampar, Malaysia   Humaira Nisar

Turku, Finland   Abdulhamit Subasi

Contents

Contributors

Anam Abid Department of Mechatronics Engineering, University of Engineering and Technology, Peshawar, Pakistan

Siti Anom Ahmad Department of Electrical and Electronic Engineering, Faculty of Engineering, Universiti Putra Malaysia, UPM Serdang, Serdang, Selangor, Malaysia

Malaysian Research Institute of Ageing (MyAgeing™), Universiti Putra Malaysia, Serdang, Serdang, Selangor, Malaysia

Rabab Al Talib Electrical and Computer Engineering Department, Effat University, Jeddah, Saudi Arabia

Alaa A. Aldoori Department of Biomedical Engineering, Al-Khwarizmi College of Engineering, University of Baghdad, Baghdad, Iraq

Mawadda Alghamdi Electrical and Computer Engineering Department, Effat University, Jeddah, Saudi Arabia

Sawal Hamid Bin Mohd Ali Department of Electrical, Electronic & Systems Engineering, Faculty of Engineering & Built Environment, Universiti Kebangsaan Malaysia, UKM Bangi, Bangi, Selangor, Malaysia

Noor Kamal Al-Qazzaz Department of Biomedical Engineering, Al-Khwarizmi College of Engineering, University of Baghdad, Baghdad, Iraq

Asmaa Alqurashi Electrical and Computer Engineering Department, Effat University, Jeddah, Saudi Arabia

Shahad Bawazeer Electrical and Computer Engineering Department, Effat University, Jeddah, Saudi Arabia

Illya Chaikovsky Glushkov Institute of Cybernetics of National Academy of Science of Ukraine, Kyiv, Ukraine

Hala Rabih Fatayerji Electrical and Computer Engineering Department, Effat University, Jeddah, Saudi Arabia

Francisco Ferrero Department of Electrical, Electronic, Communications and Systems Engineering, University of Oviedo, Gijón, Spain

Fatima Hassan Faculty of Computer Science and Engineering, GIK Institute, Topi, Pakistan

Syed Fawad Hussain Faculty of Computer Science and Engineering, GIK Institute, Topi, Pakistan

School of Computer Science, University of Birmingham, Birmingham, UK

Maimonah Akram Khudhair Department of Biomedical Engineering, Al-Khwarizmi College of Engineering, University of Baghdad, Baghdad, Iraq

Reda Jasim Lafta Department of Biomedical Engineering, Al-Khwarizmi College of Engineering, University of Baghdad, Baghdad, Iraq

Alberto López Department of Electrical, Electronic, Communications and Systems Engineering, University of Oviedo, Gijón, Spain

Danyal Mahmood Department of Electronic Engineering, Faculty of Engineering and Green Technology, Universiti Tunku Abdul Rahman, Kampar, Malaysia

Saeed Mian Qaisar Electrical and Computer Engineering Department, Effat University, Jeddah, Saudi Arabia

Mohammad Hasan Moradi Biomedical Engineering Department, Amirkabir University of Technology, Tehran, Iran

Humaira Nisar Department of Electronic Engineering, Faculty of Engineering and Green Technology, University Tunku Abdul Rahman, Kampar, Malaysia

Jorge J. Palacios-Venegas Biofeedback Center®. Computational Neurosciences Laboratory, Mexico City, Mexico

Anton Popov Electronic Engineering Department, Igor Sikorsky Kyiv Polytechnic Institute, Kyiv, Ukraine

Faculty of Applied Sciences, Ukrainian Catholic University, Lviv, Ukraine

Tan Ysin Ren Department of Electronics Engineering, Faculty of Engineering and Green Technology, University Tunku Abdul Rahman, Kampar, Malaysia

Hannan Naseem Riaz Department of Electronic Engineering, Faculty of Engineering and Green Technology, Universiti Tunku Abdul Rahman, Kampar, Malaysia

Majed Saeed Department of Urology, Sahiwal Teaching Hospital, Sahiwal, Pakistan

Faya Saifuddin Electrical and Computer Engineering Department, Effat University, Jeddah, Saudi Arabia

Navabeh Sadat Jalili Shani Biomedical Engineering Department, Amirkabir University of Technology, Tehran, Iran

Abdulhamit Subasi College of Engineering, Effat University, Jeddah, Saudi Arabia Institute of Biomedicine, Faculty of Medicine, University of Turku, Turku, Finland

Kim Ho Yeap Department of Electronic Engineering, Faculty of Engineering and Green Technology, Universiti Tunku Abdul Rahman, Kampar, Malaysia

Zo-Afshan Department of Electrical and Computer Engineering, Air University, Islamabad, Pakistan

Chapter 1
Introduction to Non-Invasive Biomedical Signals for Healthcare

Danyal Mahmood, Hannan Naseem Riaz, and Humaira Nisar

Abstract With the advancement of medical science, new healthcare methods have been introduced. Biomedical signals have provided us with a deep insight into the working of the human body. Invasive biomedical signaling and sensing involve inserting sensors inside the human body. Non-invasive biomedical signals such as electroencephalogram (EEG), electromyogram (EMG), electrocardiogram (ECG), electrooculogram (EOG), phonocardiogram (PCG), and photoplethysmography (PPG) can be acquired by placing sensors on the surface of the human body. After the acquisition of these biomedical signals, further processing such as artifact removal and feature extraction is required to extract vital information about the subject's health and well-being. In addition to conventional signal processing and analysis tools, advanced methods that involve machine and deep learning techniques were introduced to extract useful information from these signals. There are several applications of non-invasive biomedical signal processing, including monitoring, detecting, and estimating physiological and pathological states for diagnosis and therapy. For example, detection and monitoring of different types of cancer, heart diseases, blood vessel blockage, neurological disorders, etc. In addition, biomedical signals are also used in brain control interfaces (BCI), Neurofeedback and biofeedback systems to improve the mental and physical health of the subjects.

1.1 Introduction to Biomedical Signals

With the advancement in technology in recent years, the biomedical industry has radically grown. Real-time health monitoring is now possible using smart sensing technologies. Biomedical signals are the records of physiological events including

D. Mahmood · H. N. Riaz · H. Nisar (✉)
Department of Electronic Engineering, Faculty of Engineering and Green Technology,
Universiti Tunku Abdul Rahman, Kampar, Malaysia
e-mail: humaira@utar.edu.my

© The Author(s), under exclusive license to Springer Nature Switzerland AG 2023
S. Mian Qaisar et al. (eds.), *Advances in Non-Invasive Biomedical Signal Sensing and Processing with Machine Learning*, https://doi.org/10.1007/978-3-031-23239-8_1

neural activities, cardiac rhythms, and tissue imaging [1]. Biomedical signals can be divided into two categories depending upon the source of energy for measurement, active and passive biomedical signals. In active biomedical signals, the source of energy for measurement is driven by the subject himself. There are further two types of signals in the active category i.e., electrical such as EEG, ECG, etc., and non-electrical signals such as blood pressure, temperature, etc. In passive biomedical signals, the source of energy for measurement is from outside the subject such as X-Ray, MRI, etc. Biomedical signals can also be divided into sub-categories depending upon the nature of the signals such as electrical, mechanical, and chemical biomedical signals. Electrical biomedical signals originate from neural cells such as EEG, from muscles such as EMG and ECG, and other sources such as EOG. Like electrical biomedical signals, strong magnetic field from outside the subject's body can also be used to scan different organs of the subject. These scans are known as MRI scans. These include motion and displacement signals, pressure and tension, blood flow signals, etc. Another category of biomedical signals is the chemical signals which measure the chemical change in the subject's body such as PPG, level of glucose, blood oxygen levels, etc. Mechanical biomedical signals such as blood pressure and phonocardiogram can also be measured. Furthermore, there are acoustic biomedical signals as well such as PCG and respiratory sounds. Optical biomedical signals include endoscopy while there are thermal biomedical signals as well such as the heatmap of the subject.

In this chapter, the focus will be on electrical and magnetic biomedical signals which are recorded by the sensors placed outside the subject's body. These biomedical signals are then used for the diagnosis and monitoring and progression of various diseases. The improvements in signal processing methods and electronics have encouraged the use of biomedical signals for prognosis and diagnosis.

Sensors of different types are used to measure and record biomedical signals. Some sensors are implanted or inserted inside the subject to record these signals e.g., implanted EEG and endoscopy. While some sensors record these signals from outside the subject's body e.g., MRI, and X-Ray. The recorded signals are used for the improving people's health. Engineers have developed many devices that process these signals and present the results in an easy-to-understand way. Heart rate monitoring devices have enabled us to examine irregularities in the beating rhythms of the heart [2]. Body glucose monitoring devices help diabetic patients to monitor and manage their blood sugar levels without any help and supervision from healthcare providers. Emotiv MN8 is a wearable device that monitors brain activities to measure stress and attention.

In this chapter, a brief introduction to important biomedical signals followed by their acquisition techniques will be provided. Afterwards, processing and analyzing these signals will be discussed followed by the application of these signals for rehabilitation such as brain-computer interface (BCI) and neurofeedback & biofeedback systems. Finally, a brief conclusion of this chapter will be provided.

1.2 Invasive and Non-Invasive Procedures

Biomedical signals can be divided into two types depending upon the nature and procedure of signal acquisition. In the invasive method of obtaining biomedical signals, sensors are inserted inside the human body. In other words, invasive tests are performed by penetrating the body using medical tools [3]. On the other hand, the non-invasive technique of acquiring biomedical signals does not involve any skin breaking. These tests are performed by placing sensors on the surface of the human body from outside the skin [4].

Non-invasive methods are much simpler and have low risk. No surgery is required for the placement of sensors. Once the sensors are placed, the collected data is processed to get the required information. These techniques are cheaper and user-friendly and involve low risk which makes them more acceptable to the subject instead of invasive techniques. One of the main advantages of using a non-invasive method over an invasive method is that, for an invasive method, a professional specialist is required to perform the procedure. While in the case of non-invasive techniques, scientists have developed many user-friendly devices which can be worn by the subject themselves with minimal supervision and the data can be easily recorded [5].

Both invasive and non-invasive techniques have some advantages and disadvantages. One of the main disadvantages of non-invasive methods is their low signal-to-noise ratio (SNR). To overcome this problem, the data is recorded under specific conditions to avoid noise and enhanced noise removal procedures are applied before using the data for analysis. Non-invasive methods generally yield less information rather than invasive techniques. Invasive sensors can be of different types such as single electrodes or multi-electrode arrays (MEA) [6]. Depending upon the type of the sensor, more precise information can be collected. For example, if the brain signals are recorded by inserting sensors inside the brain, the resulting information will be much more reliable, precise, and detailed rather than trying to collect the same data from outside the scalp of the subject. At the same time, invasive techniques are more laborious and have a higher risk factor.

Invasive methods require trained professionals to insert sensors inside the body by operations or by inserting the sensor into a body opening. For example, for bone conduction hearing devices, surgery is performed to implant a device inside the skin of the subject and for endoscopy, a long tube with a camera is inserted to examine the inside of the subject's body. Similarly, EEG can be collected invasively where EEG electrodes are surgically implanted on the surface or inside the brain. On the other hand, the non-invasive method includes X-rays, MRI, ECG, EEG, etc. In terms of biomedical signaling, EEG is one of the examples, in which the signals can be recorded in both invasive and non-invasive ways. The invasive EEG will have high spatial resolution and fewer artifacts with more risk while non-invasive EEG will have high temporal resolution with more artifacts and less risk.

1.3 Non-Invasive Biomedical Signals

1.3.1 Electroencephalography (EEG)

EEG is an electrophysiological signal that records brain activity in terms of electrical potentials. It is a non-invasive technique to record the potential differences formed by the ionic currents between the brain neurons [7]. In 1875, Richard Canton performed the first neurophysiological recordings of animals. In 1924, Hans Berger a German psychiatrist recorded the first EEG of human subjects.

To record the EEG signals, the sensors, also known as EEG electrodes, are placed over the scalp of the subject at specific locations. Reference electrodes are required to record EEG data. EEG data for the required site is then collected as a potential difference between the two electrodes. These reference electrodes are generally placed beside the ear of the subject. EEG activity is quite small, measured in microvolts. The location of EEG electrodes is governed by international standards such as 10–5, 10–10, and 10–20 systems among which the international 10–20 system of electrode placement is most used as shown in Fig. 1.1. This system of electrode placement is designed in such a way that the distance between the electrodes is either 10% or 20% of the total front-to-back or left-to-right distance of the skull [8].

The human brain is divided into four different lobes based on its location and tasks that it performs. The frontal lobe is responsible for concentration, attention, working memory, and executive planning. The temporal lobe is responsible for language and memory, object recognition, music, and facial recognition. The parietal lobe is responsible for problem-solving, attention, and association. The occipital lobe controls visual learning and reading [9].

EEG is a complex time-series non-stationary signal which represents the electrical activity of the brain. The EEG signal varies from 0.1 to more than 100 Hz and can be decomposed into different frequency bands such as delta (0.5–4 Hz), theta (4–8 Hz), alpha (8–13 Hz), beta (13–30 Hz), and gamma (30–100 Hz). Each frequency band represents some specific physiological functions. Delta frequency band represents sleep, unawareness, deep unconsciousness, and complex

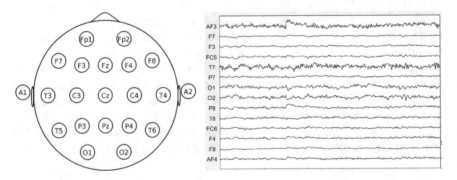

Fig. 1.1 International 10–20 system of EEG electrodes placement and 14 channel EEG data

problem-solving abilities of the brain. Theta frequency band represents the deep states, creativity, distractibility, anxiety, and depression. Alpha frequency band represents memory recall, alertness, peacefulness, relaxation, and meditation. The beta frequency band represents the thinking, alertness, attention, focus, and excitement of the subject. The Gamma frequency band represents the learning, problem-solving cognitive capabilities, and mental sharpness of the subject [9].

EEG electrodes are very sensitive and are prone to noise and have low SNR. Due to this, the EEG recordings are taken very carefully in silent rooms. Many artifacts still manage to appear into the recordings. Filtering and artifact removal techniques are utilized to remove such noises from the data. This extra procedure makes the EEG system complex and computationally expensive. The main advantage of EEG is its high temporal resolution, and the most important limitation of non-invasive EEG is its poor spatial resolution. The EEG is recorded non-invasively, by using electrodes placed over the scalp, however, the actual brain activity occurs several centimeters below the electrodes. This means that the cortical current must travel through different resistances including the scalp itself to be detected by the electrode. This causes distortions and noise at the scalp level. Therefore, for non-invasive EEG acquisition, source localization is one of the primary steps in which the actual source of EEG in the brain is identified based on the surface EEG recording.

Event-related potentials (ERPs), also known as event-related voltage or evoked potentials coming from EEG data are time-locked to sensory, motor, and cognitive events. ERPs can be used to classify and identify perceptual, memory, and linguistic processes. ERPs originate from synchronous activations of the neuronal population during some specific task or information processing. The ERPs are usually observed by averaging EEG signals. Averaging makes the ERPs less effective to background noise in the EEG data and thus it can extract vital information about the event-related activity which is otherwise difficult to differentiate in the ongoing EEG activity.

The human brain can develop different neurological and physiological diseases. Different techniques can be used to modulate EEG signals to enhance cognitive performance of subjects. Music can be used to regulate EEG signals to achieve calmness and relieve stress [10]. On the other hand, EEG can be used for the diagnoses of neurological diseases such as epilepsy, Parkinson's disease, multiple sclerosis, and Alzheimer's disease. The most common use of EEG is to diagnose epilepsy [11] in which brain activities become abnormal. This can cause seizures and loss of awareness for some time. On the other hand, EEG is also used for diagnoses and cure of many physiological disorders such as depression, post-traumatic stress disorder (PTSD), attention deficit hyperactivity disorder (ADHD), and autism. Different applications of EEG include but are not limited to diagnosing and checking the status of brain injury, brain infections, tumors, etc. EEG can also be used to identify the reason for symptoms such as syncope, memory loss, confusion, or seizures. EEG is also used to diagnose sleep disorders in which the EEG recordings must be taken while the subject is sleeping to analyze any disorders.

Fig. 1.2 Sample MEG scan

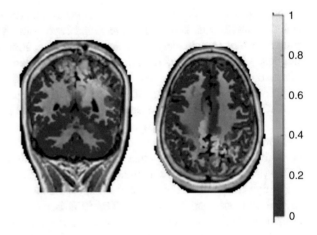

1.3.2 Magnetoencephalography (MEG)

MEG is a brain imaging technique that measures tiny magnetic fields inside the subject's brain. Superconducting detectors and amplifiers (SQUIDs) are highly sensitive devices that are used to detect magnetic fields of the brain without the emission of magnetic field or radiation. It generates a magnetic source image (MSI) to classify the specific part of the brain that is causing seizures.

Some of the advantages of MEG are its non-invasive nature, sensitivity and accuracy, and safety. MEG can also record the brain activities when it is actively functional. MEG can be used to either detect the brain's impulsive activity like a seizure or for mapping motor, sensory areas, memory, vision, and other functions of the brain. Due to the high sensitivity of the devices, the imaging is done in a specially designed shielded room with a video and intercom system to communicate with the subject and technicians. Electrodes are placed over the scalp of the subject while the head of the subject will remain in the helmet like MEG scanner. Movement of the head during the test may cause noise or artifacts in the recorded image so it is important to remain still during the test. While the technician may ask the subject to move certain body parts to measure the response in the brain. The sample MEG scan can be seen in Fig. 1.2.

MEG scan can be used by doctors to identify the source of seizures in the brain and determine if the subject requires seizure surgery or not. Generally, MEG is accompanied by EEG and magnetic resonance imaging (MRI) which creates an anatomical image of the brain.

1.3.3 Electromyography (EMG)

EMG is used to diagnose the health of muscles and motor neurons that controls the contraction of those muscles [12]. Muscles contract when the motor neurons from the brain send electrical signals to them. The EMG activity is directly proportional

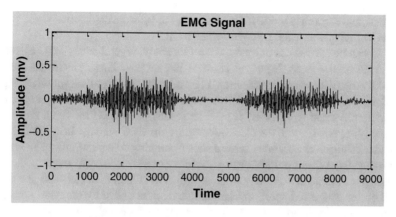

Fig. 1.3 Sample EMG signal

to the number of contracted muscles as well as the strength of the contracted muscle. Generally, the range of the electrical signals captured by the electrodes is in microvolts. Non-invasive sticky electrodes are placed near the muscles over the skin to record their electrical activity. EMG is a process of translating these electrical activities into graphs.

The non-invasive nature of EMG allows us to monitor physiological processes without affecting movement patterns. To prepare the skin for high-quality EMG recordings, the area must be cleaned, and any residual makeup or dirt must be removed. To get valid and reliable EMG data, EMG electrodes are placed over the muscle group of interest. This requires a certain level of anatomic knowledge. To collect the EMG data, a reference electrode is required. EMG data for the required site is then collected as a potential difference between the two electrodes. The recommended reference sites are elbow, hip, and collar bones. Figure 1.3 shows an example of an EMG signal. The noise can be induced in EMG recordings from the surrounding power sources. To minimize such noises, the distance between the EMG sensors and the amplifier is kept minimum [13].

EMG is used to diagnose several muscle and nerve disorders. It is used to test if the muscle correctly responds to the nerve signal or not. Some of the common problems diagnosed by the EMG test are muscle weakness, muscle cramps, numbness in arms, legs, hands, feet, or face, and muscle paralysis [14]. Facial EMG (fEMG) is used for the detection of facial emotions.

1.3.4 Electrocardiography (ECG)

ECG is a test that is performed to check the electrical activity and rhythm of the heart. A heart specialist might recommend taking an ECG test to check any unusual activity in the heartbeats of the subject. Sticky sensors are placed over the skin of the subject which detect the electrical activity produced by the contraction and expansion of the heart muscles [15]. The detected electrical activities are then recorded, and a graph is plotted. The doctor or the heart specialist then looks at these graphs to find any unusual behavior of the heart.

ECG can be carried out in many ways. Generally, several sticky ECG electrodes are placed on the arms, legs, and chest of the subject. These electrodes are connected by the ECG machine via wires. Figure 1.4 (a) displays a sample ECG signal. The duration of the test is normally around 5 min after which the subject is free to go. There are three types of ECG tests. A resting-state ECG in which the subject must be lying down while the electrodes record the ECG signals. In stress ECG, the subject is required to do some exercise such as running on a treadmill. In an ambulatory ECG test, a small portable and wearable machine is used to monitor the ECG for a longer period such as a day or more [16]. The selection of the ECG test type is based on the suspected heart problem and is recommended by the heart specialist. For example, if the heart problem symptoms appear during a workout or some physical activity, a stress ECG test might be conducted while if the symptoms are unpredicted or random, an ambulatory ECG test will be more suitable [17]. In the case of ambulatory ECG tests, the machine records and stores the collected data which can be later accessed by the specialist once the test is complete.

ECG devices record the electrical activities of the heart. These electrical activities are generated due to the contractions of the beating heart. The ECG machine records and prints or displays the electrical activity and rhythm of the subject on a graph. The spikes in the ECG graph represent one complete heartbeat. Each heartbeat is composed of several spikes in which the first peak is a P wave which represents contracting atria, the largest one known as the R or QRS complex, occurs due to the contracting of ventricles. Before and after the QRS complex, inverted peaks can be seen which are known as Q and S waves respectfully. The last spike is the T wave which occurs because of the relaxation of ventricles again as shown in Fig. 1.4 (b). There should be regularity in the spikes of ECG data. The distance between these spikes represents heart rate. Irregularities in these spikes can be a sign of a problem. Abnormalities in these rhythms indicate some heart disorders such as arrhythmia often known as heart attack which causes damage to the heart due to the lack of oxygen to the heart muscles. Similarly, the distance between the spikes should not be too short, or too long. If the spikes are too close, it can be a sign of tachycardia. Other tests might be required to confirm any heart problem.

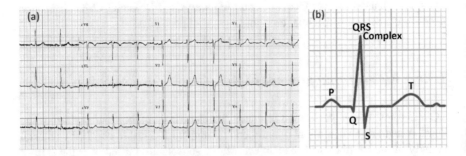

Fig. 1.4 (a) Sample ECG signal (b) Components of ECG signal

Due to the non-invasive nature of the ECG test, there is very little risk in performing the ECG. During the stress ECG, the subject is required to be monitored all the time and if the subject feels unwell, the test is immediately stopped. The removal of sticky electrodes might cause some discomfort, and, in some cases, a mild rash can be felt after the removal of the electrodes.

ECG is often performed along with other tests to diagnose potential heart problems such as chest pain, palpitations, dizziness, and shortness of breath. If the subject feels irregularities in the heartbeat or the heart beats too slowly or quickly, it is possibly due to arrhythmias. Coronary heart disease can occur if there is any blockage in the blood supply of the heart. This can happen due to the build-up of fats in the blood vessel connected with the heart. If the supply of blood is suddenly stopped, it might cause a heart attack. Thickened walls of the heart might cause cardiomyopathy.

1.3.5 Electrooculography (EOG)

EOG measures the resting potential between the front and the back of the human eye. Due to the neurons and ion channel, the back of the retina creates a negative pole. The EOG measures this potential difference by placing pair of electrodes near the eye (up and down or right and left) [18]. The electrodes are divided into two groups: horizontal and vertical electrodes. The horizontal electrodes are placed near the outer edges of the eyes. The vertical electrodes are placed above and below the eyes. A ground electrode is placed on the forehead as shown in Fig. 1.5 (a). This arrangement of EOG electrode placement allows us to examine the full movement of the eye. The movement of the human eye will change the effective distance between the poles and the electrodes. One electrode will become nearer to the negative side of the retina while the other will become nearer to the positive side. This change can be sensed by the electrodes as an electrical activity and hence can be recorded and plotted.

The potential difference changes with the change in the exposure to light. EOG is used to evaluate the efficiency of the pigment epithelium. In this test, a subject

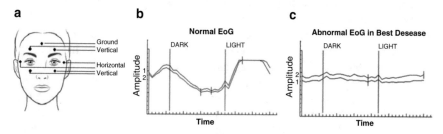

Fig. 1.5 (a) EOG electrode position, (b)Normal EOG signal, (c) Abnormal EOG signal with Best disease

with EOG electrodes is requested to sit (resting state) in a dark room with his/her eyes open. In this phase, the subjects adapt to the darkness in such a way that their EOG voltage decreases at the start and reaches a minimum value after some time. Then the lights in the room are turned on and the subject remains sitting there for another several minutes. In this phase, the EOG voltage will increase and eventually reaches a maximum point. Once the subject adapts to the lighting condition, the voltage will decrease again. The comparison of voltages in the dark and light phases is known as Arden Ratio (AR). Generally, the AR should be around 2.0, if the AR decreases to 1.8 or less, there are chances that the subject has the best disease, which is an inherited retinal disease causing macular degeneration and may cause loss of central vision, as well as the ability to perceive colors and details [19]. Figure 1.5 (b) shows a normal EOG signal while Fig. 1.5 (c) displays an abnormal EOG signal with the best disease where AR is less than 1 [20].

Due to its non-invasive nature, portability, cheap price, and low risk of EOG, its applications are limitless [21]. The application of EOG in the diagnoses of diseases related to human eyes is just one example. Other applications of EOG include Human-Computer Interface (HCI). Many EOG-controlled assistive devices are available such as controlling wheelchair-using eye movement, video games controlled by eyes, etc.

1.3.6   Phonocardiogram (PCG)

PCG measures and plots the sounds and murmurs generated by the heart of the subject using a machine known as a phonocardiograph. The machine has a sensor that is placed over the chest of the subject to detect the sound and murmurs coming from the heart. These sounds are recorded, plotted on the screen, and can be listened to directly using a headphone. Figure 1.6 displays an example of PCG recording. The high resolution of phonocardiography makes this procedure very useful. These sounds and plots are then listened to or viewed by the specialist to diagnose any heart disease [22].

From ancient times, it is known that the heart makes a sound while beating. Robert Hooke proposed the idea of developing an instrument to record these sounds back in the seventeenth century. In the 1930s and 1940s, phonocardiography monitoring and recording equipment were developed. In the 1950s, the PCG was standardized in the first conference held in Paris [23]. NASA used the PCG system made by Beckman Instruments to monitor the heartbeat of astronauts in space.

The vibrations made by the opening and closure of the beating heart valves, and the movement of heart walls generates sounds. PCG records two sounds in each heartbeat. The first sound appears at the closure of atrioventricular valves during systole while the second sound appears at the end of systole when aortic and pulmonary valves close. PCG is used for recording subaudible echoes and murmurs of the heart. On the other hand, a stethoscope is unable to detect such minor sounds. Hence a stethoscope cannot be used for a more precise diagnosis of heart disease.

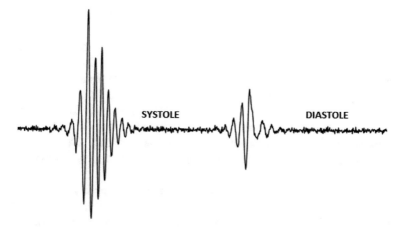

Fig. 1.6 Sample PCG Signal

Some of the common uses of PCG are the detection of the rheumatic valvular lesion in which the valves of the heart are possibly damaged or not functioning well. The murmur of the aortic stenosis can also be detected using PCG in which the high pressure of blood through small openings of the aortic valve causes turbulence and hence cause intense vibrations. The non-invasive nature of PCG is very beneficial to diagnose several diseases related to the heart with a very low factor of risk. The murmur of mitral and aortic regurgitation in which the blood flows backward from the mitral and aortic valves during systole and diastole can also be detected by using PCG. Similarly, it is also used to detect the murmur of mitral stenosis in which the pressure difference causes difficulty while the blood passes from the left atrium to the left ventricle [24].

1.3.7   Photoplethysmography (PPG)

PPG is a simple, non-invasive, and low-cost procedure, commonly used for monitoring heart rate. In PPG, a light source generally in the infrared range is used with a photodetector over the skin of the subject to measure the volumetric alterations of blood flows. The light is emitted on the tissue by the light source which is reflected and measured by the photodetector. This measurement is proportional to the volumetric variation of blood circulation. Recently, wearable PPG devices have been introduced. Depending upon the type of the device, these can be worn on different parts of the body such as the forehead, earlobe, forearm, fingertip, and ankle [25].

Several factors may affect the response of PPG such as the geometry of the sensors being used, the intensity of the light source, ambient light, and photodiode sensing power. Other than that, the oxygen concentration and organ characteristics can also change the PPG recordings. Similarly, some cardiovascular factors may also alter the PPG readings. This is the reason that different PPG devices are designed to use in different parts of the body. The basic working of PPG is shown in Fig. 1.7 (a). One of the main advantages of PPG over traditional heart monitoring devices such as ECG is its cheap cost and simplicity. Instead of using multiple electrodes on the chest and other body parts in the case of ECG, a single PPG sensor is required to monitor heart rate.

A PPG signal has two parts, a pulsatile or AC component which is due to the heartbeats and causes synchronous variations in blood volume. The other part is the DC component which is superimposed on the AC component. The DC component of PPG is due to respiration and thermoregulation [26]. A sample PPG signal is shown in Fig. 1.7 (b).

Portable and wearable PPG devices have the potential for early detection of cardiovascular diseases. PPG devices are widely used in various clinical applications. Some of the common applications of PPG are monitoring blood pressure and oxygen saturation, heart rate, respiration, vascular assessment, arterial diseases or compliance and aging, microvascular blood flow, thermoregulation, and orthostasis [27, 28].

1.3.8 Magnetic Resonance Imaging (MRI)

MRI generates a three-dimensional anatomical image of the required organ of the subject. The non-invasive and high-resolution MRI allows the specialists to examine the organs, tissues, and skeleton system of the subject and diagnose several diseases. The working principle of MRI is that it detects the change in direction of the rotational axis of protons found in the living tissues using powerful magnets and radiofrequency [29]. Physicians can differentiate different types of tissues from the magnetic features of the MRI image. Figure 1.8 shows an MRI machine and an MRI image of a muscle.

To get an MRI image, the subject is placed inside a large tube-like magnet. The magnetic field aligns the water molecules inside the body for a fraction of time while radio waves are used to create a cross-sectional image of these aligned

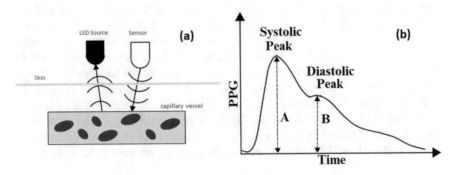

Fig. 1.7 (a) PPG sensor working principle (b) Sample PPG signal

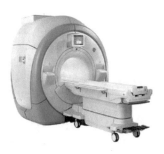
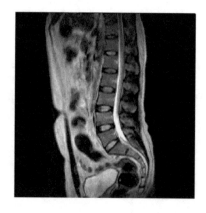

Fig. 1.8 MRI Machine and Sample MRI image of a muscle

molecules. Sometimes, gadolinium is injected as a contrast material into the vein in the hand of the subject to enhance a variety of details. To ensure the best quality of the image, the subject must not move otherwise the MRI image might get blurred.

MRI of different body parts can be taken to diagnose different disorders. MRI of the brain might be required for the detection of stroke, tumors, or disorders in the spinal cord. In the 1990s, functional MRI (fMRI) was invented which is a non-invasive brain imaging technology. fMRI can detect brain activities by measuring changes in the blood flow within a specific part of the brain. This can be used to analyze the function of different brain regions. fMRI can detect which parts of the brain are activated during specific tasks such as lifting the leg and even just thinking about something. fMRI is being used by researchers to diagnose, better understand, monitor, and treat several diseases such as post-concussion syndrome, schizophrenia, tumors, etc.

MRI of the heart can be used to examine the working of the heart, functionality of heart chambers, and magnitude of damage after heart disease or blockages in the blood vessels of the heart. Similarly, MRI of internal organs such as kidneys, uterus, liver, etc. can be used for the detection and examination of tumors or abnormalities in them. It can also be used for the detection of breast cancer.

An MRI machine contains very strong magnets, the metal in the body of the subject might be dangerous. Metals that are not attracted to the magnets can still modify the MRI image. So, it is required to remove any metal item before taking the test [30]. Other than that, a doctor might avoid taking MRI if the subject has some kidney or liver problem and/or the subject is pregnant or breastfeeding [31].

1.4 Biomedical Signal Processing

Biomedical signal processing deals with extracting significant and useful information from the biomedical signals for medical purposes [32]. As the non-invasive techniques of the biomedical signal acquisition have a low peak signal-to-noise ratio (PSNR), advanced signal processing methods are developed and used to extract the required user information. A full-time check on patients' heartbeat, blood pressure sugar levels, and neural activity can extensively improve medical diagnosis. This monitoring is not only used to know the status of the patient's body but also to diagnose diseases in the body. With the help of biomedical signal processing, biologists can develop methods for the detection, monitoring, and cure of diseases. Proper processing and analysis of biomedical signals can provide numerous advantages in the field of medicine. The four steps involved in the processing of signals are:

1.4.1 Signal Acquisition

The first step is a signal acquisition which deals with capturing a signal from the subject. A hardware device is used to capture biomedical signals from the subject body. Analog signals are recorded and transformed into digital signals.

1.4.2 Signal Visualization and Annotation

Visualizing the recorded biomedical signals gives significant information which can effectively boost the analyzing procedures. Currently, periodograms and spectrograms are used for visualization and analyses [33]. A periodogram determines the frequency spectrum of a biomedical signal and is the most used tool for visualization. A spectrogram is a visual representation of signal strength over time at various frequencies. A spectrogram is a 2-dimensional graph where the color represents the signal strength. Modern tools e.g., MATLAB, LABVIEW provide built-in apps to visualize and analyze the data in time as well as a frequency domain.

1.4.3 Artifacts Removal and Preprocessing

Artifact Removal is a preprocessing step that involves removing any artifact, error, or noise from the recorded data before processing and analysis of biomedical signals. Different biomedical signals have different types of noise. For example, power line noise can be found in PCR and EEG data. In ECG data, baseline wanders artifact can be found which is a low-frequency data superimposed on the recorded ECG signal. Similarly in MRI data, motion artifacts and external magnetic field artifacts are very common. In addition, the noise can be found in the recorded biomedical signals due to faulty or improper use of the acquisition instrument such as dislocation of electrodes/sensors. Noise in the recorded signals might also be found in the acquisition that does not follow the standard procedures while recording the data such as recording from unclean skin, unwanted movements of body parts while recording, interference of electrodes, and impedance from power sources. Non-invasive biomedical signal acquisition techniques often yield low PSNR. These artifacts or noise can interfere with the diagnostic system and may result in improper classification or detection of diseases. Different artifact removal methods are available based on the type of artifacts in the signals [34]. Some artifacts or noise such as powerline interference and DC component in the recording can be removed by using the filtration method. To remove more complicated artifacts or noise, many filtration and machine learning models are available. After that, various preprocessing steps are implemented which include dealing with missing values, data normalization, outlier removal, etc. before using the recorded biomedical signal.

1.4.4   Feature Extraction

Feature extraction is a process in which raw data is used to extract useful information that can be processed by machine learning or deep learning models. The model uses these features to classify the data. Raw data is not useful until feature extraction is done. Features can be extracted manually as well as automatically. Feature extraction is generally based upon the required classification. For instance, Nawaz et al. [35] provided a comparison between different methods for feature extraction for the classification of emotions using EEG data. For manual feature extraction, Fast Fourier transform (FFT) is widely used in biomedical signal processing [36]. The FFT involves the conversion of a time domain signal into a frequency domain signal. FFT can achieve high efficiency because a smaller number of calculations are required to evaluate a waveform. For automatic feature extraction, the wavelet scattering method is used which creates the representation of a signal into a function called waves. A wavelet can acquire both local as well as temporal spectra. Two types of wavelet transformation, discrete and continuous wavelet transforms are often considered while extracting features automatically [37]. Discrete wavelets transform gives back data of equal length as that of input while the continuous transform returns an array with high dimensions data as compared to the input. Other than these methods, statistical feature extraction also plays an important role in the signal analysis [38]. Some commonly used statistical features are mean, variance, skewness, and kurtosis.

In Fig. 1.9, we can see all the steps and observe that after feature extraction we can use these features for multiple purposes. Medical diagnoses are made very easy with visualization and manipulation of features using digital tools. Machine learning is used to identify various patterns in the signal which can lead to major discoveries.

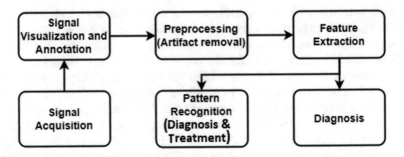

Fig. 1.9 Flow of biomedical signal processing

1.5   Machine Learning in Biomedical Signal Analysis

After the first mathematical modeling of neural networks in, machine learning was invented. In 1943, Warren McCulloch published a paper in which he mathematically mapped decision-making and thought processes in human cognition [39]. Alan Turing proposed a "Turing Test" in 1950 which can classify any system to be intelligent or unintelligent [40]. The idea behind this test is that a machine can be considered intelligent if it can convince humans that the machine is also a human. After this point, many machine learning models and processes started to appear, and a new era of smart and intelligent machines was started.

Machine Learning (ML) enables software and applications became more efficient in predicting outcomes and results using trained data. The concepts of machine learning are used in various fields like health care, finance, marketing, new developments in cyber security, and other significant fields [41]. Machine learning has proven its application in various domains, and it is also widely used in biomedical signal processing and healthcare. It can be beneficial in extracting, analyzing, and visualizing various signals as well as for the detection and classification of biomedical signals such as ECG, EMG, EEG, etc. [42]. Deep neural networks (DNN) have enabled us to achieve more accurate and robust results of detection and classification of biomedical signals. Applications of DNN in biomedical signal processing includes classification of ECG signals [43], brain tumor classification [44], missing data prediction in ECG signals [45], and many more. Convolutional Neural networks (CNN) have also played an important role in this filed such as drowsiness detection [46], detection of congestive heart failure [47], classification of EEG data listening to different kinds of music [48], EEG signal classification for emotion recognition [49] etc.

With the advancement in medical science and the increase in environmental pollution, many new diseases have been detected. Some mild intensity of diseases can be cured by simple over the counter medicines. But other diseases require proper diagnoses, clinical surgeries, and treatments. To correctly cure any disease, proper diagnoses must be carried out for which correct evaluation of symptoms and biomedical signals from the human body is required. Machine Learning may assist in making the right decision for the diagnosis and treatment of diseases. To develop automated symptoms and disease diagnostic systems, the contribution of machine learning is very important, e.g., for the segmentation of skin lesions, tumors, cancer cells, etc. Normal practice is the observation by radiologists or other specialists that puts a high burden on them in terms of time and cost and it also results in inter and intra-rater variability. Hence developing automated systems using machine learning can decrease the burden on radiologists and specialists.

After analysis, the next step is a prediction of the right treatment for the patients. This prediction could be challenging if developers have not designed an intelligent system. Machine learning allows the development of efficient and reliable systems for the prediction of diseases as well as medicines. For analysis and diagnosis of disease in the human body, different models of machine learning can be used. There are two main types of machine learning algorithms, supervised and non-supervised learning models. In supervised learning models such as support vector machine (SVM), naïve Bayes (NB), and K-nearest neighbor (KNN), the models are trained on a labeled dataset containing the ground truth. The dataset provided to the model contains data from diseased and healthy subjects. The model is trained in such a way that once it is trained, it can predict that either the subject has the disease or not. In medical science, the availability of labeled datasets is very limited as it requires a lot of time and effort by healthcare professionals and specialists. To overcome such problems, unsupervised ML models such as K-means, Gaussian mixture, and neural networks can be trained without the need for the labeled dataset. These models extract features from the non-labeled dataset and classify them based on those features extracted [50].

The impact of ML cannot be denied in health care and medicine because of its capability for disease detection, management, and treatment [51]. Disease diagnosis through machine learning techniques can reduce the risk of losing patients' life. Advanced algorithms are used nowadays for a prior diagnosis of epilepsy, heart attack, and other fatal diseases. It is now easy to handle big data through ML as many advancements and modifications have been made. The processing, analyzing, and characterizing of biomedical signals is now done efficiently using ML approaches. Biomedical signals such as MRI, (CT), (PET), whole slide images (WSIs), ECG, EEG, EMG, etc. are very important and significant for analyzing and determining the current condition of some diseases in the human body. The diagnosis of diseases in a traditional way in which health specialists visually inspect the biomedical signals can induce a risk of human error and ambiguities. ML methods remove these limitations providing low-risk systems. Signal feature extraction is one of the techniques in ML that provides systematic visualization of biomedical signals. Modern ML methods provide advantages in noise reduction, artifact removal, and early detection of diseases. ML can be used for the classification and clustering of biomedical signals and images. For small dataset, classical ML is used and optimized by following the conditions that suit microcontrollers that are inbuilt into biomedical signal processing devices. This requires the correct selection of ML algorithms that are done by experts in ML.

1.6   Brain-Computer Interface BCI)

Research and advancements in BCI began in the 1970s by Jacques Vidal at the University of California, Los Angeles (UCLA). He published his studies of controlling external objects using EEG signals in 1973 and stamped the name brain control interface [52]. Cogent Negative variation (CNV) was a major part of his publications. He calculated the evoked electrical activity of the cerebral cortex from the skull using EEG [53]. In 1988, Farwell and Donchin [54] added another achievement in establishing direct communication between a computer and the brain of an individual. After these initial establishments, a lot of progress was made by developers. In 1990, research was done on bidirectional adaptive BCI controlling computer buzzers. These studies and research opened the path for the concept of BCI technologies to restore brain functionality.

The brain-computer interface, often called the brain interface machine, provides a direct communication door between the brain's electrical activity and an external device [55]. The physical implementation of the BCI ranges from non-invasive to invasive methods [56]. BCI system acquires brain signals from the subject, processes these signals which might contain preprocessing such as noise reduction, feature extraction according to the application of BCI, and classification of the brain signals into useful commands, and returns a feedback information to the subject as per application to enhance certain brain functions.

There are a lot of applications of BCI in medical, educational, and other fields which makes it an important topic for research and development. The medical application can be divided into 3 parts, prevention, detection, and rehabilitation. In prevention, BCI techniques are used to prevent a subject from certain diseases or habits such as smoking and alcohol. This is done by first training a subject specific classifier that learns the EEG pattern of smoking and neutral cue and then the subject is asked to deactivate their real-time EEG activity patterns of smoking cue calculated using a previously constructed classifier [57]. The possible loss of function and decrease in alertness level resulting from smoking and or alcohol drinking can be prevented. Similarly, in detection, BCI can be used for forecasting and detecting health issues such as abnormal brain structure. Diseases such as stroke can be detected before time so that the subject can gather proper medical help. Rehabilitation is another important medical application of BCI in which the subjects who suffer from mobility disorders after strokes and other traumatic brain disorders can be trained to regain their previous level of these functions by helping to guide activity-dependent brain plasticity using EEG to indicate to the current state of brain to the subject and enable the subject to subsequently lower abnormal activity [58]. EEG-based BCI uses brain signals to control robotic arms, artificial limbs, wheelchairs, and other prosthetic devices [59]. The BCI approach allows the disabled individual to use their limbs and voice once again to communicate with the world [60].

The applications of BCI are not limited to the medical field but smart environment such as smart homes, safer transportation, and brain-controlled home appliances is also a major use of BCI [61]. The use of BCI to monitor the stress and attention of the driver and assist drivers during transportation in reducing the risk of accidents on roads [62]. Furthermore, marketing and advertisements have also been an interest of researchers. BCI-based advertisement is being implemented in which the attention and watching activity of the subject is analyzed and the most effective advertisements are displayed to the audience.

Moreover, in the educational field, BCI techniques such as neurofeedback training are being used to enhance the performance of the subject's brain including improvement in alertness, focus, and cognitive skills of the subject. The entertainment industry is also using BCI to enhance the user's involvement in games. BCI is being used to control toys and video games that attract more and more users to try and use them. BCI is being used in security as well, where cognitive biometrics (such as brain signals) are used as sources of identity information, reducing vulnerabilities and the chance of being hacked [63].

BCI techniques have some challenges that need to be resolved for user acceptance. The usability of BCI has certain challenges such as the training process which is necessary to discriminate between classes. In the training process, the subject is taught to use the system as well as control the brain feedback signal. After training, the BCI system would be able to classify or do certain functions as per the subject's requirements. Noise in the recordings of brain activities can reduce the performance of the BCI system. For this, the subject must be careful while using BCI. Time consumption also played an important role in the acceptability of BCI in normal life as the training process can be very long. Other than that, there are a few technical issues such as the non-linearity of the brain signals. Thus, the noise or artifact removal process is computationally expensive.

1.7 Neurofeedback & Biofeedback Systems

Hans Berger, a German researcher was the first to use EEG devices on human subjects in the 1920s, by attaching electrodes to the scalp and measuring the produced currents [64]. After this, in the 1950s and 1960s, a method of altering brain activities was formulated by Dr. Joseph Kamiya and Dr. Barry and they called it Neurofeedback [65]. The main concept behind this system is that if a subject is offered a simple reward system, he/she can control their brain waves. Dr. Kamiya used a simple bell sound based on the subject's EEG as a reward to achieve an alpha state.

Biofeedback has been found in ancient times where Indian Yogis used to practice similar yoga and transcendental meditation [66]. The modern biofeedback was first documented in 1969. The concept behind this is the feedback formalized by cybernetics during World War II [67]. Biofeedback instruments deployed modern electronic technologies in the field of psychiatry.

In the biofeedback treatment method, self-regulation of the bodily process is achieved by monitoring some aspect of the physiological functioning of the subject using electronic devices, and feedback is provided to the subject, generally in the form of audio or video, so that the subject can learn to alter that function in some way. Some subjects used biofeedback training to control heartbeat and body temperature [68]. Similarly, biofeedback training can be used to train subjects to gain control over blood pressure, skin temperature, and electrical activities of the brain.

In EMG biofeedback, electrical changes in specific muscle groups are converted into electrical signals and displayed to the subject. Similarly, thermal biomedical signals use skin temperature as feedback to train the subject to control blood flow and blood pressure. Electrodermal (EDR) biofeedback measures skin conduction and uses it as feedback to reduce the sympathetic tone of the subject [69].

Some of the common applications of biofeedback include the treatment of headaches, Cardiovascular disorders including hypertension, cardiac arrhythmias, and Raynaud's disease. Neuromuscular rehabilitation such as spasmodic torticollis, blepharospasm, and chronic pain can also be achieved by using biofeedback training [70]. Similarly, gastrointestinal disorders can also be treated using biofeedback methods [71].

Neurofeedback training is a non-invasive form of therapy used to regulate brain waves. This process has been found helpful in the treatment of various neurological disorders and psychological disorders. In neurofeedback training, EEG signals are used to detect brain activities of the subject and real-time feedback is provided to the subject to improve certain functions of the brain. Neurofeedback training is also widely used to improve brain activity to obtain cognitive and behavioral improvements [72]. Alpha neurofeedback training can be used for cognitive enhancement of healthy subjects [73]. Other applications of Neurofeedback training include improvement in cognitive processing speed and executive functions [74], decreasing anxiety [75], treatment of epilepsy disorder and ADHD [76], improvement in artistic performance [77], and improvement in intelligence testing and psychological assessments [78].

1.8   Conclusion

In this chapter, a brief introduction to non-invasive biomedical signals for healthcare is provided. Biomedical signals are the recordings of the physiological activities occurring inside a human body. These signals can be recorded from different parts of the body such as the brain, heart, eyes, etc. The use of biomedical signals has enabled professionals to get a deep insight into the working of different body parts of the subject. Non-invasive biomedical signals are usually very prone to noises. This requires some extra preprocessing steps before using the signals for analysis. First, the data is recorded with a lot of care to minimize the noise. The recorded data is then visualized, and artifact removal methods are implemented which remove the signals not associated with the activities of the observed body part. Once the signal is cleaned, the features are extracted. These features are then fed to machine learning algorithms for the analysis of different diseases and disorders. Non-invasive biomedical signals have been used to detect and prevent various diseases and disorders. ECG and PCG have been used for the detection of heart-related diseases. Similarly, EEG can be used for early diagnoses of neurological and psychological disorders. The applications of non-invasive biomedical signals are not only limited to the cure and prevention of diseases, but these signals can also be used for the improvement and betterment of human cognitive and physical health. EEG can be used to improve the cognition and mental health of the subject. PPG can be used to monitor blood pressure, heart rate, and oxygen saturation in the blood. Applications of non-invasive biomedical signals such as neurofeedback and biofeedback training enabled us to enhance mental and physical health.

1.9   Teaching Assignments

1. Describe different types of biomedical signals.
2. Differentiate between invasive and non-invasive acquisition procedures of bio-medicals signals with examples.
3. Explain different steps involved in Biomedical signal processing.
4. What are features and what is meant by feature extraction?
5. Briefly describe Brain Computer Interface and what are its applications.
6. What is biofeedback therapy?
7. What are the benefits of Biofeedback?
8. Explain how Neurofeedback training works.
9. What is neurofeedback training used for?

References

1. H.-H. Chang, J.M. Moura, Biomedical signal processing. Biomed. Eng. Design Handbook **2**, 559–579 (2010)
2. R. Delgado-Gonzalo et al., *Evaluation of accuracy and reliability of PulseOn optical heart rate monitoring device*, in *2015 37th Annual International Conference of the IEEE Engineering in Medicine and Biology Society (EMBC)*, (IEEE, 2015)
3. P. Patel, M. Sarkar, S. Nagaraj, *Ultra wideband channel characterization for invasive biomedical applications*, in *2016 IEEE 17th Annual Wireless and Microwave Technology Conference (WAMICON)*, (IEEE, 2016)
4. K.S. Litvinova et al., Non-invasive biomedical research and diagnostics enabled by innovative compact lasers. Prog. Quant. Electron. **56**, 1–14 (2017)
5. C.D. Block et al., Minimally-invasive and non-invasive continuous glucose monitoring systems: Indications, advantages, limitations and clinical aspects. Curr. Diabetes Rev. **4**(3), 159–168 (2008)
6. M.E. Spira, A. Hai, Multi-electrode array technologies for neuroscience and cardiology. Nat. Nanotechnol. **8**(2), 83–94 (2013)
7. K. Blinowska, P. Durka, *Electroencephalography (Eeg)* (Wiley encyclopedia of biomedical engineering, 2006)
8. R.W. Homan, J. Herman, P. Purdy, Cerebral location of international 10–20 system electrode placement. Electroencephalogr. Clin. Neurophysiol. **66**(4), 376–382 (1987)

9. H. Marzbani, H. Marateb, M. Mansourian, Methodological note: Neu-rofeedback: A comprehensive review on system design, Methodol-ogy and clinical applications. Basic Clin. Neurosci. **7**(2), 143–158 (2016) 10.15412

10. D. Mahmood et al., The effect of music listening on EEG functional connectivity of brain: A short-duration and long-duration study. Mathematics **10**(3), 349 (2022)

11. U. Amin, S.R. Benbadis, The role of EEG in the erroneous diagnosis of epilepsy. J. Clin. Neurophysiol. **36**(4), 294–297 (2019)

12. M. Simão et al., A review on electromyography decoding and pattern recognition for human-machine interaction. Ieee Access **7**, 39564–39582 (2019)

13. B. Farnsworth, *What Is EMG (Electromyography) and How Does It Work?*

14. E. An, *Electromyography (EMG) and Nerve Conduction Studies*

15. Y. Sattar, L. Chhabra, Electrocardiogram, in *StatPearls [Internet]*, (StatPearls Publishing, 2021)

16. J. Xue, L. Yu, Applications of machine learning in ambulatory ECG. Heart **2**(4), 472–494 (2021)

17. M. Collins et al., A review of hand-held electrocardiogram (ECG) recording devices. Eur. J. Cardiovasc. Nurs. **20**(Supplement_1), zvab060 (2021)

18. D.J. Creel, The electroretinogram and electro-oculogram: Clinical applications by Donnell. J. Creel. Webvision: The Organization of the Retina and Visual System (2015)

19. J. Seggie et al., Retinal pigment epithelium response and the use of the EOG and Arden ratio in depression. Psychiatry Res. **36**(2), 175–185 (1991)

20. L. Voxuan, Recognizing Best's disease: Two cases of this rare condition, involving a mother and son, demonstrate an assortment of diagnostic challenges. Rev. Optom. **147**(11), 87–91 (2010)

21. J. Heo, H. Yoon, K.S. Park, A novel wearable forehead EOG measurement system for human computer interfaces. Sensors **17**(7), 1485 (2017)

22. Britannica. *phonocardiography.* 2019 4 July 2022; Available from: https://www.britannica.com/science/phonocardiography

23. H.B. Sprague, History and present status of phonocardiography. IRE Trans. Med. Electron. **PGME-9**, 2–3 (1957)

24. A. Sa-Ngasoongsong et al., A low-cost, portable, high-throughput wireless sensor system for phonocardiography applications. Sensors **12**(8), 10851–10870 (2012)

25. D. Castaneda et al., A review on wearable photoplethysmography sensors and their potential future applications in health care. International journal of biosensors & bioelectronics **4**(4), 195–202 (2018)

26. J. Allen, Photoplethysmography and its application in clinical physiological measurement. Physiol. Meas. **28**(3), R1–R39 (2007)

27. A.M. Johnson, R. Jegan, X.A. Mary, *Performance measures on blood pressure and heart rate measurement from PPG signal for biomedical applications*, in *2017 International Conference on Innovations in Electrical, Electronics, Instrumentation and Media Technology (ICEEIMT)*, (IEEE, 2017)

28. S. Bagha, L. Shaw, A real time analysis of PPG signal for measurement of SpO2 and pulse rate. Internat. J. Computer Applicat. **36**(11), 45–50 (2011)

29. J.C. Richardson et al., Pharmaceutical applications of magnetic resonance imaging (MRI). Adv. Drug Deliv. Rev. **57**(8), 1191–1209 (2005)

30. S.E. Alert, Preventing *accidents and injuries in the MRI suite*

31. E.K. Weidman et al., MRI safety: A report of current practice and advancements in patient preparation and screening. Clin. Imaging **39**(6), 935–937 (2015)

32. N. Dey, *Classification and clustering in biomedical signal processing*. IGI global (2016)

33. M. Elgendi, Eventogram: A visual representation of main events in biomedical signals. Bioengineering **3**(4), 22 (2016)

34. D. Mahmood, H. Nisar, Y.V. Voon, *Removal of Physiological Artifacts from Electroencephalogram Signals: A Review and Case Study*, in *2021 IEEE 9th Conference on Systems, Process and Control (ICSPC 2021)*, (IEEE, 2021)

35. R. Nawaz et al., Comparison of different feature extraction methods for EEG-based emotion recognition. Biocybernetics and Biomedical Engineering **40**(3), 910–926 (2020)

36. S. Krishnan, Y. Athavale, Trends in biomedical signal feature extraction. Biomedical Signal Processing and Control **43**, 41–63 (2018)
37. A.A. Al-Taee et al., Feature extraction using wavelet scattering transform coefficients for EMG pattern classification, in *Australasian Joint Conference on Artificial Intelligence*, (Springer, 2022)
38. J. Rafiee et al., Feature extraction of forearm EMG signals for prosthetics. Expert Syst. Appl. **38**(4), 4058–4067 (2011)
39. W.S. McCulloch, W. Pitts, A logical calculus of the ideas immanent in nervous activity. Bull. Math. Biophys. **5**(4), 115–133 (1943)
40. A.M. Turing, J. Haugeland, *Computing Machinery and Intelligence* (Verbal Behavior as the Hallmark of Intelligence, The Turing Test, 1950), pp. 29–56
41. P.P. Shinde, S. Shah, *A review of machine learning and deep learning applications*, in *2018 fourth international conference on computing communication control and automation (ICCUBEA)*, (IEEE, 2018)
42. V. Patel, A.K. Shah, Machine learning for biomedical signal processing, in *Machine Learning and the Internet of Medical Things in Healthcare*, (Elsevier, 2021), pp. 47–66
43. S.K. Dhull, K.K. Singh, ECG beat classifiers: A journey from ANN to DNN. Procedia Computer Sci. **167**, 747–759 (2020)
44. N. Ghassemi, A. Shoeibi, M. Rouhani, Deep neural network with generative adversarial networks pre-training for brain tumor classification based on MR images. Biomedical Signal Processing and Control **57**, 101678 (2020)
45. S. Banerjee, G.K. Singh, Deep neural network based missing data prediction of electrocardiogram signal using multiagent reinforcement learning. Biomedical Signal Processing and Control **67**, 102508 (2021)
46. S. Chaabene et al., Convolutional neural network for drowsiness detection using EEG signals. Sensors **21**(5), 1734 (2021)
47. M. Porumb et al., A convolutional neural network approach to detect congestive heart failure. Biomedical Signal Process. Cont. **55**, 101597 (2020)
48. K.H. Cheah et al., Convolutional neural networks for classification of music-listening EEG: Comparing 1D convolutional kernels with 2D kernels and cerebral laterality of musical influence. Neural Comput. & Applic. **32**(13), 8867–8891 (2020)
49. S. Madhavan, R.K. Tripathy, R.B. Pachori, Time-frequency domain deep convolutional neural network for the classification of focal and non-focal EEG signals. IEEE Sensors J. **20**(6), 3078–3086 (2019)
50. A. Anuragi, D.S. Sisodia, Empirical wavelet transform based automated alcoholism detecting using EEG signal features. Biomedical Signal Process. Cont. **57**, 101777 (2020)
51. M. Fatima, M. Pasha, Survey of machine learning algorithms for disease diagnostic. J. Intell. Learn. Syst. Appl. **9**(01), 1–16 (2017)
52. C. Marquez-Chin, N. Kapadia-Desai, S. Kalsi-Ryan, *Brain–Computer Interfaces* (Springer, 2021), pp. 51–65
53. J.J. Vidal, et al., Biocybernetic control in man-machine interaction: final technical report 1973-1974. California univ los angeles school of engineering and applied science (1974)
54. L.A. Farwell, E. Donchin, Talking off the top of your head: Toward a mental prosthesis utilizing event-related brain potentials. Electroencephalogr. Clin. Neurophysiol. **70**(6), 510–523 (1988)
55. C. Guger, B.Z. Allison, A. Gunduz, Brain-computer interface research: A state-of-the-art summary 10, in *Brain-Computer Interface Research*, (Springer, 2021), pp. 1–11
56. S. Waldert, Invasive vs. non-invasive neuronal signals for brain-machine interfaces: Will one prevail? Front. Neurosci. **10**, 295 (2016)
57. J. Bu, X. Zhang, BCI-based neurofeedback training for quitting smoking, in *Brain-Computer Interface Research*, (Springer, 2021), pp. 13–23
58. J.J. Daly, J.R. Wolpaw, Brain–computer interfaces in neurological rehabilitation. The Lancet Neurology **7**(11), 1032–1043 (2008)

59. M.M. Moore, Real-world applications for brain-computer interface technology. IEEE Trans. Neural Syst. Rehabil. Eng. **11**(2), 162–165 (2003)
60. J.J. Shih, D.J. Krusienski, J.R. Wolpaw, Brain-computer interfaces in medicine, in *Mayo Clinic Proceedings*, vol. 87, (Elsevier, 2012), pp. 268–279
61. M.C. Domingo, An overview of the internet of things for people with disabilities. J. Netw. Comput. Appl. **35**(2), 584–596 (2012)
62. J.-R. Wang, S. Hsieh, Neurofeedback training improves attention and working memory performance. Clin. Neurophysiol. **124**(12), 2406–2420 (2013)
63. D.T. Karthikeyan, B. Sabarigiri, Enhancement of multi-modal biometric authentication based on iris and brain neuro image coding. Int. J. Biom. Bioinform.(IJBB) **5**, 249 (2011)
64. R. İnce, S.S. Adanır, F. Sevmez, The inventor of electroencephalography (EEG): Hans Berger (1873–1941). Childs Nerv. Syst. **37**(9), 2723–2724 (2021)
65. C. Kerson, *A Neurofeedback Story* (Neurofeedback. The First Fifty Years, 2019), p. 229
66. J. Blumenthal, *Relaxation therapies and biofeedback: Applications in medical practice*, in *Consultation Liaison Psychiatry and Behavioural Medicine*, (WB Saunders, Philadelphia, 1988), pp. 272–283
67. R.R. Kline, *The cybernetics moment: Or why we call our age the information age* (JHU Press, 2015)
68. P.M. Lehrer, Biofeedback training to increase heart rate variability. Principl. Pract. Stress Manag. **3**, 227–248 (2007)
69. A.M. Freedman, H.I. Kaplan, B.J. Sadock, *Comprehensive textbook of psychiatry* (1975), pp. 1350–1350
70. J.P. Hatch, R.J. Gatchel, R. Harrington, Biofeedback: Clinical applications in medicine, in *Handbook of Psychology and Health*, (Routledge, 2021), pp. 37–73
71. A.L. Davidoff, W.E. Whitehead, Biofeedback, relaxation training, and cognitive behavior modification: Treatments for functional GI disorders, in *Handbook of Functional Gastrointestinal Disorders*, (2020), pp. 361–384
72. R. Nawaz, H. Nisar, Y.V. Voon, Changes in spectral power and functional connectivity of response-conflict task after neurofeedback training. IEEE Access **8**, 139444–139459 (2020)
73. R. Nawaz et al., The effect of alpha neurofeedback training on cognitive performance in healthy adults. Mathematics **10**(7), 1095 (2022)
74. E. Angelakis et al., EEG neurofeedback: A brief overview and an example of peak alpha frequency training for cognitive enhancement in the elderly. Clin. Neuropsychol. **21**(1), 110–129 (2007)
75. J.V. Hardt, J. Kamiya, Anxiety change through electroencephalographic alpha feedback seen only in high anxiety subjects. Science **201**(4350), 79–81 (1978)
76. H. Heinrich, H. Gevensleben, U. Strehl, Annotation: Neurofeedback–train your brain to train behaviour. J. Child Psychol. Psychiatry **48**(1), 3–16 (2007)
77. J. Raymond et al., Biofeedback and dance performance: A preliminary investigation. Appl. Psychophysiol. Biofeedback **30**(1), 65–73 (2005)
78. L. Thompson, M. Thompson, A. Reid, Neurofeedback outcomes in clients with Asperger's syndrome. Appl. Psychophysiol. Biofeedback **35**(1), 63–81 (2010)

Chapter 2
Signal Acquisition Preprocessing and Feature Extraction Techniques for Biomedical Signals

Abdulhamit Subasi and Saeed Mian Qaisar

Abstract The primary purposes of the biomedical signals are the detection or diagnosis of disease or physiological states. These signals are also employed in biomedical research to model and study biological systems. The objective of the signal acquisition, pre-conditioning and feature extraction is to attain a precise realization of model or recognition of decisive elements or malfunctioning of human corporal systems using machine or deep learning. Furthermore, it allows future clinical or physiological events to be predicted using machine and deep learning. The obtained biological signal is frequently a complex combination of noise, artifacts, and signal. Instrumentation using sensors, amplifiers, filters, and analog-to-digital converters can produce artifacts. The muscular activities can introduce interference and the powerline and electromagnetic emissions are considered as the primary sources of noise. A good choice of signal collection and processing techniques may be made as a consequence of intended design specifications. This chapter aims to familiarize scientists and biomedical engineers with potential feature extraction methods and in comprehending the fundamentals of the signal acquisition and processing chain.

2.1 Introduction

The biomedical and healthcare industries have undergone a transformation thanks to recent technology advances. The cloud computing of biomedical data, collected by using wire-free wearables and the Internet of Medical Things (IoMT), has

A. Subasi
College of Engineering, Effat University, Jeddah, Saudi Arabia

Institute of Biomedicine, Faculty of Medicine, University of Turku, Turku, Finland
e-mail: abdulhamit.subasi@utu.fi

S. Mian Qaisar (✉)
Electrical and Computer Engineering Department, Effat University, Jeddah, Saudi Arabia
e-mail: sqaisar@effatuniversity.edu.sa

resulted in real-time and portable health monitoring solutions [1]. Numerous medical conditions are diagnosed and distinguished using biomedical signals. Few examples are the identification and categorization of epilepsy, brain tumors, emotions, lie detection, head injuries, blood oxygen levels, glucose levels, strokes, psychiatric illnesses, sleep disorders, cerebral anoxia, cardiac diseases, lung diseases, behavioral disorders, drug effect monitoring, alertness monitoring, and anesthesia depth control.

The signal is a physical quantity that carries information. Signals in the physical and biological realms can be categorized as stochastic or deterministic. Unlike a deterministic signal, a stochastic signal cannot be defined by a mathematical function. The timing of a discharge capacity or a pendulum's location are two instances of predictable signals. The quantity of particles released by a radioactive source or the result of a noise generator are two examples of typical random processes. Although they frequently include both a deterministic and a random component, physiological signals can be classified as stochastic signals. The random component might be more evident in some signals while deterministic impacts are more dominant in others. The Electroencephalogram (EEG) is a type of stochastic signal where the random component is significant. An Electrocardiogram (ECG) can represent a different class of signals since it has a strong deterministic component connected to the transmission of electrical activity in the heart's structures, along with some random components resulting from biological noise.

Biomedical signals are measured and recorded using a variety of sensors. The sensing can be carried out with and without a physical body contact. In the first case, to effectively capture the biomedical signals, certain sensors are implanted to the body of intended subjects, such as endoscope, ECG electrodes and EEG headset. However, in the second case, such as Magnetic Resonance Imaging (MRI), Positron Emission Tomographic (PET) Scanners, and X-ray sensors the information is acquired without by scanning and without a physical contact with the subject's body [2, 3].

The acquired biomedical signals are processed and analyzed using the sophisticated signal processing techniques, transformation approaches, and decomposition algorithms [4]. In certain approaches the features are extracted from the incoming signals. Onward, the most pertinent features can be selected by using the dimension reduction techniques [5, 6]. Finally the selected feature set is processed by single or ensemble machine learning algorithms for the diagnosis, decision making, and prediction [7]. However, in certain approaches the incoming signals are directly conveyed to the deep learning stage. In this case feature extraction, diagnosis/decision making/prediction is merged in deep learning stage. Therefore, the hand-crafted feature engineering is not needed and this task is done by the machine. However, the processing complexity and computing resources requirement is usually superior in this case compared to the prior approach [8].

The stages involved in contemporary features extraction and machine learning based biomedical signal processing and classification chains are the transduction, analog conditioning, analog-to-digital conversion, pre-processing, features selection and classification. The signal transduction process involves the transformation of physical phenomena to electrical signals. Onward these signals are conditioned by amplifying, baseline restoration and analog-filtering to prepare them for an effective interface with the analog to digital converters. The digitized version of information is then pre-processed to diminish any noise and interferences. Onward, the transformation and decomposition mechanisms are used for getting a detailed insight of the incoming signal. Afterward, the features are selected and then processed by the classifier for intended outcome [5].

In this chapter, the principle of signal acquisition and pre-processing stages is described. Moreover, a brief introduction to important biomedical signals features extraction techniques is presented. Finally, a conclusion is made.

2.2 The Biomedical Signal Acquisition and Processing

The biomedical sector's growth has been completely transformed by technological advancements. When it comes to the creation of mobile and remote healthcare systems, communication technology has made enormous strides. These are built on cloud-connected biomedical wearables and cloud-based applications powered by the Internet of Medical Things (IoMT). The initial stage in employing electronic devices and computers to process and analyze biomedical information is to sense and convert biological occurrences into electrical signals. It is achieved by using a variety of contact based and contactless biomedical sensing mechanisms [1]. Designing a low-cost, long-term biomedical information collection system that can offer continuous signal monitoring for illness detection and therapy is desirable in practice. A potent tool for clinical and status monitoring, medical diagnosis, and communication with healthcare systems is biological sensing. In this setting, there have been further developments in wearable biomedical sensors. These can measure the vital signs of the intended subjects such as the electrocardiogram (ECG), electromyography (EMG), blood pressure, blood oxygenation, and other parameters. By measuring, conditioning, converting them from analog to digital domain and wirelessly reporting biological data including cardiac and neurological signals, a biomedical sensor can also offer a scalable and affordable solution for clinical applications.

A variety of sensors are employed for measuring and recording the biomedical signals. The sensing can be carried out with and without a physical body contact. In the first case, to effectively capture the biomedical signals, certain sensors are implanted to the body of intended subjects, such as endoscope, ECG electrodes and EEG headset. However, in the second case, such as Magnetic Resonance Imaging (MRI), Positron Emission Tomographic (PET) Scanners, and X-ray sensors the information is acquired without by scanning and without a physical contact with the subject's body [2, 3].

The sensed biomedical signals possess a crucial information regarding the intended patient's health conditions. The interferences and physiological artifacts can alter these signals. It can decrease the effectiveness of diagnosis. The power line

interference and baseline wander are the mainly present types of noises in the biomedical signals [9, 10]. The baseline wander and other artifacts are introduced by
respiration and activity of human muscles. These are mainly the low-frequency artifacts [10]. The electromagnetic interference of the alternating supply causes the
power line interference to be introduced. It is necessary to remove these undesirable
signal components in order to diagnose biological disorders with accuracy.
Numerous amplification and filtration approaches have been proposed to achieve
this goal.

The sensed and conditioned version of the biological signals is onward converted
from the analog to digital domain. The principle of analog to digital conversion is
depicted in the following sub-section.

2.2.1   The Analog to Digital Conversion

In comparison to analog processing, the Digital Signal Processing (DSP) offers
certain benefits [11]. Because of this, the majority of activities involved in processing of the biomedical signals and images have moved from the analog to the digital
domain in recent years. In this scenario, the Analog to Digital Converters (ADCs)
are becoming a significant influence on the performance of the entire system [12].

Recent applications like the brain-to-computer interface, man-machine interface,
positron emission tomography, biological sensors networks, prosthesis control, and
bioinformatics require out of the shelf solutions. Several developments in the field
of A/D conversion have been made in this regard. There is a wealth of available literature in this area [13]. This chapter's major goal is to quickly recapitulate the key
ideas of the A/D conversion.

By first sampling $x(t)$ in time and then rounding the sample amplitudes (quantization), the A/D conversion is accomplished. The phrase "rounding off" in this context refers to assessing sample amplitudes by contrasting them with selected
reference thresholds.

A discrete representation of an analog signal is created by sampling. To accomplish this in the time domain, multiply the continuous time signal $x(t)$ by the sampling function $s_F(t)$. According to [14], Eq. (2.1), represents the generalized $s_F(t)$.

$$S_F\left(t\right)=\sum_{n=-\infty}^{\infty}\delta\left(t-t_n\right).\qquad(2.1)$$

The Dirac function $\delta(t-t_n)$ and the sampling instant sequence $\{t_n\}$ are used here.
As a result, Eq. (2.2) may be used to represent a sampled signal, $x_s(t)$.

$$x_S\left(t\right)=\sum_{n=-\infty}^{\infty}x\left(t\right).\delta\left(t-t_n\right)=x\left(t_n\right).\qquad(2.2)$$

The sampling is the convolution of the spectra of the analog signal and the sampling function in the frequency domain. Equation (2.3) can be used to express, $S_F(f)$, the spectra of sampling function.

$$S_F\left(f\right) = \sum_{n=-\infty}^{\infty} e^{-j2\pi f t_n}.$$ (2.3)

Finally, Eq. (2.4) may be used to describe the sampled signal Fourier transform $(X_s(f))$.

$$X_S\left(f\right) = X\left(f\right) * S_F\left(f\right).$$ (2.4)

Here, the input analog signal spectrum is denoted by $X(f)$. The traits of "$\{t_n\}$" have a direct impact on the sampling procedure. The sampling procedure is largely divided into the uniform and non-uniform categories depending on how "$\{t_n\}$" is distributed [14].

The uniform sampling is the base of mostly existing biomedical signal processing chains. This is the traditional sampling method, which Shannon first suggested in 1949 [11]. Shannon required a universal method for turning an analog signal into a series of integers in order to create his distortion theory, which is how he came up with the classical sampling theorem [11]. The majority of current digital signal processing (DSP) theory is built on this sampling theorem, which makes the assumptions that the input signal is bandlimited, the sample is regular, and the sampling rate complies with the Shannon sampling criteria.

The classical sampling method is a wholly predictable and periodic one, theoretically. The sample instants in this instance are evenly spaced. As a result, the time difference T_s between two successive samples is special. T_s is referred to as the sample period in literature. The periodicity of the sampling process is a product of T_s' singularity. This characteristic has led to several names for this sampling procedure, including periodic and equidistant. The sampling model has the following mathematical definition.

$$t_n = nT_S, n = 0, 1, 2, \ldots.$$ (2.5)

In this instance, $s_F(t)$ may be written as a series of evenly spaced infinite delta impulses. Equation (2.6) expresses the procedure.

$$S_F\left(t\right) = \sum_{n=-\infty}^{\infty} \delta\left(t - nT_S\right).$$ (2.6)

Following Eq. (2.6), Eqs. (2.2), (2.3) and (2.4) become as follow in this case.

$$x_s\left(t\right) = \sum_{n=-\infty}^{\infty} x\left(t\right).\delta\left(t - nT_S\right) = x\left(nT_s\right).$$ (2.7)

$$S_F(f) = \frac{1}{T_s} \sum_{n=-\infty}^{\infty} \delta(f - nF_S). \tag{2.8}$$

$$X_s(f) = \frac{1}{T_s} \sum_{n=-\infty}^{\infty} X(f - nF_S). \tag{2.9}$$

The Fourier transform's frequency shifting feature, which states that $X_s(f)$ is generated by shifting and repeating $X(f)$ forever at the integral multiples of F_s, is used to achieve Eqs. (2.8) and (2.9), where $F_s = 1/T_s$ is the sampling frequency (cf. Equation 2.9). The original signal spectrum is recognized as a picture of these repeating duplicates.

According to Shannon's research, $x(t)$ can be entirely reconstructed if its ordinates are provided at a succession of locations spaced $1/(2.f_{max})$ seconds apart and there are no frequencies greater than fmax. The following condition on the sampling frequency F_s is essentially used.

$$F_s \geq 2.f_{max}. \tag{2.10}$$

Shannon first suggested this F_s criteria, and Nyquist later expanded on it. This is the basis for the term "Nyquist sampling frequency," which refers to sampling at a frequency that is precisely equal to two twice the maximum frequency (f_{max}).

$$F_{Nyq} = 2.f_{max}. \tag{2.11}$$

The spectral images (cf. Equation (2.9)) do not alias in the $x_s(t)$ spectrum since condition (2.10) is satisfied. The Poisson formula, which asserts that filtering $x_s(t)$ via an ideal low pass filter yields $x(t)$, may be used to recover $x(t)$ from $x_s(t)$.

$$x(t) = \sum_{n=-\infty}^{\infty} x(n.T_s). \frac{\sin(\pi.F_s(t - nT_s))}{\pi.F_s(t - nT_s)}. \tag{2.12}$$

The sampling function that is given by Eq. (2.6) is the one that is used the most frequently in practical applications. Although this sampling procedure is theoretically abstracted in Eq. (2.6). Purely deterministic sampling was never feasible in real-world applications. The non-uniformity in the process is due to the real sampling instants, which are constantly out of phase with where they should be on the time axis [11, 13].

After sampling, the second main step in A/D conversion is the quantization. There are several ways to implement the quantization process, which yields a variety of quantized signal properties. Generally speaking, the distribution mechanism for the reference thresholds determines whether the quantization process is deterministic or random. The references are preserved in fixed places for deterministic quantization, but they are changed at random for randomized quantization [13].

Traditionally, a uniform sampling and uniform deterministic quantization technique are used to carry out the A/D conversion. The reference thresholds in this case are uniformly distributed, which implies that each threshold's subsequent amplitude difference is unique. This is referred to as uniform quantization. The quantization procedure in this situation is evident from Fig. 2.1. Where, q is the quantization step.

The only error that a theoretical ADC may introduce is the quantization error Qe. This inaccuracy occurs because the output is a series of limited precision samples but the analog input signal can take on any value within the ADC amplitude dynamics [13]. The ADC resolution in bits determines the samples' accuracy (cf. Fig. 2.2).

The dynamic range of an M-bit resolution converter may be described by Eq. (2.13) in the situation of uniform deterministic quantization if the ADC voltage changes between $[-Vmax; Vmax]$.

$$2^M = \frac{2.V_{max}}{q}.$$ (2.13)

In this case, the upper bound on Q_e is given by Eq. (2.14) [13].

$$Q_e \leq \frac{LSB}{2}.$$ (2.14)

Where, LSB is the converter least significant bit, which is clear from the transfer function of an ideal M-bit ADC, shown in Fig. 2.3.

In Fig. 2.3, q is the weight of an LSB in terms of voltage. The process of calculating q is straightforward from Eq. (2.13).

Authors examined the real Qe spectrum in [13]. They have demonstrated that for each sample point, the Qe can occur within the range of ½ q. Qe's more information may be found in [13].

Fig. 2.1 Uniform deterministic quantization: original and quantized signals

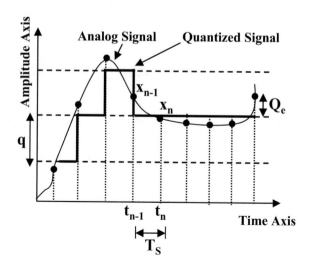

Fig. 2.2 M-bit resolution
A/D conversion process

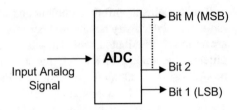

Fig. 2.3 Ideal M-bit ADC
quantization error

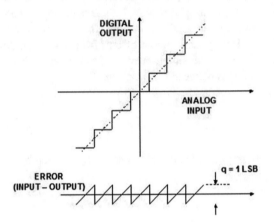

Qe may be represented as a sawtooth waveform by supposing that it is a white noise process and that it is uncorrelated to the input signal. Equation (2.15) provides Qe as a function of time based on this supposition.

$$Q_e(t) \leq s, \qquad \frac{-q}{2.s} < t < \frac{q}{2.s}. \tag{2.15}$$

Where, s is the waveform slope (cf. Fig. 2.4). The MS (Mean Square) value of $Q_e(t)$ can be calculated by employing Eq. (2.16).

$$MS(Q_e(t)) = \frac{s}{q} \int_{\frac{q}{2s}}^{\frac{-q}{2s}} (s.t)^2 .dt. \tag{2.16}$$

After simple integration and simplification, Eq. (2.16) results into Eq. (2.17).

$$MS(Q_e(t)) = \frac{(q)^2}{12}. \tag{2.17}$$

Finally, the RMS (Root Mean Square) value of $Q_e(t)$ is given by Eq. (2.18).

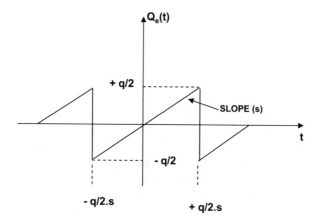

Fig. 2.4 Quantization error as a function of time

$$RMS\left(Q_e\left(t\right)\right) = \frac{q}{\sqrt{12}}. \tag{2.18}$$

In the $[-\infty; \infty]$ Hz frequency band, the $Qe(t)$ generates harmonics [13]. The desired spectral band typically is between $[0; F_s/2]$, where F_s is the sampling frequency of the system. The in-band spectral width BW_{in} is the term used in literature to refer to the bandwidth $[0; F_s/2]$ [13]. The harmonics of the spectrum go far beyond than BW_{in}. The higher order harmonics, however, are all folded back into BW_{in} as a result of spectral periodization, and they add up to roughly generate an RMS $(Q_e(t))$ equal to $q/\sqrt{12}$ [13].

2.2.2   The Digital Filtering

The signal is further denoised in the digital domain before it is converted to digital form. While reducing artifacts and noise, it enables emphasis on the signal's pertinent contents. Filtering, a method that alters the relative amplitudes of a signal's frequency components or may even completely delete specific frequency components, is useful in a range of significant applications [14]. The conventional digital filtering is a time-invariant operation. They use a fixed order filter with a set sample rate to process the input signal [12]. A wide variety of filters, including Chebyshev, Butterworth, Bessel, windowed sinc, moving average, etc., are described in literature. To acquire the required results for a given application, a suitable filter should be carefully designed.

Analog and digital are mainly two primary categories of filters. An analog filter creates the desired filtering effect by utilizing electrical components such operational amplifiers, resistors, and capacitors. The signal being filtered is an electrical voltage or current that is the exact physical equivalent of the quantity at all times. A digital processor is used by a digital filter to compute the values of digitized signals. The calculator might be a general-purpose computer or a specialized digital signal processor. Instead of being represented by a voltage or current in a digital filter, the signal is instead represented by a series of numerical values.

There are several situations in which analog filters ought to be utilized. This has more to do with general aspects that can only be accomplished with analog circuits rather than the actual filtering performance. The primary benefit is speed; analog is quick, whereas digital is slow. The amplitude and frequency dynamic range is analog's second intrinsic advantage over digital.

The analog filters are being quickly replaced by the digital ones as a result of recent technical breakthroughs. This is because, for a given task, digital filters might produce results that are far superior than those of their analog counterparts [14]. Digital filters provide programmability, temperature resistance, smaller attainable pass band ripples, linear phase characteristics, sharper achievable roll-off and stop band attenuation, the ability to obtain greater SNR, and other benefits over analog filters [14].

The implementation of the digital filters might be either recursive or non-recursive. The terms Infinite Impulse Response (IIR) and Finite Impulse Response (FIR) are also widely used to refer to the recursive and non-recursive filters, respectively. The FIR filters are the linear phase filters and possess the unconditional stability. These are the key benefits of the FIR filters over IIR filters [12]. They are preferred for several applications because to these qualities, including equalizers, multirate processing, wavelets, etc.

If h_k is the FIR filter impulse response, then in time domain the filtering is performed by convolving h_k with the digitized input signal x_n. The process can be formally represented as follow.

$$y_n = h_k * x_n = \sum_{k=0}^{P} h_k . x_{n-k}. \tag{2.19}$$

The filtered signal in this case is y_n. The filter coefficients are indexed by k. The number of earlier input samples utilized to generate the current output is called the filter order, or P. The filtering process in the frequency domain may be stated as follows, just as the convolution in the time domain becomes the multiplication in the frequency domain [14]. Here, the DFTs of y_n and x_n are calculated to provide $Y(f)$ and $X(f)$, respectively. The DFT of h_k is computed to produce the FIR filter frequency response, $H(f)$. h_k, by using time domain convolution, or $H(f)$, by using frequency domain multiplication, affects the input signal spectrum. It highlights some frequency components and attenuating others.

$$Y(f) = H(f).X(f). \tag{2.20}$$

2.2.3 The Windowing

Often, a waveform is a small piece of a much larger time series. EEG and ECG waveforms are biomedical waveforms that endure the full life of the person. Only a fraction of these waveforms may be kept in computer memory due to how the waveform is truncated. In most cases, a rectangular window is created by simply cutting out a part of the whole waveform and storing it in memory without additional shaping. Now just the windowed part of the waveform is subject to examination. Other window shapes, usually referred to as tapering functions, are sometimes advised. The waveform must be multiplied by the correct shape to use them. By applying the Fourier transform to the window itself, the frequency properties of the window are included in the resultant frequency spectrum, allowing us to draw the conclusion that all windows generate artifacts. The triangular windows, Hanning, Blackman, Kaiser, and Hamming are the most well-known. Below are their equations in [15, 16]:

Triangular window:
for odd n:

$$w(k) = \begin{cases} 2k/(n-1) & 1 \le k \le (n+1)/2 \\ 2(n-k-1)/n+1 & (n+1)/2 \le k \le n \end{cases} \tag{2.21}$$

for even n:

$$w(k) = \begin{cases} (2k-1)/n & 1 \le k \le n/2 \\ 2(n-k+1)/n & n/2+1 \le k \le n \end{cases} \tag{2.22}$$

Hamming window:

$$w(k+1) = 0.54 - 0.46(2\pi k/(n-1))k = 0,1,\ldots,n-1 \tag{2.23}$$

The most effective window is frequently found by testing with real data, or we might consider which spectral properties are significant to us. The rectangular window is chosen if there are two narrowband signals that are closely spaced apart since it has the smallest mainlobe. The sidelobes of the strong signal must not overwhelm the weak signal in order to resolve a fairly spaced strong and weak signal. In this situation, a window with quick sidelobe decay is desirable. The optimal option may be a window with moderately fading sidelobes and a relatively thin main lobe when there are two quite strong signals, one nearby and one farther away from a weak signal [15, 16].

2.3   The Features Extraction Techniques

In the categorization of biomedical signals, the feature extraction phase is crucial. Since there are so many data points in the EEG signals, distinct and useful characteristics may be retrieved from them using a variety of feature extraction techniques. Biomedical signals' behavior is characterized by these distinct and illuminating features, which may point to a particular action or activity. By highlighting distinctive and educational elements, biomedical signs can be identified. Frequencies and amplitudes can be utilized to depict the signal patterns employed in biological signal analysis. These features may be extracted using a variety of techniques, which is another stage of signal processing that facilitates and augments the effectiveness and efficiency of the post classification stage [17]. Since all waveforms have a finite duration and frequency, an efficient biomedical signal decomposition is required for the integration of the time, frequency, and space dimensions. Utilizing temporal-frequency (TF) methods, which can spot changes in both time and frequency, biomedical signals could be analyzed [16, 18, 19].

It is crucial to deal with smaller data sets that identify the proper signal characteristics in order to obtain greater performance. Feature extraction, the process of converting signals into a pertinent feature vector, is typically how features are gathered into a feature vector. A signal classification framework examines a signal's distinguishing characteristics and establishes the signal's class based on those characteristics [16, 20]. Time-frequency approaches dissect signals in the time and frequency domains, as has been discussed in this Chapter. Examples include the empirical wavelet transform (EWT), discrete wavelet transform (DWT), short-time Fourier transform (STFT), wavelet transform (WT), and empirical mode decomposition (EMD). The most crucial information from the original vector should be preserved when the feature extraction procedure reduces the original data to a smaller dimension. As a result, it is crucial to pinpoint the primary traits that, given the structure of the collection, define the whole thing. Different statistical characteristics may be derived from each sub-sample data point as the most typical values characterize the distribution of the biological signals. The minimum, maximum, mean, median, mode, standard deviation, variance, first, third, and inter-quartile range (IQR) are some of the frequently used features of biological signals [16, 20].

2.3.1   The Spectral Analysis

A waveform's representation in the frequency domain can frequently be more helpful than one in the time domain. As a consequence, by examining a range of biological signals in the frequency domain, we can find fascinating and beneficial traits for diagnosis. Common examples of biological signals and signs include the heart rate, EMG, EEG, ECG, eye movements, acoustic heart sounds, and stomach sounds [15]. The frequency content of a waveform is determined using spectral analysis. It demonstrates to be a practical method for categorizing a range of biological data. This technique was developed to more accurately depict the biomedical signals activity than could simple be depicted by analytical techniques like one-dimensional histograms of the sample data. Given the periodic nature of many biological rhythms, signal decomposition in terms of sine and cosine functions was shown to be favorable. It was also a workable option in terms of computing. The fundamental result of Fourier transform spectral analysis is a collection of coefficients that describe the power spectrum and connect the signal to sines and cosines at various frequencies. A frequency band's power may be rapidly ascertained using the power spectrum. This characteristic can help us identify whether the EEG data contains an alpha rhythm or other rhythms [16, 21].

There are several spectrum analysis techniques accessible, each with its own set of benefits and drawbacks. These methods are divided into two categories: Both conventional techniques (Fourier transform) and contemporary techniques based on model parameter estimates [15]. Because no assumptions about parametric modelling are made, spectral analysis based on the Fourier transform is frequently referred to be nonparametric [16, 22].

2.3.1.1   The Fourier Transform (FT)

One of the most popular spectrum estimating techniques utilized today is the traditional Fourier transform (FT) approach. The sine and cosine functions have a single frequency of energy, which is the foundation of the Fourier transform. The basic idea is to divide a waveform into many sinusoids of various frequencies. The amplitude of these sinusoids is related to the frequency component of the waveform at these frequencies [15]. A series of sines, cosines, and their multiples can be used to depict any periodic waveform. It can alternatively be represented by a single sine wave with its versions with different amplitudes, frequencies and phases. In the first situation, we must multiply the waveform with the sine and cosine families and integrate over time to obtain the correct amplitude of the frequency components [15, 16]. The two equations below provide an explanation for this process.

$$a(m) = \frac{2}{T} \int_{\frac{T}{2}}^{-\frac{T}{2}} x(t) \cos\left(2pmf_T t\right) dt. \tag{2.24}$$

$$b(m) = \frac{2}{T} \int_{\frac{T}{2}}^{-\frac{T}{2}} x(t) \sin\left(2pmf_T t\right) dt. \tag{2.25}$$

where m is a collection of numbers, $m = 1, 2, 3,...$, identifying the family member and creating harmonically related frequencies, mf_T, and T is the period or whole time duration of the waveform, $f_T = 1/T$.

Fourier series analysis is sometimes referred to as harmonic decomposition since waveforms are represented by harmonically linked sine waves. Only for m/T values that match the waveform for $m = 1$ do the sinusoids have valid frequencies. For $m > 1$, harmonics are greater multiples. The Fourier transform and Fourier series combine to provide a bidirectional transform for periodic functions. In other words, after a waveform has undergone the Fourier transform to produce sinusoidal components, those components may be utilized to recreate the original waveform [15, 16]:

$$x(t) = \frac{a(0)}{2} + \sum_{m=1}^{\infty} a(m)\cos(2\pi mf_T t) + b(m)\sin(2\pi mf_T t). \tag{2.26}$$

$$x(t) = \frac{a(0)}{2} + \sum_{m=1}^{\infty} c(m)\sin(2\pi mf_T t + \theta_m). \tag{2.27}$$

where $c(m) = \sqrt{a^2(m) + b^2(m)}$ and $\theta_m = tan^{-1}(b(m)/a(m))$.

But for the majority of actual waveforms, there are not many sinusoidal components with appreciable amplitudes, thus a finite summation in Eq. (2.27) is frequently fairly correct. Waveforms can be symmetric or antisymmetric with respect to the y-axis or $t = 0$. An even function is one in which $x(t) = x(-t)$ and around $t = 0$, the waveform exhibits mirror symmetry. An odd function, with zero values for all $b(m)$ terms, results by multiplying an even function with an odd function (see Eq. (2.25)). Multiplications using cosines result in an odd function when the waveform is antisymmetric near $t = 0$, $x(t) = -x(t)$, zeroing all $a(m)$ coefficients (see Eq. (2.24)). Half-wave symmetric functions contain a(m) and b(m) terms that, for even m, are both equal to zero. These functions can be odd or even and have the condition $x(t) = x(T - t)$ [15]. These symmetry qualities may be helpful in lowering the complexity and computation time when computing the coefficients by hand [16].

The continuous analysis we just reviewed is followed by the discrete-time Fourier series analysis. There are several similarities between the equations for continuous-time and discrete-time Fourier series analysis. Summation is used in place of integration, and complex variable notation and Euler's identity are used to represent sinusoidal terms [16]:

$$ejx = \cos x + j \sin x. \tag{2.28}$$

where j represents $\sqrt{-1}$ since i is reserved for current in engineering. The expression for the discrete Fourier transform now becomes:

$$X(f) = \sum_{n=0}^{N-1} x(n) e^{\left(\frac{-j2\pi f_n}{N}\right)} = \sum_{n=0}^{N-1} x(n)\sin(2\pi mf_T t + \theta_m). \tag{2.29}$$

If N is the total number of points, f is the harmonic number, or family member (the length of the digital data).

For the sake of calculation, $f = -N/2,..., N/2-1$ must have both positive and negative values for $X(f)$. Negative frequencies, which have no physical significance, are linked to negative values. The formula for the inverse Fourier transform is as follows:

$$x(n) = \frac{1}{N} \sum_{n=0}^{N-1} X(m) e^{\left(\frac{j2\pi m_n}{N}\right)}.$$
(2.30)

2.3.1.2 The Parametric Model Based Methods

The Fourier transform is used to produce power spectra, which represents the most reliable spectral estimators. Though they are not necessary, assumptions or information about the characteristics of the waveform may be helpful when choosing windows and averaging strategies. Furthermore, estimate distortion could result from assuming that the waveform beyond the window equals zero. Some of the drawbacks and distortions created by traditional approaches are supposed to be addressed by modern spectrum analysis techniques. They work well when analyzing signals with a brief period. The waveform of interest and maybe the mechanism that created it should be known to modern approaches. When that happens, these techniques can make assumptions about the waveform beyond the window, which improves spectral resolution, especially for waveforms with a lot of noise. The spectral resolution, however, will be greatly influenced by how well the selected model fits the situation [16, 23].

Additionally, the popularity of distinct linear model types, which may be separated by the properties of their transfer functions, might be partially explained by the availability of computationally advantageous methods for parameter assessment. But up to now, the main focus has been on autoregressive modelling [16, 21].

The following model types are among the most common:

- autoregressive (AR),
- moving average (MA), and
- autoregressive moving average (ARMA).

It is necessary to have some understanding of the potential spectrum form in order to select the optimal model. The formula for an AR model is:

$$y(n) = -\sum_{k=1}^{p} a(k) y(n-k) + v(n).$$
(2.31)

In (2.31), $v(n)$ is noise, p is the filter order and $a(k)$ are parameters of the model. $E[v^2(n)] = \sigma_v^2$ is variance of noise. $y(n-k)$ and $y(n)$ are respectively the previous and computed outcomes.

In the numerator and denominator of an AR model transfer function, there is a constant and a polynomial. The AR model is hence commonly called an all-pole model. The transfer function, H(z), of an AR model is obtained using the Z-transform:

$$H(z) = \frac{1}{A(z)} = \frac{1}{1 + a_1 z^{-1} + \ldots + a_p z^{-p}}. \qquad (2.32)$$

The model is determined by the positions of the poles and zeroes. In the spectrum, the valleys correspond to the zeros, whilst the peaks correspond to the poles. Therefore, when analyzing spectra with strong peaks and no discernible troughs, the AR model performs well.

On the other hand, spectra with troughs but no significant peaks can be estimated using the moving average method. There is just one polynomial for the numerator in the transfer function of the MA model. As a result, it is commonly referred to as an all-zero model. The equation below describes the MA model:

$$y(n) = -\sum_{k=1}^{q} b(k) v(n-k) \qquad (2.33)$$

where q is a model's order and $v(n)$ is the input noise function.

When high peaks and deep troughs are expected in the spectrum, a model that combines elements of the AR and MA models may be used. Since a transfer function with polynomials in both the numerator and the denominator is most likely present in an ARMA model, it is commonly referred to as a pole-zero model. An ARMA model's equation is given as:

$$y(n) = -\sum_{k=1}^{p} a(k) y(n-k) + \sum_{k=1}^{q} b(k) v(n-k). \qquad (2.34)$$

The rational transfer function can define the ARMA model just as effectively,

$$H(z) = \frac{B(z)}{A(z)} = \frac{b_0 + b_1 z^{-1} + \cdots + b_q z^{-q}}{1 + a_1 z^{-1} + \cdots + a_p z^{-p}}. \qquad (2.35)$$

Since solving a linear matrix problem is often involved in determining AR parameters, the process is extremely effective. The assessment techniques for computing the parameters of the ARMA and MA models, on the other hand, need a lot more computations. Additionally, these two methods may not converge at all or may converge incorrectly [16, 21].

Although this is not the case for the great majority of ARMA techniques, ARMA approaches should evaluate the AR and MA parameters simultaneously in order to get the best performance The MA approach also cannot be used as a high-resolution spectral estimator since it has trouble modelling narrow-band spectra properly. It cannot be utilized to calculate the power spectrum of biological signals as a result.

Although the autocorrelation sequence estimation aspect of the AR spectral approach is frequently used to characterize it, techniques that work directly on waveform's finite data segments yield superior results [15, 16]. The most common methods for directly extracting the parameters and accompanying power spectrum of the AR model from the waveform are:

- Yule-Walker,
- Burg,
- Covariance, and
- Modified covariance methods.

It is natural to wonder which AR spectral estimation approach is ideal for biological signal processing given the variety of options available. It is also necessary to address the problem of choosing the model order p. One of the various design aspects that must be taken into account is the sample rate [16, 21].

The most suitable strategy is decided by the desired spectrum shape since various approaches stress certain spectral features. The Yule-Walker method, for instance, generates the least-resolved spectra and hence offers the greatest smoothing. Contrarily, the modified covariance approach produces the sharpest spectral peaks, making it simpler to identify sinusoidal waveform components [23]. The spectra generated by the covariance and Burg methods are equivalent. The modified covariance technique could, however, not provide a stable AR model with all of the poles inside the unit circle [24]. Fortunately, stability has little impact on spectrum analysis, but it must be taken into account when creating an AR-based classifier. Evidently, Burg's method yields a trustworthy AR model [16, 21].

In addition to choosing the model type, we also need to decide on the model order, indicated by p and/or q. When choosing the order of the models, it may be helpful to comprehend the data generating process. Several guidelines are available to assist with this [15]. For instance, selecting a p number that is too high leads to phony spectral peaks, while selecting a p value that is too low leads to an incredibly smooth spectrum with poor resolution [21]. To allow the model spectrum to solely suit the signal spectrum while rejecting noise, the model's order must be high enough [15]. Actually, the vast majority of investigations have relied on a predetermined model sequence. Even lower model orders offer some amount of noise and artifacts resistance while offering sufficient spectral resolution for categorization of signal spectra [25]. The fifth- or sixth-order AR model has been effectively used in several studies [26, 27]. A higher model order is required if we wish to represent the power spectrum more accurately. For each spectral peak of interest, the model order is increased by two, and this number creates a lower bound for p. N/3 allows for the freely chosen upper limit of the model order [23]. However, the chosen model order is frequently a lot smaller than N/3 [16, 21].

2.3.1.3 The Subspace Based Methods

From noise-distorted data, the powers and frequency of signals are calculated using subspace-based methods. These methods make advantage of the eigen-decomposition of the correlation matrix of the noise-corrupted signal, and they perform best with noise-corrupted signals composed of a number of discrete sinusoids [28–32]. The PSD, $A(f)$, is computed as [16]:

$$A(f) = \sum_{k=0}^{m} a_k e^{-j2\pi fk} \tag{2.36}$$

Where, m is the eigen-filter order and a_k present the model parameters. Additionally, assuming white noise, the polynomial is represented in terms of the input signal's autocorrelation matrix R.

$$R = E\left\{ x(n)^* . x(n)^T \right\} = SPS^\# + \sigma v^2 I. \tag{2.37}$$

Where, $x(n)$ is the observer signal, S is the direction matrix. $(m + 1)L$, L is the matrix dimension, R is the autocorrelation matrix of dimension $(m + 1)(m + 1)$, and P is the signal power matrix. The size of P is $(L)(L)$. sv^2 is the power of noise and I denotes the identity matrix. * presents the complex conjugate and # is the complex conjugate transposition.

$$S = [Sw1\, Sw2 ... SwL], \tag{2.38}$$

When the signal frequencies are represented by $w_1, w_2,...,w_L$::

$$Swi = [1\, ejwi\, ej2wi ... ejmwi]T\ i = 1, 2,..., L. \tag{2.39}$$

The estimated autocorrelation matrix R is often created using the autocorrelation lags in real-world applications:

$$\hat{R}(k) = \frac{1}{N} \sum_{n=0}^{N-1-k} x(n+k).x(n) \quad k = 0, 2,.......m \tag{2.40}$$

where N is the number of signal samples and k is the autocorrelation lag index. The following is the calculated autocorrelation matrix:

$$\hat{R}(k) = \begin{bmatrix} \hat{R}(0) & \hat{R}(1) & \hat{R}(2) & \cdots & \cdots & \hat{R}(m) \\ \hat{R}(1) & & & \cdots & \cdots & \hat{R}(m-1) \\ \hat{R}(2) & & & \cdot & & \hat{R}(m-2) \\ & & \cdot & \cdot & \cdot & \\ & & \cdot & \cdot & \cdot & \\ \hat{R}(m) & \hat{R}(m-1) & \cdots & \cdots & \cdots & \hat{R}(0) \end{bmatrix}. \tag{2.41}$$

Equation (2.42) may be written as: multiplying by the eigenvector of the autocorrelation matrix a:

$$\hat{R}a = SPSa + sv^2 a. \tag{2.42}$$

Where, a is the eigenvector of autocorrelation matrix (R's). a is composed of $[a_0, a_1, ..., a_m]^T$. The needed polynomial is only used by the subspace-based techniques, which also use it to compute the spectrum, as they only use the eigenvector corresponding to the least eigenvalue [33]. Therefore, $S\#a = 0$. Equation (2.42) changes to (2.43) when the eigenvector is considered to reside in the noise subspace:

$$\hat{R}a = sv^2 a. \tag{2.43}$$

with the restriction that $a = 1$, where σv^2 is the noise power, which corresponds to the subspace-based modelling minimal eigenvalue associated with the eigenvector a. Under the supposition of white noise, it follows that all eigenvalues in the noise subspace must be equal.

$$\lambda_1 = \lambda_2 = \lambda_3 = ... = \lambda_k = \sigma v^2. \tag{2.44}$$

where $i = 1, 2,..., K$ denotes the noise subspace dimension and λ_i represents the noise subspace eigenvalues [16, 34].

2.3.2 The Time-Frequency Analysis

The Fourier transform of a musical phrase "tells us what notes are played, but it is very difficult to determine when they are performed" [35]. The inverse Fourier transform can, however, uniquely reconstruct the waveform, therefore the frequency spectrum must contain frequency timing information. Since particular time events are dispersed throughout all phase components, turning a local feature in time into a global feature in phase, this information is really encoded in the transform's phase portion, which is challenging to understand and retrieve. For nonstationary signals having time-dependent spectral components, the Fourier transform is hence inappropriate [15, 36]. In order to display the frequencies at each time instant, methods for extracting both time and frequency information from a waveform were created. Understanding nonstationary biological signals has been substantially facilitated by the use of combined time-frequency information [16, 21].

2.3.2.1 The Short-Time Fourier Transform

A simple and well-liked Time-Frequency Analysis (TFA) approach is the short-time Fourier transform (STFT), which is based on a common sliding-window methodology. When the non-stationary signal is split into a number of quick data segments, stationarity is presumed in the sliding-window approach. In other words, the spectrum of any given short data segment remains constant, but the signal's spectrum evolves with time. The sliding window approach allows for the application of common spectrum estimate techniques to each of these segments, including the periodogram, Welch's method, and AR technique. After that, a spectral power distribution in the combined time-frequency domain may be created by concatenating the spectral estimates from all windows. Time resolution and frequency resolution are the two most important TFA methods' features. A time-frequency distribution's (TFD) ability to distinguish between two closely spaced signal components in the time domain or frequency domain is referred to as its time resolution and frequency resolution, respectively. The uncertainty principle of the TFA governs the trade-off between time-resolution and frequency resolution in STFT (and all other sliding-window approaches). According to the uncertain principle, it is impossible to determine a signal's precise time-frequency representation since both time resolution and frequency resolution cannot be reduced to arbitrary tiny values [37].

Because it is straightforward, computationally effective, and yields a consistent time-frequency spectrum, STFT is a well-liked technique for evaluating non-stationary data. The decomposition must choose between time and frequency resolution, which is the main problem. For transitory signals, it could be difficult to handle this compromise adequately [16, 38, 39].

The initial time-frequency methods involved segmenting the waveform into a number of brief, succeeding, and perhaps overlapping portions, and then performing the Fourier transform on each one of them. The time-dependent character of the signal was then shown by the resulting series of spectra. A window function is used to trim the waveform, successfully separating the data portions from the waveform of interest. This method, known as the short-time Fourier transform (STFT), has been effectively employed in a number of biological applications since the Fourier Transform is applied to data portions that are significantly shorter than the entire waveform. The sliding window function w(t) is added to the Fourier transform equation to construct the STFT equation, resulting in the two-dimensional function X(t, f) that is defined as follows:

$$X(t,f) = \int_{-\infty}^{+\infty} x(\tau)w(\tau-t)e^{-j2\pi f\tau}d\tau \tag{2.45}$$

where $x(t)$ is the waveform, and τ is the variable that moves the window through it. The following definition identifies the equation's discrete form:

$$X(n,m) = \sum_{k=1}^{N} x(k)\left[W(k-n)e^{-\frac{j2\pi km}{N}} \right]. \tag{2.46}$$

Since the spectrogram of the waveform $x(t)$ is equal to the squared STFT magnitude in Eq. (2.47), the STFT produces a time-frequency representation or distribution of the waveform.

$$P(t,f) = |X(t,f)|2 \tag{2.47}$$

This results in a nonnegative, real-valued distribution being represented by the spectrogram [15, 16]. The spectrogram has two significant drawbacks: Finding the ideal window length for data segments and balancing time and frequency are two important first steps. The frequency resolution is decreased when the data length, N, is shortened to enhance temporal resolution. Loss of low frequencies that are not fully incorporated into the data segment may result from cutting the data segment short. As a result, the frequency resolution decreases when a narrower window is utilized to increase temporal resolution, and vice versa.

2.3.2.2 The Wavelet Transform

The fixed-length window's fixed time-frequency resolution over the entire time-frequency domain is the STFT's biggest flaw. To improve the time-frequency resolution for various spectral components of a signal, the time-frequency domain window size should be adjusted. One effective window selection method uses an adaptable and changing temporal window that is long at low frequencies and short at high frequencies. In fact, the continuous wavelet transform's window selection strategy is another widely used time-frequency analysis technique (CWT). CWT can handle the issue of fixed time-frequency resolution in STFT depending on the time-frequency characteristics of the signal and the real demands. Long windows are used by CWT in the low-frequency range, whereas short windows are used in the high-frequency region [37].

Each transform should provide more details, which often results in a fresh interpretation of the original waveform. The time-frequency problem has not been fully resolved despite the use of several time-frequency approaches. Another technique for defining the time-frequency features of a waveform is the wavelet transform. But now the waveform is separated into scale segments, not time segments [15, 16].

The Fourier transform was used to decompose the waveform $x(t)$ in a vast range of sinusoidal functions:

$$X\left(\omega_m\right) = \int_{-\infty}^{+\infty} x(t) e^{-j\omega_m t} dt \tag{2.48}$$

Due to their popularity and the fact that they have energy at just one frequency, sine functions are a great option for examining the frequency characteristic of a waveform known as the frequency spectrum. Practically every function family may be utilized to assess or examine a waveform's unique feature or behavior. Finite-length probing functions are suitable for sliding over the waveform $x(t)$, just like the sliding window function $w(t)$ is used to perform the STFT. The following convolution characterizes a transform with a sliding weighing function in general:

$$X\left(t,m\right) = \int_{-\infty}^{+\infty} x(\tau) f\left(t-\tau\right)_m d\tau \tag{2.49}$$

where m is the family number and $f(t)_m$ denotes a family of functions. Note that the waveform was multiplied with the probing functions in the final two equations before being averaged to accomplish the comparisons described above. This transform is bidirectional because the family of functions, which must be large, should be able to show all characteristics of the waveform $x(t)$ by producing a redundant set of descriptions $X(t,m)$, which is more than enough to reconstruct $x(t)$. Unless it is occasionally employed for noise reduction, this redundancy is practically useless. Take note that while the STFT and all distributions are redundant, the Fourier transform is not [15, 16].

Wavelets have two parameters, one for sliding through time and the other for scaling it. In order to properly characterize transitory signals, oscillating functions with their energy focused on time are called wavelets. Band-pass filtering is one of the mathematical properties that a wavelet function must possess. To obtain adequate localization in both time and frequency, which is the aim of wavelet analysis. The exploration of the coexistence of fine structures and global waveforms in signals is made possible by two extra degrees of freedom, sliding and scaling. The fundamental concept of analyzing signals at many scales with increasing levels of resolution is embodied in a multi-resolution analysis [21]. The subject of filter banks, which is closely related to wavelet analysis, is covered in a number of good works that provide thorough explanations of wavelet analysis using mathematics [16, 40, 41].

The wavelet transform has been digitalized and is known as the discrete wavelet transform (DWT). It frequently accomplishes coefficient frugality by limiting the scale and sliding variation to powers of two; for this reason, it is also referred to as the dyadic wavelet transform and has the same name (DWT). However, by correctly reconstructing the original signal using the discrete coefficients of the dyadic wavelet transform [42]. Even with the DWT, a non-redundant bi-lateral transform is feasible if the wavelet belongs to an orthogonal family [15, 16].

The two wavelet parameters are sampled dyadically as: $s = 2^{-j}$, $\tau = k2^{-j}$. where j and k are both integers. The discretized probing function the becomes:

$$\psi_{j,k}(t) = 2^{j/2}\psi\left(2^{j}t - k\right). \tag{2.50}$$

The signal $x(t)$ can be decomposed by using DWT. The process is given as:

$$\omega_{j,k} = \int_{-\infty}^{+\infty} x(\tau)\psi_{j,k}(t)d\tau. \tag{2.51}$$

The wavelet series expansion, also known as the inverse DWT, is used to recover the original signal.

$$x(t) = \sum_{j=-\infty}^{\infty} \sum_{k=-\infty}^{\infty} \omega_{j,k}\psi_{j,k}(t). \tag{2.52}$$

where the set of orthonormal basis functions $\psi_{j,k}(t)$ is present. The sum of two indices, j and k, which stand for the scaling and sliding of the basis functions j, k, determines the wavelet series expansion $\psi_{j,k}(t)$. As a result, we provide a novel idea known as the scaling function, which makes it easier to apply and calculate the DWT. The coarser resolutions are generated after the fine resolutions, using the original waveform's smoothed version rather than the waveform itself. This smoothed form is created using the scaling function, often known as the smoothing function [15, 16].

2.3.2.3 The Empirical Wavelet Analysis

The Empirical Wavelet Transform (EWT), created by the authors of [43], is a time frequency approach for signal decomposition utilizing an adaptive wavelet depending on information content. In order to generate the proper wavelet filter bank, the EWT first identifies local maxima in the signal's Fourier spectrum. Next, it separates the spectrum into its component parts using the identified maxima.

It works in the three steps listed below [16].

1. Use FFT to identify the applied signal's frequency components.
2. By accurately segmenting the Fourier spectrum, the various kinds are produced.
3. To each segment that was discovered, apply the wavelet and scaling algorithms. The segmentation of the Fourier spectrum is the most crucial step in applying this approach to the data under analysis.

The empirical wavelets ($\Psi(w)$) are comprised of band-pass filters. The empirical scaling function $\phi(w)$ may be written as follows [43].

$$\psi_n(w) = \begin{cases} 1 & if\ (1+\gamma)\Omega_n \le |w| \le (1-\gamma)\Omega_{n+1} \\ \cos\left[\dfrac{\pi}{2}\beta(\gamma,\Omega_{n+1})\right] & if\ (1-\gamma)\Omega_{n+1} \le |w| \le (1+\gamma)\Omega_{n+1} \\ \sin\left[\dfrac{\pi}{2}\beta(\gamma,\Omega_n)\right] & if\ (1-\gamma)\Omega_n \le |w| \le (1+\gamma)\Omega_n \\ 0 & if \qquad\qquad otherwise \end{cases} \tag{2.53}$$

and,

$$\varnothing_1(w) = \begin{cases} 1 & if\ w \le (1-\gamma)\Omega_1 \\ \cos\left[\dfrac{\pi}{2}\beta(\gamma,\Omega_1)\right] & if\ (1-\gamma)\Omega_1 \le |w| \le (1+\gamma)\Omega_1 \\ 0 & if \qquad\qquad otherwise \end{cases} \tag{2.54}$$

The function $\beta(x)$ is an arbitrary $C^k[(0,1)]$ function defined by Eq. (2.55). Where $x = \dfrac{1}{2\gamma\Omega_n}(|\Omega| - (1-\gamma)\Omega_n)$. γ is a parameter to guarantee no overlap between two consecutive transition regions.

$$\beta(x) = \begin{cases} 1 & if\ x \ge 1 \\ 0 & if\ x \le 0 \\ \beta(x) + \beta(1-x) = 1 & if\ \forall x \in [0,1] \end{cases} \tag{2.55}$$

Numerous functions fulfil these properties, the widely utilized in the literature is:

$$\beta(x) = x^4\left(35 - 84x + 70x^2 - 20x^3\right). \tag{2.56}$$

A description of the EWT for the conventional wavelet transform is provided. The inner product with the empirical scaling function provided below yields the detailed coefficients, whereas Equation's inner product with the scaling function yields the approximate coefficients (2.58). where the signal's, $x(t)$, Fast Fourier Transform is shown by $(X(w))$ [16].

$$W_x(n,t) = x(t), \psi_n = IFFT\left(X(w) \times \psi_n(w)\right) \tag{2.57}$$

$$W_x(1,t) = x(t), \varphi_1 = IFFT\left(X(w) \times \varphi_1(w)\right) \tag{2.58}$$

2.3.2.4   The Empirical Mode Decomposition

The authors of [44] created the Empirical Mode Decomposition (EMD). The zero-mean sum of AM-FM components is used in EMD to represent any signal. The algorithm, despite its remarkable accomplishment, has difficulty understanding of analytical formulations. The authors of [45] proposed a number of modifications to the initial idea. If the signal $x(t)$ comprises two sequential extrema, a (local) high-frequency component or detail connected to the oscillation terminating at the two minima and proceeding to the maximum, that largely exists in between them can be utilized to define $x(t)$. The method may then be used on the residual, which contains all local trends, to iteratively recover a signal's constituent components. This can be done in an acceptable manner for all oscillations that make up the complete signal. The following is a summary of the effective EMD algorithm:

1. List all x(t)'s extrema
2. Use interpolation to connect minima to maxima), producing envelopes
3. Determine the mean of envelopes, $m(t)$
4. Use $d(t) = x(t) - m(t)$ to extract the detail
5. Repeat the loop with the residue

The aforementioned method must be refined in reality by a filtering technique by first iterating steps 1–4 on the detail signal $d(t)$, till the latter may be deemed zero-mean according to some stopping condition [32]. After determining the associated residual and referring to the detail as an Intrinsic Mode Function (IMF), step 5 is complete. The number of extrema diminishes as one residual is added to the next, and the decomposition is said to be complete with a finite number of modes overall. On "spectral" arguments, modes and residuals are heuristically represented. Even with harmonic oscillations, the high vs. low frequency differentiation, which is analogous to the wavelet transform, is only useful locally. To choose modes, adaptive and completely automatic time-variant filtering is employed [16, 45].

2.4   Conclusion

To sum up, with the recent technological advancements, the biomedical sector is evolving. The cloud assisted mobile healthcare solutions are in trend these days. Their success is mainly based on the revolutionized advancement in the communication technology, wire-free biomedical implants, Internet of Medical Things, cloud computing and artificial intelligence. The identification or diagnosis of physiological or pathological states is an important use of biomedical signals. In order to simulate and investigate biological models, these signals can also be used. Another usage is in the development of prosthetics and man-machine interface. Certain other usages are the identification and categorization of epilepsy, brain disorders, emotions, lie detection, head injuries, blood oxygen levels, glucose levels, strokes, psychiatric illnesses, sleep disorders, cerebral anoxia, cardiac diseases, lung diseases, behavioral disorders, drug effect monitoring, alertness monitoring, and anesthesia depth control. The goal of the signal collecting, and processing chain is to use machine or deep learning to realize a model precisely or recognize critical components or malfunctions in human bodily systems. Additionally, it enables the prediction of future clinical or physiological occurrences using machine and deep learning. The acquired biological signal is typically a complicated mixture of signal, noise, and artifacts. Artifacts can be produced by instruments that use sensors, amplifiers, filters, and analog-to-digital converters. While power lines and electromagnetic radiation are thought to be the main sources of noise, muscle activity has the potential to add interference. The planned design standards might lead to a wise decision about the signal gathering and processing methods. For biomedical engineers and scientists, it is mandatory to understand the processes of signal acquisition, conditioning and features extraction. In this framework, the principles of signal acquisition and pre-processing have been introduced in this chapter. Additionally, this chapter also tries to acquaint the readers with various key feature extraction approaches, used in the biomedical signal processing chains.

2.5   Assignments for Readers

- Describe your thoughts and key findings about the use of biomedical signal processing in the healthcare sector.
- Mention the important processes that are involved in the biomedical signal acquisition process.
- Describe the key steps used in the analog-to-digital conversion process.
- Describe your thoughts about the use of pre-conditioning in the biomedical signals processing chain.
- Describe how the spectral analysis can complement the time-domain signal analysis.
- Describe the key difference between spectral and time-frequency analysis.
- Identify the feature extraction techniques, presented in this chapter.
- Present a brief comparison between the feature extraction techniques, described in this chapter.

References

1. M. Masud et al., A lightweight and robust secure key establishment protocol for in-ternet of medical things in COVID-19 patients care. IEEE Internet Things J. **8**(21), 15694–15703 (2020)
2. S.M. Qaisar, A custom 70-channel mixed signal ASIC for the brain-PET detectors signal read-out and selection. Biomed. Phys. Eng. Express **5**(4), 045018 (2019)
3. M.A. Naser, M.J. Deen, Brain tumor segmentation and grading of lower-grade glioma using deep learning in MRI images. Comput. Biol. Med. **121**, 103758 (2020)

4. K.J. Blinowska, J. Żygierewicz, *Practical Biomedical Signal Analysis Using MATLAB®* (CRC Press, 2021)
5. S.M. Qaisar, S.I. Khan, K. Srinivasan, M. Krichen, Arrhythmia classification us-ing multi-rate processing metaheuristic optimization and variational mode decomposi-tion. J. King Saud Univ.-Comput. Inf. Sci. (2022)
6. N. Salankar, S.M. Qaisar, EEG based stress classification by using difference plots of varia-tional modes and machine learning. J. Ambient. Intell. Humaniz. Comput., 1–14 (2022)
7. A. Subasi, S. Mian Qaisar, The ensemble machine learning-based classification of motor imag-ery tasks in brain-computer interface. J. Healthc. Eng. **2021** (2021)
8. J. Gröhl, M. Schellenberg, K. Dreher, L. Maier-Hein, Deep learning for biomedi-cal photo-acoustic imaging: A review. Photo-Dermatology **22**, 100241 (2021)
9. S.M. Qaisar, A two stage interpolator and multi threshold discriminator for the brain-PET scanner timestamp calculation. Nucl. Instrum. Methods Phys. Res. Sect. Accel. Spectrometers Detect. Assoc. Equip. **922**, 364–372 (2019)
10. S. Mian Qaisar, Baseline wander and power-line interference elimination of ECG sig-nals using efficient signal-piloted filtering. Healthc. Technol. Lett. **7**(4), 114–118 (2020)
11. A.V. Oppenheim, J.R. Buck, R.W. Schafer, *Discrete-time signal processing*, vol 2 (Prentice Hall, Upper Saddle River, NJ, 2001)
12. S.M. Qaisar, Efficient mobile systems based on adaptive rate signal processing. Comput. Electr. Eng. **79**, 106462 (2019)
13. W. Kester, *Data Conversion Handbook* (Newnes, 2005)
14. S. Mian Qaisar, L. Fesquet, and M. Renaudin, "Adaptive rate sampling and filtering based on level crossing sampling," EURASIP J. Adv. Signal Process., vol. 2009, pp. 1–12, 2009
15. J. Semmlow, Biosignal and biomedical image processing: MATLAB-based applications (2004)
16. A. Subasi, *Practical Guide for Biomedical Signals Analysis Using Machine Learning Techniques, A MATLAB Based Approach, First* (Elsevier, 2019)
17. A. Graimann, B. Allison, G. Pfurtscheller, Brain–computer interfaces: A gentle introduction, in *Brain-Computer Interfaces*, (Springer, 2009), pp. 1–27
18. J. Kevric, A. Subasi, Comparison of signal decomposition methods in classifica-tion of EEG signals for motor-imagery BCI system. Biomed. Signal Process. Control **31**, 398–406 (2017)
19. S. Sanei, *Adaptive Processing of Brain Signals* (John Wiley & Sons, 2013)
20. S. Siuly, Y. Li, Y. Zhang, *EEG Signal Analysis and Classification* (Springer, 2016)
21. L. Sörnmo, P. Laguna, *Bioelectrical Signal Processing in Cardiac and Neurological Applications*, vol 8 (Academic, 2005)
22. G. Dumermuth, H. Flühler, Some modern aspects in numerical spectrum analysis of multi-channel electroencephalographic data. Med. Biol. Eng. **5**(4), 319–331 (1967)
23. S.L. Marple, S.L. Marple, *Digital Spectral Analysis: With Applications*, vol 5 (Prentice-Hall Englewood Cliffs, NJ, 1987)
24. C.W. Therrien, *Discrete Random Signals and Statistical Signal Processing* (Prentice Hall PTR, 1992)
25. F.L. da Silva, E. Niedermeyer, F. da Silva, EEG analysis: Theory and practice; computer-assisted EEG diagnosis: Pattern recognition techniques. Electroenceph-alogr. Basic Princ. Clin. Appl. Relat. Fields, 871–919 (1987)
26. B.H. Jansen, J.R. Bourne, J.W. Ward, Autoregressive estimation of short seg-ment spectra for computerized EEG analysis. I.E.E.E. Trans. Biomed. Eng. **9**, 630–638 (1981)
27. C.W. Anderson, E.A. Stolz, S. Shamsunder, Multivariate autoregressive models for classifi-cation of spontaneous electroencephalographic signals during mental tasks. I.E.E.E. Trans. Biomed. Eng. **45**(3), 277–286 (1998)
28. A.L. Swindlehurst, T. Kailath, A performance analysis of subspace-based meth-ods in the presence of model errors, part I: The MUSIC algorithm. IEEE Trans. Signal Process. **40**(7), 1758–1774 (1992)

29. L. Swindlehurst, T. Kailath, A performance analysis of subspace-based meth-ods in the presence of model errors: Part II-multidimensional algorithms. IEEE Trans. Signal Process. **41**(9) (1993)
30. B. Friedlander, A.J. Weiss, Effects of model errors on waveform estimation using the MUSIC algorithm. IEEE Trans. Signal Process. **42**(1), 147–155 (1994)
31. B. Friedlander, A sensitivity analysis of the MUSIC algorithm. IEEE Trans. Acoust. Speech Signal Process. **38**(10), 1740–1751 (1990)
32. M. Viberg, Subspace-based methods for the identification of linear time-invariant systems. Automatica **31**(12), 1835–1851 (1995)
33. B. Porat, B. Friedlander, Analysis of the asymptotic relative efficiency of the MUSIC algo-rithm. IEEE Trans. Acoust. Speech Signal Process. **36**(4), 532–544 (1988)
34. A. Subasi, E. Erçelebi, A. Alkan, E. Koklukaya, Comparison of subspace-based meth-ods with AR parametric methods in epileptic seizure detection. Comput. Biol. Med. **36**(2), 195–208 (2006)
35. A.B. Hubbard, *The World According to Wavelets: The Story of a Mathematical Tech-Nique in the Making* (AK Peters/CRC Press, 1998)
36. S.M. Qaisar, L. Fesquet, M. Renaudin, An adaptive resolution computationally efficient short-time Fourier transform. Res. Lett. Signal Process. **2008** (2008)
37. L. Hu, Z. Zhang, *EEG Signal Processing and Feature Extraction* (Springer, 2019)
38. B. Marchant, Time–frequency analysis for biosystems engineering. Biosyst. Eng. **85**(3), 261–281 (2003)
39. A. Subasi, M.K. Kiymik, Muscle fatigue detection in EMG using time–frequency methods, ICA and neural networks. J. Med. Syst. **34**(4), 777–785 (2010)
40. M. Basseville, I.V. Nikiforov, *Detection of Abrupt Changes: Theory and Applica-Tion*, vol 104 (Prentice Hall Englewood Cliffs, 1993)
41. F. Gustafsson, F. Gustafsson, *Adaptive filtering and change detection*, vol 1 (Citeseer, 2000)
42. G. Bodenstein, W. Schneider, C. Malsburg, Computerized EEG pattern classifica-tion by adaptive segmentation and probability-density-function classification. De-scription of the method. Comput. Biol. Med. **15**(5), 297–313 (1985)
43. J. Gilles, Empirical wavelet transform. IEEE Trans. Signal Process. **61**(16), 3999–4010 (2013)
44. N.E. Huang et al., *The empirical mode decomposition and the Hilbert spectrum for nonlinear and non-stationary time series analysis*, vol 454 (1998), pp. 903–995
45. G. Rilling, P. Flandrin, P. Goncalves, *On empirical mode decomposition and its algorithms*, vol 3 (2003), pp. 8–11

Chapter 3
The Role of EEG as Neuro-Markers for Patients with Depression: A Systematic Review

Noor Kamal Al-Qazzaz and Alaa A. Aldoori

Abstract Depressive symptoms may include feelings of melancholy, lack of interest, and difficulty remembering and focusing. The existing techniques of detecting depression need a lot of interaction with humans, and the findings are highly reliant on the knowledge and skill of the doctor doing them. Electroencephalography (*EEG*) is a potential tool that reveals interesting information that can be used in diagnosis and evaluation of human beings' brain abnormalities with excellent time resolution; however, detecting depression is a challenge for engineers and scientists to support personalized health care. However, *EEG* may provide an idea of cognitive decline toward depression classification. To create a neurophysiological diagnostic index for therapeutic use that is sensitive to the severity of depression, it may be possible to combine the *EEG* with other biological, cognitive markers, and imaging methods. The goal of the current study is to emphasize baseline *EEG* activity in depressed individuals, beginning with *EEG* signal collection and continuing through *EEG* data preprocessing steps for signal augmentation, linear and nonlinear properties. The subsequent focus will be on *EEG* signal extraction to account for the large swings of *EEG* signals, followed by classification approaches to differentiate the severity of depression. Therefore, the present review has examined the role of *EEG* signal processing and analysis in helping medical doctors and clinicians to determine suitable planning and optimal, more effective treatment programs.

N. K. Al-Qazzaz (✉) · A. A. Aldoori
Department of Biomedical Engineering, Al-Khwarizmi College of Engineering, University of Baghdad, Baghdad, Iraq
e-mail: noorbme@kecbu.uobaghdad.edu.iq

3.1   Introduction

The World Health Organization (WHO) estimates that 322 million individuals, or 4.4 percent of the global population, suffer from depression [1, 2]. It is one of the major mental illnesses that contribute to disability. Depression raises the chance of suicide significantly, which adds to the burden on patients, their families, and society [2] in addition to a number of physical problems.

Due to a lack of understanding, incompetent medical personnel, a lack of funding, and inaccurate diagnoses, a surprising 50% of patients with depression go untreated. A detailed understanding of the etiology and pathophysiology of the illness is urgently required, as is the development of a precise and effective method for identifying depression. If identified properly and with quick recognition, this disease can be easily treated [2].

One type of mental illness, known as major depressive disorder (MDD), has a significant impact on the patient, the healthcare system, and the economy Depression has been recognized as a substantial global source of impairment and disability among persons of working age [3], with a tendency to worsen physical and cognitive impairments and limit performance on professional duties. According to predictions made by MDD, adjusted life years in high-income nations would be considerably influenced by the disease by 2030 [4], which will cause major productivity losses due to presenteeism and absenteeism (failing to show up for work due to illness) (being present at work while sick). According to a 2003 World Health Organization study on mental health, employees with depression have an average yearly health care spend that is 4.2 times higher than that of a typical beneficiary [4–6].

To demonstrate the spatiotemporal feature of *EEG*, researchers have used non-invasive electroencephalography (*EEG*). When analyzing emotions, there are signs of sadness, seizures, Alzheimer's, Parkinson's disease, and more [2, 7–11].

In order to help the reader identify gaps, areas of agreement, key references, and other details that will help future research, this article highlights various gaps and difficulties in depression studies that have emerged in recent years while also providing a concise summary of each of these works. In order to do this, a methodical mapping process was undertaken, which included a review of the literature on non-invasive *EEG* depression markers that was mainly published between 2018 and 2022.

3.2   Brain Structure and Depression

The electroencephalogram (*EEG*) is a conductivity monitoring tool which records extremely irregular electrical activity of brain impulses and offers crucial information about various areas of the brain [9]. It offers methods for capturing brain electrical activity over time that are both non-invasive and affordable [12]. It is extensively used for doctors to study how the brain works and to identify physical disorders. Since *EEG* is reliable, it is also employed in *EEG* biometrics for *person* verification [8, 13–19]. Furthermore, the *EEG* method is the most accurate due to its simplicity and high *temporal* resolution when compared to other methods for detecting depression (such as audio [20], facial [21], and MRI [22]).

Both depression and bipolar illness are signs of a brain problem. The aberrant structure of *EEG* signals manifests as variances in signal patterns for different patient states, allowing for the exact diagnosis of brain disorders, and the *EEG* responds to the biotic activities of the brain [9]. Fine contrasts between the chaotic and composite nature of normal and sad *EEG* data represent diverse brain processes in the depressive and normal groups that are challenging to show graphically [23].

3.2.1 Brain Structure

The brain is a remarkable organ that controls all bodily functions and processes environmental data. The brainstem, cerebellum, and cerebrum, all of which are located inside the skull, make up this structure [24]. One of the most crucial areas of the brain is the cerebrum. It is capable of doing complex tasks such as predicting touch, visuals, audio, speaking, mental skills, training, and correct motion control. The cerebrum is divided into two hemispheres, each of which has its own fissures and governs the opposing side of the body. Each hemisphere has four lobes: frontal, temporal, parietal, and occipital. The frontal lobe is in charge of consciousness, processing complex inputs as well as the senses of sound and scent are within the purview of the temporal lobe, the parietal lobe is in charge of managing objects and processing sensual information, and the occipital lobe is in charge of processing information related to the sense of sight [25]. The voltage differential between a scalp electrode and an ear lobe reference electrode is isolated during *monopolar* recording. On the other hand, *bipolar* electrodes record the voltage variation between two scalp electrodes [23].

3.2.2 Depression Types

There are several different types of depressive diseases Fig. 3.1. It's helpful to be aware of the many illnesses and their distinctive symptoms because symptoms can range from mild to severe [26].

3.2.2.1 Major Depression Disorder (MDD)

Major depressive disorder (MDD), one of most prevalent kind of depression, is characterized by a pervasive sensation of melancholy. Depressed mood, decreasing interests, diminished cognitive ability, and vegetative signs such irregular eating and

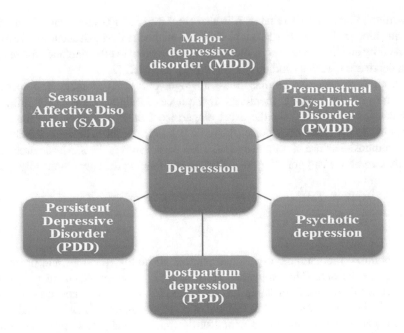

Fig. 3.1 Depression types

sleeping schedules are the hallmarks of MDD. One in six persons will experience MDD at some point in their lives, which affects almost twice as many women as males [26].

3.2.2.2 Premenstrual Dysphoric Disorder (PMDD(

Premenstrual dysphoric disorder is now considered to affect 3 *to* 8% of women of reproductive age who fit the rigorous criteria (PMDD).Studies show that the number of people who have clinically severe dysphoric premenstrual disorder is likely to be higher. Even if a woman doesn't have more than the arbitrary number of five indicators on the PMDD list, 13 to 18 percent of women of childbearing age may be unable to work or feel uncomfortable because of premenstrual dysphoric symptoms [27].

3.2.2.3 Psychotic Depression

The intensity of major depression was once thought to range from mild to severe, with psychotic depression being at one extreme. Experience gained later showed that psychosis is a distinct characteristic that may coexist with mood disorders of various degrees of severity. Poorly understood are trauma-related temporary or mild schizophrenia, emotional incongruent features, and psychotic symptoms. While much is understood more about effects of extreme mood delusions and hallucinations on the progression and responsiveness to treatment of depression, there is still more to learn [28, 29].

3.2.2.4   Postpartum Depression (PPD)

The phrase "postpartum depression" refers to a wide range of mood disorders that arise after a baby is born. It's important to distinguish between the two because they may require quite different treatment options or none at all. Postpartum depression (PPD) affects 10–15% of new moms, however many instances go unreported [30]. Postpartum depression should not be confused with postpartum blues, which are transitory mood symptoms that occur within the first week to ten days following birth and normally go away within a few days [31].

3.2.2.5   Persistent Depressive Disorder (PDD)

There are four diagnostic subgroups for persistent depressive disorder (PDD), which is defined as a depressed illness lasting at least two years (dysthymia, chronic major depression, recurrent major depression with incomplete remission between episodes, and double depression). In the Western world, persistent types of depression account for a considerable number of depressive disorders, with lifetime prevalence rates ranging from 3 to 6 percent [32].

3.2.2.6   Seasonal Affective Disorder (SAD)

Seasonal Affective Disorder (SAD) is a recurrent major depressive disorder with a *seasonal pattern* that often begins in the fall and lasts through the winter. The "winter blues," also known as S-SAD, is a subsyndromal variation of SAD. SAD is less likely to cause depression in the spring and early summer. A low mood and a lack of energy are the most common symptoms. Females, those under the age of 35, those living far from the equator, and those with a family history of depression, bipolar disease, or SAD are the most vulnerable [33].

3.2.3   Effect of Depression on the Brain

Three regions of the brain are involved in memory and emotion regulation: the amygdala, located in the basal ganglia, the hippocampus, located in the temporal lobe (the frontal portion of the temporal lobe),are all affected by depression and bipolar disorder [34]. The hippocampus controls the release of the stress hormone cortisol and preserves memories. When someone is depressed, their body releases cortisol; however, when too much cortisol is released and carried to the brain, it causes problems. In persons with MDD, prolonged exposure to high cortisol levels can prevent the growth of new neurons. It also affects memory issues by shrinking the neurons in the hippocampus. The prefrontal cortex, which is located in the *frontal lobe*, is important for emotion regulation, decision-making, and memory formation. When cortisol levels in the brain become too high, the prefrontal cortex shrinks. The amygdala is a structure in the temporal lobe's frontal region that controls emotional responses. Because of the constant exposure to a high cortisol ratio, the amygdala in depression and bipolar disorder patients grows larger and more active. Sleep difficulties and other activity patterns can result from an enlarged and manic amygdala, as well as erratic activity in other parts of the brain. Cortisol levels usually rise in the morning and fall at night. The cortisol ratio is usually higher in MDD patients, even at night [23].

3.3 Depression Diagnosis

Currently, the diagnosis of depression may be made using a variety of symptoms that aid physicians in evaluating many aspects of depressive functioning. The biomarkers, psychological evaluations, and physiological measurements are the most often utilized symptom-based diagnostic tools.

3.3.1 Biomarkers

A biomarker may be used to study the biology of depression as well as to predict or evaluate the risk of developing the disease, which are both necessary steps in the process of finding a *clinical* diagnostic or *therapeutic* intervention monitoring that may modify or stop the condition [35, 36]. A trait that can be reliably tested and evaluated as a predictor of physiological processes, pathologic processes, or responses to a *therapeutic* intervention is referred to as a biomarker [37]. Markers should not be mistaken with symptoms of a particular illness. Ideal candidates for the biomarker should be people who are at risk of depression and those who can recognize neuropathological processes even before a clinical diagnosis.

Figure 3.2 depicts the classification of biomarkers that Lopresti et al. [38] suggested. The classification of biomarkers comprises prognostic biomarkers, which are used to forecast how the illness will progress, diagnostic biomarkers, which are used to identify if a disease is present or not, therapy biomarkers, which may be useful in determining the best therapeutic option for a specific patient from a variety of therapeutic options, treatment-response biomarkers (also known as mediators), which are used to gauge treatment progress, and prediction biomarkers. Additional categories for biomarkers include trait, state, and endophenotype ones [39]. In

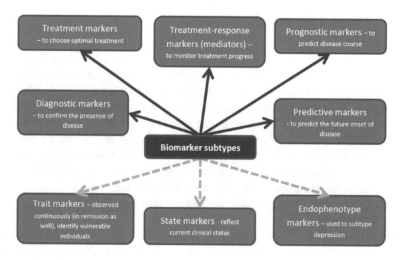

Fig. 3.2 Biomarkers subtypes

addition to the acute stage of the illness, trait biomarkers are those that can be reliably found before the onset of the disease or even in remission. Because of the final characteristic, they somewhat resemble predictive biomarkers [37].

3.3.2   Psychological Assessments

According to the Diagnostic and Statistical Manual of Mental Disorders (DSM-5) published by the American Psychiatric Association (APA) [40], Depressive disorders include but are not limited to Major Depressive Disorder (MDD), Disruptive Mood Dysregulation Disorder (DMDD), Persistent Depressive Disorder (Dysthymia), Premenstrual Dysphoric Disorder (PDD), Substance/Medication-Induced Depressive Disorder (S/M-IDD), and Depressive Disorder Due to Other Medical Conditions (DDOC) [40, 41]. The genesis of MDD is linked to genetic, biochemical, hormonal, immunological, neurological, and environmental variables, as well as acute life events and neuroendocrine systems, according to [42]. While other varieties of depression have many of the same symptoms as MDD, they differ in a number of ways. DMDD, for example, is a *non − episodic* disorder that affects adolescents and teenagers. Obstinately irritable, displeased moods, as well as recurring temper outbursts, are symptoms. Dysthymia is a type of depression that lasts for a long time. During the last week or two before the menstruation begins, PDD produces extreme irritation and anxiousness [43]. The long-term type of MDD known as S/M-IDD (Drug/Medication-Induced Depressive Disorder) is brought on by or follows substance misuse. Depressive disorder caused by another medical condition might be brought on by ongoing diseases and persistent bodily suffering (DDDAMC) [23].

3.3.3 Physiological Measurements

Reducing the number of failed therapy trials could enhance MDD treatment. This outcome is expected if predictive measurements are used to accurately predict treatment results. The predictive measures must be sufficiently sensitive to changes in illness states, according to the definition [44–46]. These should also be suitable for therapeutic applications, like precise therapy forecasts for certain patients. The development of *EEG/ERP* metrics for assessing the efficacy of MDD treatments will be the main topic of this section. The *EEG* and *ERP* data that have shown significant associations with the *R* or *NR* subgroups will be explained, along with the values that were extracted from those data. Examples include *EEG* theta accordance, asymmetries, *antidepressant treatment response* (*ATR*) score, and alpha and theta activations [47].

For MDD patients it was discovered that the *ERP* elements, *P*300 levels, and latencies were related with therapeutic efficacy [47, 48]. The Loudness Dependence Auditory Evoked Potential (*LDAEP*) *ERP* type explains how one *EPR* component (*N*100/*P*200) varies when the auditory input becomes louder. It's thought to measure the amount of *serotonergic* neurotransmission in the primary auditory cortex. Lower *LDAEP* readings suggested higher chemical (serotonin) levels in the brain, and vice versa. The following subsections discuss related studies [47].

An auditory evoked potential (*AEP*) is an *ERP* component that is obtained by grand averaging numerous auditory stimuli of a single type *AEP*. *AEPs* have been found to have a beneficial relationship with cognitive capacities and brain auditory processes [49, 50]. In addition, a delay in the *P*300 component has been linked to depression [51]. Similar findings were reported in other investigations that only demonstrated a delay in *P*300 in MDD patients compared to controls [50, 52]. During *LORETA* analysis, there was also a drop in *P*300 intensity in the right hemisphere [53]. When compared to healthy controls, depressive individuals had longer *P*300 latencies for *visually evoked stimuli* [54]. The *P*300 delay returns to normal after 4 *weeks* of antidepressant use [47]. Furthermore, the normal *P*300 amplitude predicted electro-convulsive treatment response [55]. In contrast, there were no discernible variations in *P*300 amplitude between those who responded to the therapy, those who did not react, and the controls [56].

3.4 EEG-Based Depression Recognition Neuromarker

Neurological illnesses are challenging to accurately diagnose due to the absence of recognized biomarkers and the patient's subjectivity while responding to psychological evaluation questionnaires [57]. Research has examined the use of non-invasive *EEG* in order to search for biomarkers for the purpose of diagnosis or therapy prediction in light of this [58–61]. The search for non-invasive indicators of depression using *EEG* is crucial as it might help with more accurate illness diagnosis, which is now done through questionnaires that are vulnerable to professional and patient subjectivity. But it's also problematic because depression has a vast variety of signs and symptoms [62] and a high level of comorbidity, particularly with anxiety [63], resulting in contradictory biomarker findings. Given the intricacy of depression, it's critical in order to keep up with the most recent findings of research on depression biomarkers [61].

EEG and *ERP* has role based prognostic biomarkers for MDD are discussed in [47]. Referenced *EEG* (*rEEG*) and *ERP* biomarkers *P*300, theta band activations, theta *QEEG* cordance, and asymmetrical alpha power [64]. The *P*300's potential clinical use as a marker for persons with present major depressive disorder in [65]. Previous studies have demonstrated that the Alpha and Theta frequency bands can provide information on the diagnosis and treatment of depression [66, 67], Gamma bands were not widely recognized in depression diagnosis [68].

In contrast, by giving some notable data on gamma pulses, [69] declares gamma waves as a depression diagnostic biomarker [70] *EEG* characteristics, including *linear* and *nonlinear* biomarkers and the Phase Lagging Index (*PLI*) at the patient's resting state, are used to identify depression. The *frontal Theta asymmetry* was used as a biomarker for depression by [67]. According to [71] multi-modal should be employed to diagnose MDD since depression affects not only mood but also psychomotor and cognitive processes [72]. looked at brainwaves as a possible biomarker for MDD risk assessment. The neural activities aren't just valuable in detecting depression, but also provide the groundwork for effective and dependable depression therapy. Compared to neuroimaging approaches, *EEG*-based depression biomarkers offer significant advantages [23].

3.4.1 EEG and the Brain

Due to the complex nature of electric brain activity that recorded as an *EEG*, it is necessary to characterize *EEG* fluctuations to understand its nature. Clinical *EEG* waveforms generally have physiological amplitudes of between (10 *and* 100) μv and frequencies between (1 *and* 100) Hz. According to their frequency ranges, *EEG* may be divided into five rhythms.

Alpha waves (α) are rhythmic waves that occur in awake, relaxed adults with their eyes closed and are associated with intelligence, memory, and cognition [73]. They have a frequency range of (8 *to* 13) Hz and a normal voltage range of (20 *to* 200) μV, and they vanish in pathological conditions like coma or sleep [74]. It is visible at the back of the head and reflects activity in the *frontal*, *parietal*, and *occipital* regions of the scalp [75].

Beta waves (β) have smaller amplitudes ranging from of (5 − 10) μv, and frequencies that are greater than those of waveforms, in the range of (13 − 30) Hz [73]. Records from the *frontal* and *parietal* lobes of the scalp [75].

Theta waves (θ) have a frequency range of (4 *to* 7) Hz and are most prevalent during sleep, as well as during emotional stress, arousal in adults and older children, and idleness. It has an amplitude range of $(5 - 10)$ µv and is recorded from the scalp's *temporal* and *parietal* area [73]. Based on their activities, people exhibit two different forms of *theta*. It has been connected to endeavors including concentration, focus, mental effort, and stimulus processing [75].

Delta waves (δ) have an amplitude range of $(20 - 200)$ µv and a lowest frequency of less than 3.5 Hz. Deep sleep, infancy, and severe organic brain illnesses are times when it happens [73].

Gamma waves (γ) have frequencies between 30 *and* 100 Hz [73]. In the case of *cross − model* sensory processing, during *short − term memory* to recognize noises, objects, and tactile sensations, and in the pathological situation brought on by cognitive decline, especially as it related to band [75] recordings from the somatosensory cortex were made.

It is interesting to note that *alpha* and *beta* wave activities rise linearly throughout the lifespan while *delta* and *theta* wave activities decrease with age [76]. *Delta* current density and glucose metabolism have an antagonistic connection in the event of cerebrovascular illness, such as stroke, and this relationship changes as a result of depression in the sub-genual prefrontal cortex [77].

An individual's morphological *EEG* when they are healthy, *K − complex* is transient complex waveforms that have amplitude of about 200 µv and a slow frequency of 14 Hz. During sleep, it happened suddenly or in reaction to a quick stimulation and was linked with sharp components [78, 79].

Lambda wave is a monophasic, positive, sharp waves with an amplitude of less than 50 µv appeared posteriorly in the occipital lobes. It has to do with eye movements and visual exploration together [78]. *Mu* rhythm is located in the middle of the scalp, it appears as a cluster of waves with an arcade or comb form and amplitude less than 50 µv with a frequency range of $(7 to 11)$ Hz. When there is thinking, preparedness, and contralateral movement of tactile stimulus, it manifests as blocks [78]. Spike is a transient, pointed peak, propagation duration $(20 - 30)$ msec [78].

Sharp waves are transitory, sharp peak, propagation duration $(70 - 200)$ msec [78]. Spike and wave rhythm consists of a series of surface sluggish, negative waves with a range of frequencies $(2.5 - 3.5)$ Hz and amplitude of up to 1000 µv. It can sometimes manifest as complex waves and polyspikes [78]. Sleep spindle is an episodic rhythm occurred over the *fronto − central* area of the brain during sleep at a frequency of 14 Hz and an amplitude of 50 µv [78]. Vertex sharp transient, also known as a *V − wave*, is a response to sensory events experienced during sleep or awake and has an amplitude of roughly 300 µv [78].

3.4.2   Experimental EEG Protocol for Recognizing Depression

The *experimental* protocol for *EEG* depression detection includes a standard set of regulations, including the participants, subject selection criteria, *EEG* recording length, and other details.

In terms of the participants, there can be anywhere from one and two hundred, with a median of 30 people, depending on the study [41, 80–83], however other researches have been involved more than 50 participants [84–91]. Research with limited number of individuals have been illustrated challenges in determining the accuracy and in getting the final the findings [92–94].

Regarding participant gender, the majority of studies involve both male and female individuals [95]; however, only a small number of studies exclusively use female participants to detect severe depressive disorder using *EEG*. Men and women must both participate in studies since there is a chance that they will view depression in different ways [23].

Healthcare professionals and researchers frequently utilize the *Beck Depression Inventory* (*BDI*) [96] as a screening tool before making a diagnosis of depression or anxiety. Patients with MDD are chosen for this exam based on many *multiple − choice questions*. Patients having a *BDI − II* score of greater than 13 are categorized as depressive subjects. A high overall *BDI − II* score demonstrates the severity of depression. Many research employ the *BDI* to choose subjects [90, 92–94, 97].

The Diagnostic and Statistical Manual of Mental Disorders (*DSM − IV*), developed by the American Psychiatric Association (*APA*), has also been used in several research to quantify various mental illnesses [40]. A *DSM − IV*-based questionnaire is used as a preliminary *psychometric* test to evaluate depression in *EEG* -based diagnoses and most articles used it as a preliminary *EEG* test [90, 91, 98].

3.4.3 EEG Publicly Available Dataset for Depression Diagnosis

Due to the sensitive nature of the data and privacy and confidentiality concerns, few public datasets for *EEG* -based depression diagnosis are accessible.

The Healthy Brain Network (*HBN*) public data biobank was established by the Child Mind Institute [99]. *HBN*'s major goal is to create a data collection that correctly captures the broad range of variance and impairment that defines developmental psychopathology [99].

The National Institute of Mental Health has made the Establishing Moderators/Mediators for a Biosignature of Antidepressant Response in Clinical Care (*EMBARC*) dataset accessible to the general public (*NIMH*). Using *EEG* in the resting state and an algorithm for machine learning, it may be possible to determine the neurological signal of antidepressant medication response [100].

In the Depression public dataset, which is utilized in this study, motor activity recordings of 23 *unipolar* and *bipolar* depressed patients and 32 healthy controls are included [101].

Trans Diagnostic Cohorts [102] is assessed the effectiveness of brief transdiagnostic cognitive-behavioral group therapy (*TCBGT*) in treating individuals with anxiety and depression. Instead of focusing on a single element, they conceptualize mental illness in terms of domain-wide inequalities [103].

Patient Repository for *EEG* Data and Computational Tools is a sizable, open-access dataset (*PREDICT*) contains *EEG* data [104]. There are numerous data repositories that house patient-specific information and imaging data. The Patient Repository for *EEG* Data + Computational Tool (*PRED + CT*) website is among the few that offer *EEG* -based patient-specific data [23].

3.4.4   Function of EEG in Depression Detection and Classification

For additional signal processing to extract significant indicators and depression classification, noise from the collected *EEG* dataset is need to be eliminated. The four basic phases in processing *EEG* signals are *EEG* signal capture, preprocessing, feature extraction, and classification.

3.4.4.1   *EEG* Signal Acquisition Stage

The *EEG* is a medical equipment that records data from the scalp using conductive material and metal electrodes and displays the electrical activity of brain neurons [105]. A *low − pass, high − pass*, and notch filter can be found in one of the most used *EEG* devices [106]. With a 50 Hz or 60 Hz notch filter, the usual frequency range for *EEG* recordings in depressed individuals is 0.3 Hz to 70 Hz [112]. The application determines the sampling frequency [23, 107]. The American *EEG* Society has recognized the worldwide federation's 10–20 system for recording the *EEG* of depressed patients while they are peacefully resting with their eyes closed [107–109]. For *EEG* recordings on depressive individuals, researchers have employed 19 electrodes [108–110].

3.4.4.2   Preprocessing Stage

Preprocessing is essential to distinguish vital information from tainted *EEG* signals since these artifacts reduce the quality of the genuine *EEG* signals [111].

A *low − pass, high − pass*, and notch filter can be found in the most widely used *EEG* device to enhance the performance of *EEG* signals [112].

A 12 *bit A/D* converter digitizes the signal to increase its accuracy. It is determined by the application whether the sample frequency is 128 Hz, 173 Hz, or 256 Hz. The *EEG* signal will then be captured, typed down, and presented on a computer screen for further examination [23, 107].

The frequencies of *EEG* signals and the majority of artifacts overlap. The *EEG* signal was contaminated by both physiological and non-physiological [113–117]. Because noise has a direct influence on the characteristics of the *EEG* signal, several signal processing algorithms have been developed to overcome this problem and obtain relevant data from the recorded *EEG* 3 signal

A collection of recorded *EEG* signals are divided into their sources using the blind source separation *higher order statistical* technique known as independent component analysis (*ICA*) [118–120].

To process non-stationary signals, such as *EEG*, the *Wavelet* transform (*WT*) method was developed [121–124].

Combining *ICA* and *WT* to create an *ICA − WT* hybrid strategy was done by Nazareth et al. and other researchers [125]. Additionally, the WT can divide *EEG* signals into various sub-bands [126– 131]. Electrooculography (*EOG*) and muscular activity (*EMG*) artifacts have been successfully eliminated using the *ICA − WT* approach [11, 132]. So, the signal is prepared for the following step (i.e., feature extraction stage).

3.4.4.3   Features Extraction Stage

To identify depression and create a relevant diagnostic index using *EEG*, feature extraction is used to the denoised *EEG* signal from the preceding stage. In this stage, linear and nonlinear algorithms are used to retrieve the pertinent data from the *EEG* of depressed patients.

3.4.4.3.1   Linear Spectral Features

It is simple to examine the power amplitudes for each band using linear spectral analysis, a direct information source acquired by *EEG* from the frequency domain. Alpha denotes mental sluggishness and relaxation [133, 134], whereas beta is related to expectancy [134], anxiety and introverted concentration [135]. Moreover, theta is considered for emotional processing [136, 137] and gamma is associated to attention, sensory systems [134] and may be related to mood swings [69]. However, delta is related to deep sleep [134].

The engineering way to diagnose depression is to explore essential biomarkers which would be applied to classification algorithms using power spectral features [138–140].

Recent research by Lee et al. [141] indicates that depressive individuals have lower beta waves in the central-left side of the brain than emotionally stable individuals and greater alpha waves on the left side of the brain. Last but not least, Dolsen et al. [142] found that depressed participants who had suicidal thoughts showed greater alpha activity during the whole night of sleep compared to those who had low suicidal thoughts.

Band power has thus been extensively examined and is simple to incorporate into classifiers that distinguish between depressed and healthy people. Regarding this, Fitzgerald evaluated some data in a high impact research [69] that suggests monopolar depressive individuals have elevated gamma activity.

On the other hand, although additional research is required to fully understand the role that delta and theta waves play in depression, they do appear to be worthy of consideration [138, 143]. Regarding theta, it appears to be a useful characteristic in diagnostic tools [139, 140, 144], but nothing is known about the mechanics underlying it. Furthermore, the beta wave appears to be more correlated with the anxiety and ruminative thoughts that are prevalent in depressed patients but may not be as critical for a precise diagnosis [61].

3.4.4.3.2 Nonlinear Features

Since many years ago, nonlinear dynamic methods have been extensively employed to examine the *EEG* signal. The *complex dynamic* information that is reflected from the cerebral cortex and captured by *EEG* devices has been studied by researchers using *EEG* [145, 146]. Brain behavior can be categorized as nonlinear because brain neurons are regulated by nonlinear phenomena including threshold and saturation processes [147, 148].

The Correlation Dimension (*CD*) and Maximum Lyapunov Exponent are the first nonlinear approaches that were used to analyze *EEG* in order to quantify depression based on *EEG* data as biomarkers (*MLE*). In order to determine how many independent variables are required to characterize a dynamic system, Grassberger and Procaccia adopted the *CD* method in 1983 [144, 149]. The *CD* method indicated the degree of freedom of a signal, with lower values indicating a reduced degree of unpredictability in the signal. On the other hand, Wolf used *MLE* as a dynamic metric to assess the adaptability of the system in 1985 [150, 151]. Fractal dimension (*FD*), Lempel-Ziv Complexity (*LZC*), which measures a signal's complexity and was first developed by Lempel and Ziv in 1976, can be used to predict the early identification of depression [152, 153]. It is shown that sad people have generally lower LZC values. In addition, Higuchi's Fractal Dimension (*HFD*), proposed by Higuchi [157], reveals the fractal dimension of a signal [89, 154] and Detrended Fluctuation Analysis (*DFA*), presented by Peng et al. [156], indicates long-time correlations of the signal [58]. Entropy approaches, such as sample entropy (*SampEn*) and Kologorov entropy, Tsallis Entropy (*TsEn*), approximation Entropy (*ApEn*), *SampEn*, and multiscale Entropy (*MSE*) [148, 158–163], have been used to address the complexity or irregularity in the system's capacity to generate information.

Researchers [47, 140] have used *nonlinear* features, such as *DFA*, to train a classifier and discriminate between healthy and depressed people. In comparison to healthy persons, depression significantly lowers *DFA*, according to Bachmann et al. [154].

In terms of signal complexity, HFD tends to be greater in depressed brains [58, 154], indicating a complex signal consistent with lower DFA findings.

The results utilizing DFA and HFD are consistent with the *CD* signaling a chaotic signal. Regarding LZC, it appears that the methodology may have skewed the findings because Kalev et al. [155] used a multiscale approach and observed various effects depending on the frequency whereas Bachmann et al. [154] found no difference.

3.4.4.4 Dimensionality Reduction Stage

Principal Component Analysis (*PCA*) [164] is one of many techniques that may be used to do dimensionality reduction in order to choose the ideal collection of features for automatic depression detection [165–167]. H. Cai et al., however, have utilized four feature selection techniques for this purpose, including Wrapper Subset, Correlation Attribute, Gain Ratio Attribute, and PCA [168].

The strategy of minimal-redundancy-maximum-relevance feature selection has been used in [149]. Additionally used in [169] is the sequential backward feature selection (SBFS) algorithm, while [170] applies differential evolution, a population-based adaptive global optimization algorithm.

3.4.4.5 Depression Classification Techniques

EEG is a very accurate classification method whose accuracy is directly connected to the quality of extracted features, and dimensionality reduction and classifiers are proposed to enhance *EEG* classification. Because of its accuracy and applicability in various research, linear Discriminant analysis (*LDA*) and Support Vector Machine (*SVM*) classifiers are the most prominent approaches used to categorize brain illnesses such as dementia and epilepsy [165, 166].

Different categories of machine learning based algorithms have been explored for *EEG* based depression diagnosis such as *SVM* based classifiers (Least Square-Support Vector Machine (*LS − SVM*) [171], *SVM* with different kernels [168], Linear and Quadratic Discriminant analysis based classifiers (*LDA*) and (*QLDA*) respectively, Ensemble architectures (*Bagging*, Rus-Boost (*RB*), GentleBoost (*GB*), and Random Forest (*RF*)), Logistic Regression (*LR*)), *K*-Nearest Neighbors (*KNN*) and its variants, Tree-based (Decision Tree (*DT*), *J*48, complex-tree), and others (Gaussian Mixture Model (*GMM*), BayesNet) [98, 168, 169, 172, 173].

3.5 Discussion

The literature has been used in this study to distinguish between the various depression- based *EEG* subtypes. Large-scale research is needed to discover trustworthy biomarkers that can aid in the diagnosis of depression, which is seen as a significant clinical challenge. Recent studies have looked into the potential for linear and nonlinear *EEG* -based biomarkers to be a distinguishing factor between various MDD episodes and depression severity scales.

The accurate sub-types of depression are the next significant challenge for depression-based *EEG*. Although it was a good effort, none of the machine learning models worked the best for all patients. Therefore, employing *EEG* -based data-driven methods, the answer to this significant issue can be investigated.

There has been a lot of interest in the identification and diagnosis of depression. Combining reliable markers with diagnostic criteria could achieve this. The detection of both episodes and subtypes of depression may be aided by neuropsychological tests and biomarkers evaluated against several depressive signs. We desperately require a marker for diagnosing depression that is precise, specific, and economical. *EEG* is a desirable technology for the early diagnosis and categorization of depression kinds and stages due to its low cost and non-invasive nature. The use of *EEG* as a neuro-marker to aid in the diagnosis of depression was the main topic of this review. Neurologists' subjective training makes it difficult to assess an *EEG* objectively, which leaves room for error. Additionally, it takes a lot of time and might not be able to pick up on little *EEG* changes, whereas computerized *EEG* signal analysis could streamline medical professionals' tasks and aid in more objective decision-making. Table 3.1 compares *EEG* acquisition devices, preprocessing, feature extraction, dimensionality reduction, and classification techniques used in research to diagnose depression.

In fact, BPFs and notch filters have been employed extensively in the preprocessing step [154, 174]. As shown in Table 3.1, [168, 171] frequently employs linear spectral components such as power *gamma*, *beta*, *alpha*, *theta*, and *delta*. *Nonlinear* entropy investigations, however, have produced good performance findings [170, 175].

They used a combination of classification algorithms to see if they could enhance the performance, sensitivity, and specificity of the best clinical diagnosis for early detection and classification of depression, based on its applicability in a variety of disciplines and empirically strong performance. *SVM*, on the other hand, is the most widely used machine learning-based algorithm that produces great performance outcomes for diagnosis [171] (refer to Sect. 3.1). *KNN* technology is widely used and produces excellent results. For the aim of classification, probabilistic models like *LR*, for instance, have received a lot of attention. *DT* is the most used algorithm for tree-based classifiers. Overall, *SVM* and *KNN* perform the best in terms of multiple performance measures, getting good classification results (around 99 percent) in the majority of the experiments.

Table 3.1 Comparative approaches used in depression diagnosis form *EEG* -based signals

Studies	Preprocessing methods	Features methods	Dimensionality reduction technique	Classification Techniques	Best results
X. Ding et al. [174]	Notch filter, BPF	FFT Absolute power of (*gamma, beta, alpha, theta, delta*)	---		
M. Bachmann et al. [154]	BPF	Spectral asymmetry index (*SAI*), Alpha power variability (*APV*), Relative gamma power (*RGP*), *DFA, LZC*	---	*LR*	LR (92)
M. Sharma et al. [171]	Notch filter	*DWT*, relative-wavelet energy (*RWE*), Wavelet-entropy (*WE*)	*t*-test	*LS-SVM*, Complex tree, *LD, LR, KNN*, bagged	LS- SVM (99.54)
H. Cai et al. [168]	BPF, Kalman	Relative and absolute *centroid* frequency, relative and absolute power, *C₀, CD*, entropy	Correlation-based Method, wrapper based method, *PCA*	*SVM* (RBF), RF, *LR, KNN, DT*	DT (76.4)
S. Mahato et al. [176]	BPF	Asymmetry and paired asymmetry from sub-bands (*gamma*1, *gamma*2, *beta, alpha, theta, delta*), *DFA, SE*	ReliefF	Bagging, *SVM* (kernels such as polynomial,	*SVM* (96.02)
H. Cai et al. [149]	FIR, Kalman with DWT adaptive-Predictor filter (APF)	Relative and absolute power, *Hjorth* parameters (*activity, mobility, complexity*), *Shannon* entropy, *SE, CD*, peak, *Kurtosis, Skewness*	Minimal-redundancy-maximal-relevance	*KNN, SVM*, Classification- tree	KNN (79.27)
H. Akbari et al. [177]	LPF	Recurrence phase space (*RPS*) + geometrical *nonlinear* features	*GA*, Ant colony optimization, Grey wolf optimization, particle-swarm optimization	*SVM* (RBF), *KNN*	SVM (99.30)

(continued)

Table 3.1 (continued)

Studies	Preprocessing methods	Features methods	Dimensionality reduction technique	Classification Techniques	Best results
Y. Li et al. [170]	Notch filter, LPF, HPF	AR model + max-power spectrum density, and sum power, C_0, CD, Kolmogorov-entropy (KE), Shannon entropy, permutation entropy (PE), Lyapunov exponent (LLE), singular-value deposition entropy (SVDE), variance, mean-square (MS), mean of peak-to-peak (P2P)	Differential evolution	KNN	KNN (98.40)
H. Peng et al. [178]	BPF	Phase lag index (PLI) from full-band as well four other sub-bands (alpha, beta, delta, theta)	Kendall's tau coefficient	SVM (linear kernel), KNN, DT, NB	SVM (92.73)
J. Zhu et al. [175]	LPF, HPF	AR model + power-Spectrum density (PSD), AR model + max-power spectrum density, sum power, C_0- complexity (C_0), correlation-dimension (CD), Kolmogorov-entropy (KE), Shannon entropy, permutation entropy (PE), singular-value deposition entropy (SVDE), mean-square (MS), mean of peak-to-Peak (P2P)	Correlation feature selection	LR, KNN, RF, SVM, BayesNet, NB, J48	KNN (92.65)
R. A. Movahed et al. [169]	LPF, HPF	Synchronization likelihood (SL), Higuchi-fractal dimension (HFD), Detrended-fluctuation analysis (DFA), C_0-complexity (C_0), correlation-dimension (CD), Kolmogorov-entropy (KE), Shannon entropy, Lyapunov exponent (LLE), Kurtosis, Skewness, DWT + relative-wavelet energy (RWE), Wavelet-entropy (WE)	Sequential backward feature selection (SBFS)	SVM (RBF), LR, DT, NB, RB, GB, RF	SVM (99)

X. Li et al. [98]	BPF. Adaptive- noise canceller (LMS) algorithm	*AR model* + power-Spectrum density *(PSD)*, *AR model* + activity of *theta, alpha, beta, Hjorth* parameters *(activity, mobility, complexity)*,	---	Ensemble model	Ensemble model (89.02)
QuickCap™, brain products Inc., Gilching, Bavaria, Germany et al. [179]	BPF	Task-related common spatial-pattern *(TCSP)* + *WPD* + differential entropy *(DE)* from *(gamma, alpha, beta, theta, delta)*, wide band-EEG	GA	*SVM, LR, KNN*	*SVM*
H. Akbari et al. [180]	Notch filter	*EWT* + centered-correntropy *(CC)* *alpha, beta, gamma, delta, theta*	---	*KNN, SVM (RBF* kernel)	*SVM (98)*

3.6 Conclusion

Electroencephalogram has been emphasized as a study tool and prospective neuro-marker for diagnosing depression and grading its sorts in this review by offering succinct details on brain activity and how it is altered by various depression types. It should be mentioned that the review has highlighted discoveries relating to depressive illness at times. The reason for this is because there is a far larger body of information on depression sickness. The analyzed datasets were typically small as well, necessitating additional study to support the promising findings. On the other hand, the electroencephalogram has received high marks from numerous studies for its value as a clinical evaluation tool in the diagnosis of depression. Because of its low cost and accessibility, extremely sensitive electroencephalogram -based detection of depressive episodes and subtypes categorization is a generally wanted screening strategy in clinical practice. It is a promising method that can be utilized to adapt or tailor the best treatment plans for depression sufferers.

References

1. W. Depression, Other common mental disorders: global health estimates. Geneva: World Health Organization. CC BYNC-SA **3** (2022)
2. W. Liu, K. Jia, Z. Wang, Z. Ma, A Depression prediction algorithm based on spatiotemporal feature of EEG signal. Brain Sci. **12**, 630 (2022)
3. S.P. Pandalai, P.A. Schulte, D.B. Miller, Conceptual heuristic models of the interrelationships between obesity and the occupational environment. Scandinavian J. Work Environ. Health **39**, 221 (2013)
4. Y.T. Nigatu, S.A. Reijneveld, B.W. Penninx, R.A. Schoevers, U. Bültmann, The longitudinal joint effect of obesity and major depression on work performance impairment. Am. J. Public Health **105**, e80–e86 (2015)
5. S.I. Prada, H.G. Rincón-Hoyos, A.M. Pérez, M. Sierra-Ruiz, V. Serna, The Effect of Depression on Paid Sick Leave due to Metabolic and Cardiovascular Disease in low-wage workers.(Depression and Sick Leave). Gerencia y Políticas de Salud **21** (2022)
6. W.N. Burton, C.-Y. Chen, A.B. Schultz, D.W. Edington, The prevalence of metabolic syndrome in an employed population and the impact on health and productivity. J. Occup. Environ. Med. **50**, 1139–1148 (2008)
7. N.K. Al-Qazzaz, M.K. Sabir, S.H.B.M. Ali, S.A. Ahmad, K. Grammer, Electroencephalogram profiles for emotion identification over the brain regions using spectral, entropy and temporal biomarkers. Sensors **20**, 59 (2020)
8. N.K. Al-Qazzaz, S.H.M. Ali, S.A. Ahmad, Entropy-based EEG markers for gender identification of vascular dementia patients, in *Inter. Conf. Innovat. Biomed. Eng. Life Sci.*, (2019), pp. 121–128
9. N.K. Al-Qazzaz, S.H.B. Ali, S.A. Ahmad, K. Chellappan, M. Islam, J. Escudero, Role of EEG as biomarker in the early detection and classification of dementia. Scientif. World J. **2014** (2014)
10. N.K. Al-Qazzaz, S.H. Ali, S.A. Ahmad, S. Islam, K. Mohamad, Cognitive impairment and memory dysfunction after a stroke diagnosis: A post-stroke memory assessment. Neuropsychiatr. Dis. Treat. **10**, 1677 (2014)
11. N.K. Al-Qazzaz, S.H.B.M. Ali, S.A. Ahmad, M.S. Islam, J. Escudero, Discrimination of stroke- related mild cognitive impairment and vascular dementia using EEG signal analysis. Med. Biol. Eng. Comput. **56**, 1–21 (2017)

12. N.K. Al-Qazzaz, S. Ali, M.S. Islam, S.A. Ahmad, J. Escudero, EEG markers for early detection and characterization of vascular dementia during working memory tasks, in *2016 IEEE EMBS Conference on Biomedical Engineering and Sciences (IECBES)*, (2016), pp. 347–351
13. N.K. Al-Qazzaz, M.K. Sabir, A.H. Al-Timemy, K. Grammer, An integrated entropy-spatial framework for automatic gender recognition enhancement of emotion-based EEGs. Med. Biol. Eng. Comput. **60**, 1–20 (2022)
14. N.K. Al-Qazzaz, M.K. Sabir, S.H.B.M. Ali, S.A. Ahmad, K. Grammer, Complexity and entropy analysis to improve gender identification from emotional-based EEGs. J. Healthcare Eng. **2021** (2021)
15. N.K. Al-Qazzaz, M.K. Sabir, S.H.B.M. Ali, S.A. Ahmad, K. Grammer, Multichannel optimization with hybrid spectral-entropy markers for gender identification enhancement of emotional- based EEGs. IEEE Access **9**, 107059–107078 (2021)
16. P. Nguyen, D. Tran, X. Huang, W. Ma, Age and gender classification using EEG paralinguistic features, in *2013 6th International IEEE/EMBS conference on neural engineering (NER)*, (2013), pp. 1295–1298
17. N.K. Al-Qazzaz, M.K. Sabir, K. Grammer, Gender differences identification from brain regions using spectral relative powers of emotional EEG, in *IWBBIO 2019*, (2019)
18. N.K. Al-Qazzaz, M.K. Sabir, S.H.M. Ali, S.A. Ahmad, K. Grammer, The role of spectral power ratio in characterizing emotional EEG for gender identification, in *2020 IEEE-EMBS Conference on Biomedical Engineering and Sciences (IECBES)*, (2021), pp. 334–338
19. B. Kaur, D. Singh, P.P. Roy, Age and gender classification using brain–computer interface. Neural Comput. & Applic. **31**, 5887–5900 (2019)
20. S. Sardari, B. Nakisa, M.N. Rastgoo, P. Eklund, Audio based depression detection using convolutional autoencoder. Expert Syst. Appl. **189**, 116076 (2022)
21. R.P. Thati, A.S. Dhadwal, P. Kumar, A novel multi-modal depression detection approach based on mobile crowd sensing and task-based mechanisms. Multimed. Tools Appl., 1–34 (2022)
22. J.E. Siegel-Ramsay, M.A. Bertocci, B. Wu, M.L. Phillips, S.M. Strakowski, J.R. Almeida, Distinguishing between depression in bipolar disorder and unipolar depression using magnetic resonance imaging: A systematic review. Bipolar Disord. **24**, 474–498 (2022)
23. S. Yasin, S.A. Hussain, S. Aslan, I. Raza, M. Muzammel, A. Othmani, EEG based major depressive disorder and bipolar disorder detection using neural networks: A review. Comput. Methods Prog. Biomed. **202**, 106007 (2021)
24. K. Chellappan, N.K. Mohsin, S.H.B.M. Ali, M.S. Islam, Post-stroke brain memory assessment framework, in *2012 IEEE-EMBS Conference on Biomedical Engineering and Sciences*, (2012), pp. 189–194
25. G. Parker, M.J. Spoelma, G. Tavella, M. Alda, D.L. Dunner, C. O'Donovan, et al., A new machine learning-derived screening measure for differentiating bipolar from unipolar mood disorders. J. Affect. Disord. **299**, 513–516 (2022)
26. C. Otte, S.M. Gold, B.W. Penninx, C.M. Pariante, A. Etkin, M. Fava, et al., Major depressive disorder. Nat. Rev. Dis. Primers. **2**, 1–20 (2016)
27. U. Halbreich, J. Borenstein, T. Pearlstein, L.S. Kahn, The prevalence, impairment, impact, and burden of premenstrual dysphoric disorder (PMS/PMDD). Psychoneuroendocrinology **28**, 1–23 (2003)
28. S. O'Connor, M. Agius, A systematic review of structural and functional MRI differences between psychotic and nonpsychotic depression. Psychiatr. Danub. **27**, 235–239 (2015)
29. S.L. Dubovsky, B.M. Ghosh, J.C. Serotte, V. Cranwell, Psychotic depression: Diagnosis, differential diagnosis, and treatment. Psychother. Psychosom. **90**, 160–177 (2021)
30. S. Thurgood, D.M. Avery, L. Williamson, Postpartum depression (PPD). Am. J. Clin. Med. **6**, 17–22 (2009)
31. M.W. O'Hara, Postpartum depression: What we know. J. Clin. Psychol. **65**, 1258–1269 (2009)
32. K. Machmutow, R. Meister, A. Jansen, L. Kriston, B. Watzke, M.C. Härter, et al., Comparative effectiveness of continuation and maintenance treatments for persistent depressive disorder in adults. Cochrane Database Syst. Rev. (2019)

33. S. Melrose, Seasonal affective disorder: An overview of assessment and treatment approaches. Depression Res. Treatment **2015** (2015)
34. E. Sibille, Molecular aging of the brain, neuroplasticity, and vulnerability to depression and other brain- related disorders. Dialogues Clin. Neurosci. (2022)
35. V. Dorval, P.T. Nelson, S.S. Hébert, Circulating microRNAs in Alzheimer's disease: the search for novel biomarkers. Front. Molecul. Neurosci. **6** (2013)
36. J.A. Sonnen, K.S. Montine, J.F. Quinn, J.A. Kaye, J. Breitner, T.J. Montine, Biomarkers for cognitive impairment and dementia in elderly people. Lancet Neurol. **7**, 704–714 (2008)
37. A. Nobis, D. Zalewski, N. Waszkiewicz, Peripheral markers of depression. J. Clin. Med. **9**, 3793 (2020)
38. A.L. Lopresti, G.L. Maker, S.D. Hood, P.D. Drummond, A review of peripheral biomarkers in major depression: The potential of inflammatory and oxidative stress biomarkers. Prog. Neuro-Psychopharmacol. Biolog. Psychiat. **48**, 102–111 (2014)
39. A. Gururajan, G. Clarke, T.G. Dinan, J.F. Cryan, Molecular biomarkers of depression. Neurosci. Biobehav. Rev. **64**, 101–133 (2016)
40. M. Guha, *Diagnostic and Statistical Manual of Mental Disorders: DSM-5* (Reference Reviews, 2014)
41. B. Ay, O. Yildirim, M. Talo, U.B. Baloglu, G. Aydin, S.D. Puthankattil, et al., Automated depression detection using deep representation and sequence learning with EEG signals. J. Med. Syst. **43**, 1–12 (2019)
42. N. R. Council, "Depression in Parents, Parenting, and Children: Opportunities to Improve Identification, Treatment, and Prevention," (2009)
43. S. Maharaj, K. Trevino, A comprehensive review of treatment options for premenstrual syndrome and premenstrual dysphoric disorder. J. Psychiat. Practice®. **21**, 334–350 (2015)
44. N.K. Al-Qazzaz, S.H.M. Ali, S.A. Ahmad, Differential evolution based channel selection algorithm on eeg signal for early detection of vascular dementia among stroke survivors, in *2018 IEEE- EMBS Conference on Biomedical Engineering and Sciences (IECBES)*, (2018), pp. 239–244
45. N.K. Al-Qazzaz, S.H.M. Ali, S. Islam, S. Ahmad, J. Escudero, EEG wavelet spectral analysis during a working memory tasks in stroke-related mild cognitive impairment patients, in *International Conference for Innovation in Biomedical Engineering and Life Sciences*, (2015), pp. 82–85
46. N.K. Al-Qazzaz, S. Ali, S.A. Ahmad, J. Escudero, Classification enhancement for post-stroke dementia using fuzzy neighborhood preserving analysis with QR-decomposition, in *2017 39th Annual International Conference of the IEEE Engineering in Medicine and Biology Society (EMBC)*, (2017), pp. 3174–3177
47. W. Mumtaz, A.S. Malik, M.A.M. Yasin, L. Xia, Review on EEG and ERP predictive biomarkers for major depressive disorder. Biomed. Signal Process. Cont. **22**, 85–98 (2015)
48. J. Gallinat, R. Bottlender, G. Juckel, A. Munke-Puchner, G. Stotz, H.-J. Kuss, et al., The loudness dependency of the auditory evoked N1/P2-component as a predictor of the acute SSRI response in depression. Psychopharmacology **148**, 404–411 (2000)
49. C. Brush, A.M. Kallen, M.A. Meynadasy, T. King, G. Hajcak, J.L. Sheffler, The P300, loneliness, and depression in older adults. Biol. Psychol. **171**, 108339 (2022)
50. Y. Diao, M. Geng, Y. Fu, H. Wang, C. Liu, J. Gu, et al., A combination of P300 and eye movement data improves the accuracy of auxiliary diagnoses of depression. J. Affect. Disord. **297**, 386–395 (2022)
51. N.J. Santopetro, C. Brush, K. Burani, A. Bruchnak, G. Hajcak, Doors P300 moderates the relationship between reward positivity and current depression status in adults. J. Affect. Disord. **294**, 776–785 (2021)
52. A. Sommer, A.J. Fallgatter, C. Plewnia, Investigating mechanisms of cognitive control training: Neural signatures of PASAT performance in depressed patients. J. Neural Transm. **129**, 1–11 (2021)

53. L. Zhou, G. Wang, C. Nan, H. Wang, Z. Liu, H. Bai, Abnormalities in P300 components in depression: An ERP-sLORETA study. Nord. J. Psychiatry **73**, 1–8 (2019)
54. C. Nan, G. Wang, H. Wang, X. Wang, Z. Liu, L. Xiao, et al., The P300 component decreases in a bimodal oddball task in individuals with depression: An event-related potentials study. Clin. Neurophysiol. **129**, 2525–2533 (2018)
55. M. Shim, M.J. Jin, C.-H. Im, S.-H. Lee, Machine-learning-based classification between post-traumatic stress disorder and major depressive disorder using P300 features. NeuroImage: Clin. **24**, 102001 (2019)
56. N. Ramakrishnan, N. Murphy, S. Selvaraj, R.Y. Cho, Electrophysiological Biomarkers for Mood Disorders. Mood Disorders: Brain Imaging and Therapeutic Implications, 175 (2021)
57. A.J. Flórez, G. Molenberghs, W. Van der Elst, A.A. Abad, An efficient algorithm to assess multivariate surrogate endpoints in a causal inference framework. Computat. Statist. Data Analy. **172**, 107494 (2022)
58. S. Mahato, S. Paul, Electroencephalogram (EEG) signal analysis for diagnosis of major depressive disorder (MDD): A review. Nanoelectroni. Circuit. Communicat. Syst., 323–335 (2019)
59. M.J. Kas, B. Penninx, B. Sommer, A. Serretti, C. Arango, H. Marston, A quantitative approach to neuropsychiatry: The why and the how. Neurosci. Biobehav. Rev. **97**, 3–9 (2019)
60. C.-T. Ip, S. Olbrich, M. Ganz, B. Ozenne, K. Köhler-Forsberg, V.H. Dam, et al., Pretreatment qEEG biomarkers for predicting pharmacological treatment outcome in major depressive disorder: Independent validation from the NeuroPharm study. Eur. Neuropsychopharmacol. **49**, 101–112 (2021)
61. F.S. de Aguiar Neto, J.L.G. Rosa, Depression biomarkers using non-invasive EEG: A review. Neurosci. Biobehav. Rev. **105**, 83–93 (2019)
62. B.D. Nelson, E.M. Kessel, D.N. Klein, S.A. Shankman, Depression symptom dimensions and asymmetrical frontal cortical activity while anticipating reward. Psychophysiology **55**, e12892 (2018)
63. S. Glier, A. Campbell, R. Corr, A. Pelletier-Baldelli, A. Belger, Individual differences in frontal alpha asymmetry moderate the relationship between acute stress responsivity and state and trait anxiety in adolescents. Biolog. Psychol., 108357 (2022)
64. S.M. Tripathi, N. Mishra, R.K. Tripathi, K. Gurnani, P300 latency as an indicator of severity in major depressive disorder. Ind. Psychiatry J. **24**, 163 (2015)
65. N.J. Santopetro, C. Brush, A. Bruchnak, J. Klawohn, G. Hajcak, A reduced P300 prospectively predicts increased depressive severity in adults with clinical depression. Psychophysiology **58**, e13767 (2021)
66. N. Van Der Vinne, M.A. Vollebregt, M.J. Van Putten, M. Arns, Frontal alpha asymmetry as a diagnostic marker in depression: Fact or fiction? A meta-analysis. Neuroimage Clin. **16**, 79–87 (2017)
67. A. Dharmadhikari, A. Tandle, S. Jaiswal, V. Sawant, V. Vahia, N. Jog, Frontal theta asymmetry as a biomarker of depression. East Asian Arch. Psychiatr. **28**, 17–22 (2018)
68. A.M. Hunter, T.X. Nghiem, I.A. Cook, D.E. Krantz, M.J. Minzenberg, A.F. Leuchter, Change in quantitative EEG theta cordance as a potential predictor of repetitive transcranial magnetic stimulation clinical outcome in major depressive disorder. Clin. EEG Neurosci. **49**, 306–315 (2018)
69. P.J. Fitzgerald, B.O. Watson, Gamma oscillations as a biomarker for major depression: An emerging topic. Transl. Psychiatry **8**, 1–7 (2018)
70. S. Sun, J. Li, H. Chen, T. Gong, X. Li, B. Hu, "A study of resting-state EEG biomarkers for depression recognition," arXiv preprint arXiv:2002.11039 (2020)
71. P.C. Koo, C. Berger, G. Kronenberg, J. Bartz, P. Wybitul, O. Reis, et al., Combined cognitive, psychomotor and electrophysiological biomarkers in major depressive disorder. Eur. Arch. Psychiatry Clin. Neurosci. **269**, 823–832 (2019)
72. P. Fernández-Palleiro, T. Rivera-Baltanás, D. Rodrigues-Amorim, S. Fernández-Gil, M. del Carmen Vallejo-Curto, M. Álvarez-Ariza, et al., Brainwaves oscillations as a potential biomarker for major depression disorder risk. Clin. EEG Neurosci. **51**, 3–9 (2020)

73. W. J. G., Medical Instrumentation Application and Design. New York: Wiley (1998)
74. R. Lizio, F. Vecchio, G.B. Frisoni, R. Ferri, G. Rodriguez, C. Babiloni, Electro-encephalographic rhythms in Alzheimer's disease. International journal of Alzheimer's disease, vol. **2011**, 1–11 (2011)
75. D.A. Pizzagalli, Electroencephalography and high-density electrophysiological source localization, in *Handbook of Psychophysiology*, (USA), pp. 8–12
76. E. John, H. Ahn, L. Prichep, M. Trepetin, D. Brown, H. Kaye, Developmental equations for the electroencephalogram. Science **210**, 1255–1258 (1980)
77. T.R. Oakes, D.A. Pizzagalli, A.M. Hendrick, K.A. Horras, C.L. Larson, H.C. Abercrombie, et al., Functional coupling of simultaneous electrical and metabolic activity in the human brain. Hum. Brain Mapp. **21**, 257–270 (Apr 2004)
78. R. M. Rangayyan, Biomedical Signal Analysis: A Case-Study Approach Wiley-IEEE Press (2001)
79. W.O. Tatum, A.M. Husain, S.R. Benbadis, P.W. Kaplan, *Handbook of EEG Interpretation* (Demos Medical Publishing, LLC, USA, 2008)
80. U.R. Acharya, S.L. Oh, Y. Hagiwara, J.H. Tan, H. Adeli, D.P. Subha, Automated EEG-based screening of depression using deep convolutional neural network. Comput. Methods Prog. Biomed. **161**, 103–113 (2018)
81. S.D. Puthankattil, P.K. Joseph, Classification of EEG signals in normal and depression conditions by ANN using RWE and signal entropy. J. Mechan. Med. Biol. **12**, 1240019 (2012)
82. O. Faust, P.C.A. Ang, S.D. Puthankattil, P.K. Joseph, Depression diagnosis support system based on EEG signal entropies. J. Mechan. Med.Biol. **14**, 1450035 (2014)
83. S.D. Kumar, D. Subha, Prediction of depression from EEG signal using long short term memory (LSTM), in *2019 3rd International Conference on Trends in Electronics and Informatics (ICOEI)*, (2019), pp. 1248–1253
84. W. Mumtaz, A. Qayyum, A deep learning framework for automatic diagnosis of unipolar depression. Int. J. Med. Inform. **132**, 103983 (2019)
85. P. Sandheep, S. Vineeth, M. Poulose, D. Subha, Performance analysis of deep learning CNN in classification of depression EEG signals, in *TENCON 2019–2019 IEEE Region 10 Conference (TENCON)*, (2019), pp. 1339–1344
86. Y. Mohammadi, M. Hajian, M.H. Moradi, Discrimination of Depression Levels Using Machine Learning Methods on EEG Signals, in *2019 27th Iranian Conference on Electrical Engineering (ICEE)*, (2019), pp. 1765–1769
87. S.D. Puthankattil, P.K. Joseph, Half-wave segment feature extraction of EEG signals of patients with depression and performance evaluation of neural network classifiers. J. Mec. Med. Biol. **17**, 1750006 (2017)
88. J. Zhu, Y. Wang, R. La, J. Zhan, J. Niu, S. Zeng, et al., Multimodal mild depression recognition based on EEG-EM synchronization acquisition network. IEEE Access **7**, 28196–28210 (2019)
89. S. Mahato, S. Paul, Detection of major depressive disorder using linear and non-linear features from EEG signals. Microsyst. Technol. **25**, 1065–1076 (2019)
90. X. Li, R. La, Y. Wang, J. Niu, S. Zeng, S. Sun, et al., EEG-based mild depression recognition using convolutional neural network. Med. Biol. Eng. Comput. **57**, 1341–1352 (2019)
91. H. Kwon, S. Kang, W. Park, J. Park, Y. Lee, Deep learning based pre-screening method for depression with imagery frontal eeg channels, in *2019 International conference on information and communication technology convergence (ICTC)*, (2019), pp. 378–380
92. H. Mallikarjun, H. Suresh, Depression level prediction using EEG signal processing, in *2014 International Conference on Contemporary Computing and Informatics (IC3I)*, (2014), pp. 928–933
93. H. Jebelli, M.M. Khalili, S. Lee, Mobile EEG-based workers' stress recognition by applying deep neural network, in *Advances in Informatics and Computing in Civil and Construction Engineering*, (Springer, 2019), pp. 173–180

94. B. Mohammadzadeh, M. Khodabandelu, M. Lotfizadeh, Comparing diagnosis of depression in depressed patients by EEG, based on two algorithms: Artificial nerve networks and neuro-Fuzy networks. Inter. J. Epidemiol. Res. **3**, 246–258 (2016)
95. X. Zhang, B. Hu, L. Zhou, P. Moore, J. Chen, An EEG based pervasive depression detection for females, in *Joint International Conference on Pervasive Computing and the Networked World*, (2012), pp. 848–861
96. G. Jackson-Koku, Beck depression inventory. Occup. Med. **66**, 174–175 (2016)
97. T.T. Erguzel, G.H. Sayar, N. Tarhan, Artificial intelligence approach to classify unipolar and bipolar depressive disorders. Neural Comput. & Applic. **27**, 1607–1616 (2016)
98. X. Li, X. Zhang, J. Zhu, W. Mao, S. Sun, Z. Wang, et al., Depression recognition using machine learning methods with different feature generation strategies. Artif. Intell. Med. **99**, 101696 (2019)
99. L.M. Alexander, J. Escalera, L. Ai, C. Andreotti, K. Febre, A. Mangone, et al., An open resource for transdiagnostic research in pediatric mental health and learning disorders. Scientific Data **4**, 1–26 (2017)
100. W. Wu, Y. Zhang, J. Jiang, M.V. Lucas, G.A. Fonzo, C.E. Rolle, et al., An electroencephalographic signature predicts antidepressant response in major depression. Nat. Biotechnol. **38**, 439–447 (2020)
101. E. Garcia-Ceja, M. Riegler, P. Jakobsen, J. Tørresen, T. Nordgreen, K.J. Oedegaard, et al., Depresjon: a motor activity database of depression episodes in unipolar and bipolar patients, in *Proceedings of the 9th ACM Multimedia Systems Conference*, (2018), pp. 472–477
102. H. Kristjánsdóttir, P.M. Salkovskis, B.H. Sigurdsson, E. Sigurdsson, A. Agnarsdóttir, J.F. Sigurdsson, Transdiagnostic cognitive behavioural treatment and the impact of comorbidity: An open trial in a cohort of primary care patients. Nord. J. Psychiatry **70**, 215–223 (2016)
103. N. Langer, E.J. Ho, L.M. Alexander, H.Y. Xu, R.K. Jozanovic, S. Henin, et al., A resource for assessing information processing in the developing brain using EEG and eye tracking. Scientific Data **4**, 1–20 (2017)
104. J. F. Cavanagh, A. W. Bismark, M. J. Frank, and J. J. Allen, "Multiple dissociations between comorbid depression and anxiety on reward and punishment processing: Evidence from computationally informed EEG," Computational Psychiatry (Cambridge, Mass.), vol. 3, p. 1, 2019
105. S.A. Taywade, R.D. Raut, A review: EEG signal analysis with different methodologies, in *National Conference on Innovative Paradigms in Engineering and Technology New York, USA*, (2012), pp. 29–31
106. N.K. Al-Qazzaz, S.H.B. Ali, S.A. Ahmad, K. Chellappan, M.S. Islam, J. Escudero, Role of EEG as biomarker in the early detection and classification of dementia. The Scientific World J. **2014** (2014)
107. K. R. S, Handbook on Biomedical Instrumentati. New Delhi: Tata Mc Graw-Hill (1998)
108. A. Seal, R. Bajpai, J. Agnihotri, A. Yazidi, E. Herrera-Viedma, O. Krejcar, DeprNet: A deep convolution neural network framework for detecting depression using EEG. IEEE Trans. Instrum. Meas. **70**, 1–13 (2021)
109. H. Ke, D. Chen, T. Shah, X. Liu, X. Zhang, L. Zhang, et al., Cloud-aided online EEG classification system for brain healthcare: A case study of depression evaluation with a lightweight CNN. Software: Practice and Experience **50**, 596–610 (2020)
110. C. Uyulan, T.T. Ergüzel, H. Unubol, M. Cebi, G.H. Sayar, M. Nezhad Asad, et al., Major depressive disorder classification based on different convolutional neural network models: Deep learning approach. Clin. EEG Neurosci. **52**, 38–51 (2021)
111. S. Sanei, J.A. Chambers, *EEG Signal Procesing* (Wiley, USA, 2007)
112. D.V. Moretti, C. Babiloni, G. Binetti, E. Cassetta, G. Dal Forno, F. Ferreric, et al., Individual analysis of EEG frequency and band power in mild Alzheimer's disease. Clin. Neurophysiol. **115**, 299–308 (2004)

113. T.-P. Jung, S. Makeig, M. Westerfield, J. Townsend, E. Courchesne, T.J. Sejnowski, Removal of eye activity artifacts from visual event-related potentials in normal and clinical subjects. Clin. Neurophysiol. **111**, 1745–1758 (2000)

114. M. Habl, C. Bauer, C. Ziegaus, E. Lang, and F. Schulmeyer, "Can ICA help identify brain tumor related EEG signals," in Proceedings of ICA, 2000, pp. 609–614

115. C. Guerrero-Mosquera, A. M. Trigueros, A. Navia-Vazquez, EEG Signal Processing for Epilepsy (2012)

116. I. M. B. Núñez, "EEG Artifact Dtection," 2010

117. G.N.G. Molina, *Direct Brain-Computer Communication through Scalp Recorded EEG Signals* (ÉCOLE POLYTECHNIQUE FÉDÉRALE DE LAUSANNE, 2004)

118. A. Naït-Ali, *Advanced Biosignal Processing* (Springer, 2009)

119. D. Langlois, S. Chartier, D. Gosselin, An introduction to independent component analysis: InfoMax and FastICA algorithms. Tutorials in Quantitative Methods for Psychology **6**, 31–38 (2010)

120. M. McKeown, C. Humphries, P. Achermann, A. Borbély, T. Sejnowsk, A new method for detecting state changes in the EEG: Exploratory application to sleep data. J. Sleep Res. **7**, 48–56 (1998)

121. T. Zikov, S. Bibian, G. A. Dumont, M. Huzmezan, C. Ries, "A wavelet based de-noising technique for ocular artifact correction of the electroencephalogram," in Engineering in Medicine and Biology, 2002. 24th Annual Conference and the Annual Fall Meeting of the Biomedical Engineering Society EMBS/BMES Conference. pp. 98–105. (Proceedings of the Second Joint, 2002)

122. V. Krishnaveni, S. Jayaraman, S. Aravind, V. Hariharasudhan, K. Ramadoss, Automatic identification and removal of ocular artifacts from EEG using wavelet transform. Measurement Sci. Rev. **6**, 45–57 (2006)

123. P.S. Kumar, R. Arumuganathan, K. Sivakumar, C. Vimal, Removal of ocular artifacts in the EEG through wavelet transform without using an EOG Reference Channel. Int. J. Open Problems Compt. Math **1**, 188–200 (2008)

124. V. Krishnaveni, S. Jayaraman, L. Anitha, K. Ramadoss, Removal of ocular artifacts from EEG using adaptive thresholding of wavelet coefficients. J. Neural Eng. **3**, 338–346 (2006)

125. N.P. Castellanos, V.A. Makarov, Recovering EEG brain signals: Artifact suppression with wavelet enhanced independent component analysis. J. Neurosci. Methods **158**, 300–312 (2006)

126. M.T. Akhtar, C.J. James, Focal artifact removal from ongoing EEG–a hybrid approach based on spatially-constrained ICA and wavelet de-noising, in *Engineering in Medicine and Biology Society*, (EMBC 2009. Annual International Conference of the IEEE 2009, 2009), pp. 4027–4030

127. M.T. Akhtar, C.J. James, W. Mitsuhashi, Modifying the spatially-constrained ica for efficient removal of artifacts from eeg data, in *Bioinformatics and Biomedical Engineering (iCBBE), 2010 4th International Conference on*, (2010), pp. 1–4

128. J. Walters-Williams, Y. Li, A new approach to denoising EEG signals-merger of translation invariant wavelet and ICA. Int. J. Biometrics Bioinform **5**, 130–149 (2011)

129. J. Walters-Williams, Y. Li, Performance comparison of known ICA algorithms to a wavelet-ICA merger. Signal Processing: An Inter. J. **5**, 80 (2011)

130. N. Mammone, F.L. Foresta, F.C. Morabito, Automatic artifact rejection from multichannel scalp EEG by wavelet ICA. IEEE Sensor Journal **12**(3), 533–542 (2012)

131. G. Inuso, F. La Foresta, N. Mammone, F.C. Morabito, Wavelet-ICA methodology for efficient artifact removal from Electroencephalographic recordings, in *Neural Networks*, (IJCNN 2007. International Joint Conference on, 2007), pp. 1524–1529

132. N. Al-Qazzaz, S.H.B.M. Ali, S. Ahmad, M. Islam, J. Escudero, Automatic artifact removal in EEG of normal and demented individuals using ICA–WT during working memory tasks. Sensors **17**, 1326 (2017)

133. R.P. Rao, *Brain-Computer Interfacing: An Introduction* (Cambridge University Press, 2013)

134. W. Freeman, R.Q. Quiroga, *Imaging Brain Function with EEG: Advanced Temporal and Spatial Analysis of Electroencephalographic Signals* (Springer, 2012)
135. P.A. Abhang, B.W. Gawali, S.C. Mehrotra, Technical aspects of brain rhythms and speech parameters. Introduction to EEG-and Speech-Based Emotion Recognition, 51–79 (2016)
136. L. Aftanas, S. Golocheikine, Human anterior and frontal midline theta and lower alpha reflect emotionally positive state and internalized attention: high-resolution EEG investigation of meditation. Neuroscience Letters 310, 57–60 (2001)
137. L.I. Aftanas, A.A. Varlamov, S.V. Pavlov, V.P. Makhnev, N.V. Reva, Time-dependent cortical asymmetries induced by emotional arousal: EEG analysis of event-related synchronization and desynchronization in individually defined frequency bands. Int. J. Psychophysiol. **44**, 67–82 (2002)
138. M. Mohammadi, F. Al-Azab, B. Raahemi, G. Richards, N. Jaworska, D. Smith, et al., Data mining EEG signals in depression for their diagnostic value. BMC Med. Inform. Decis. Mak. **15**, 1–14 (2015)
139. H. Cai, X. Sha, X. Han, S. Wei, B. Hu, Pervasive EEG diagnosis of depression using Deep Belief Network with three-electrodes EEG collector, in *2016 IEEE International Conference on Bioinformatics and Biomedicine (BIBM)*, (2016), pp. 1239–1246
140. B. Hosseinifard, M.H. Moradi, R. Rostami, Classifying depression patients and normal subjects using machine learning techniques and nonlinear features from EEG signal. Comput. Methods Prog. Biomed. **109**, 339–345 (2013)
141. P.F. Lee, D.P.X. Kan, P. Croarkin, C.K. Phang, D. Doruk, Neurophysiological correlates of depressive symptoms in young adults: A quantitative EEG study. J. Clin. Neurosci. **47**, 315–322 (2018)
142. M.R. Dolsen, P. Cheng, J.T. Arnedt, L. Swanson, M.D. Casement, H.S. Kim, et al., Neurophysiological correlates of suicidal ideation in major depressive disorder: Hyperarousal during sleep. J. Affect. Disord. **212**, 160–166 (2017)
143. M. Liu, L. Zhou, X. Wang, Y. Jiang, Q. Liu, Deficient manipulation of working memory in remitted depressed individuals: Behavioral and electrophysiological evidence. Clin. Neurophysiol. **128**, 1206–1213 (2017)
144. J. Shen, S. Zhao, Y. Yao, Y. Wang, L. Feng, A Novel Depression Detection Method Based on Pervasive EEG and EEG Splitting Criterion, in *2017 IEEE International Conference on Bioinformatics and Biomedicine (BIBM)*, (2017), pp. 1879–1886
145. J. Jeong, Nonlinear dynamics of EEG in Alzheimer's disease. Drug Dev. Res. **56**, 57–66 (2002)
146. D.P. Subha, P.K. Joseph, R. Acharya, C.M. Lim, EEG signal analysis: A survey. J. Med. Syst. **34**, 195–212 (2010)
147. D. Abásolo, R. Hornero, C. Gómez, M. García, M. López, Analysis of EEG background activity in Alzheimer's disease patients with Lempel–Ziv complexity and central tendency measure. Med. Eng. Phys. **28**, 315–322 (2006)
148. J. Escudero, D. Abásolo, R. Hornero, P. Espino, M. López, Analysis of electroencephalograms in Alzheimer's disease patients with multiscale entropy. Physiol. Meas. **27**, 1091–1106 (2006)
149. H. Cai, J. Han, Y. Chen, X. Sha, Z. Wang, B. Hu, et al., A pervasive approach to EEG-based depression detection. Complexity **2018**, 1–13 (2018)
150. P. Grassberger, I. Procaccia, Measuring the strangeness of strange attractors. Physica D: Nonlinear Phenomena **9**, 189–208 (1983)
151. J. Wolf, B. Swift, H.L. Swinney, J.A. Vastano, Determining Lyapunov exponents from a time series. Physica D: Nonlinear Phenomena **16**, 285–317 (1985)
152. R. Ferenets, T. Lipping, A. Anier, V. Jantti, S. Melto, S. Hovilehto, "comparison of entropy and complexity measures for the assessment of depth of sedation," biomedical engineering. IEEE Transactions on **53**, 1067–1077 (2006)
153. X.-S. Zhang, R.J. Roy, E.W. Jensen, EEG complexity as a measure of depth of anesthesia for patients. IEEE Trans. Biomed. Eng. **48**, 1424–1433 (2001)

154. M. Bachmann, L. Päeske, K. Kalev, K. Aarma, A. Lehtmets, P. Ööpik, et al., Methods for classifying depression in single channel EEG using linear and nonlinear signal analysis. Comput. Methods Prog. Biomed. **155**, 11–17 (2018)

155. K. Kalev, M. Bachmann, L. Orgo, J. Lass, H. Hinrikus, Lempel-Ziv and multiscale Lempel-Ziv complexity in depression, in *2015 37th Annual International Conference of the IEEE Engineering in Medicine and Biology Society (EMBC)*, (2015), pp. 4158–4161

156. C.-K. Peng, S.V. Buldyrev, S. Havlin, M. Simons, H.E. Stanley, A.L. Goldberger, Mosaic organization of DNA nucleotides. Phys. Rev. E **49**, 1685–1689 (1994)

157. T. Higuchi, Approach to an irregular time series on the basis of the fractal theory. Physica D: Nonlinear Phenomena **31**, 277–283 (1988)

158. P. Zhao, P. Van Eetvelt, C. Goh, N. Hudson, S. Wimalaratna, and E. Ifeachor, "EEG markers of Alzheimer's disease using Tsallis entropy," in Communicated at the 3rd International Conference on Computational Intelligence in Medicine and Healthcare. pp. 25–27 (CIMED, 2007)

159. Z. Peng, P. Van-Eetvelt, C. Goh, N. Hudson, S. Wimalaratna, E. Ifeachor, "Characterization of EEGs in Alzheimer's Disease using Information Theoretic Methods," in Engineering in Medicine and Biology Society, 2007. EMBS 2007. 29th Annual International Conference of the IEEE. pp. 5127–5131 (2007)

160. P. Zhao, E. Ifeachor, "EEG assessment of Alzheimers diseases using universal compression algorithm," in proceedings of the 3rd international conference on computational intelligence in medicine and healthcare (CIMED2007). Plymouth, UK, July **25** (2007)

161. G. Henderson, E. Ifeachor, N. Hudson, C. Goh, N. Outram, S. Wimalaratna, et al., "development and assessment of methods for detecting dementia using the human electroencephalogram," biomedical engineering. IEEE Transactions on **53**, 1557–1568 (2006)

162. M. Costa, A.L. Goldberger, C.-K. Peng, Multiscale entropy analysis of complex physiologic time series. Phys. Rev. Lett. **89**, 068102 (2002)

163. M. Costa, A.L. Goldberger, C.-K. Peng, Multiscale entropy analysis of biological signals. Phys. Rev. E **71**, 021906 (2005)

164. S. Wold, K. Esbensen, P. Geladi, Principal component analysis. Chemom. Intell. Lab. Syst. **2**, 37–52 (1987)

165. A. Subasi, M. Ismail Gursoy, EEG signal classification using PCA, ICA, LDA and support vector machines. Expert Syst. Appl. **37**, 8659–8666 (2010)

166. M. KavitaMahajan, M.S.M. Rajput, A Comparative study of ANN and SVM for EEG Classification. International Journal of Engineering **1** (2012)

167. F. Vialatte, A. Cichocki, G. Dreyfus, T. Musha, T. M. Rutkowski, R. Gervais, "Blind source separation and sparse bump modelling of time frequency representation of eeg signals: New tools for early detection of alzheimer's disease," in Machine Learning for Signal Processing, 2005 IEEE Workshop on. pp. 27–32 (2005)

168. H. Cai, Y. Chen, J. Han, X. Zhang, B. Hu, Study on feature selection methods for depression detection using three-electrode EEG data. Interdisciplinary Sciences: Computational Life Sciences **10**, 558–565 (2018)

169. R.A. Movahed, G.P. Jahromi, S. Shahyad, G.H. Meftahi, A major depressive disorder classification framework based on EEG signals using statistical, spectral, wavelet, functional connectivity, and nonlinear analysis. J. Neurosci. Methods **358**, 109209 (2021)

170. Y. Li, B. Hu, X. Zheng, X. Li, EEG-based mild depressive detection using differential evolution. IEEE Access **7**, 7814–7822 (2018)

171. M. Sharma, P. Achuth, D. Deb, S.D. Puthankattil, U.R. Acharya, An automated diagnosis of depression using three-channel bandwidth-duration localized wavelet filter bank with EEG signals. Cogn. Syst. Res. **52**, 508–520 (2018)

172. C. Kaur, A. Bisht, P. Singh, G. Joshi, EEG signal denoising using hybrid approach of Variational mode decomposition and wavelets for depression. Biomedical Signal Processing and Control **65**, 102337 (2021)

173. A. Khosla, P. Khandnor, T. Chand, Automated Diagnosis of Depression from EEG Signals Using Traditional and Deep Learning Approaches: A Comparative Analysis, in *Biocybernetics and Biomedical Engineering*, vol. 42, (2021), pp. 108–142
174. X. Ding, X. Yue, R. Zheng, C. Bi, D. Li, G. Yao, Classifying major depression patients and healthy controls using EEG, eye tracking and galvanic skin response data. J. Affect. Disord. **251**, 156–161 (2019)
175. J. Zhu, Z. Wang, T. Gong, S. Zeng, X. Li, B. Hu, et al., An improved classification model for depression detection using EEG and eye tracking data. IEEE Trans. Nanobioscience **19**, 527–537 (2020)
176. S. Mahato, N. Goyal, D. Ram, S. Paul, Detection of depression and scaling of severity using six channel EEG data. J. Med. Syst. **44**, 1–12 (2020)
177. H. Akbari, M.T. Sadiq, A.U. Rehman, M. Ghazvini, R.A. Naqvi, M. Payan, et al., Depression recognition based on the reconstruction of phase space of EEG signals and geometrical features. Appl. Acoust. **179**, 108078 (2021)
178. H. Peng, C. Xia, Z. Wang, J. Zhu, X. Zhang, S. Sun, et al., Multivariate pattern analysis of EEG-based functional connectivity: A study on the identification of depression. IEEE Access **7**, 92630–92641 (2019)
179. C. Jiang, Y. Li, Y. Tang, C. Guan, Enhancing EEG-based classification of depression patients using spatial information. IEEE Trans. Neural Syst. Rehabil. Eng. **29**, 566–575 (2021)
180. H. Akbari, M.T. Sadiq, A.U. Rehman, Classification of normal and depressed EEG signals based on centered correntropy of rhythms in empirical wavelet transform domain. Health Information Science and Systems **9**, 1–15 (2021)

Chapter 4
Brain-Computer Interface (BCI) Based on the EEG Signal Decomposition Butterfly Optimization and Machine Learning

Mawadda Alghamdi, Saeed Mian Qaisar, Shahad Bawazeer, Faya Saifuddin, and Majed Saeed

Abstract The Brain-Computer Interface (BCI) is a technology that helps disabled people to operate assistive devices bypassing neuromuscular channels. This study aims to process the Electroencephalography (EEG) signals and then translate these signals into commands by analyzing and categorizing them with Machine Learning algorithms. The findings can be onward used to control an assistive device. The significance of this project lies in assisting those with severe motor impairment, paralysis, or those who lost their limbs to be independent and confident by controlling their environment and offering them alternative ways of communication. The acquired EEG signals are digitally low-pass filtered and decimated. Onward, the wavelet decomposition is used for signal analysis. The features are mined from the obtained sub-bands. The dimension of extracted feature set is reduced by using the Butterfly Optimization algorithm. The Selected feature set is then processed by the classifiers. The performance of k-Nearest Neighbor, Support Vector Machine and Artificial Neural Network is compared for the categorization of motor imagery tasks by processing the selected feature set. The suggested method secures a highest accuracy score of 83.7% for the case of k-Nearest Neighbor classifier.

M. Alghamdi · S. Mian Qaisar (✉) · S. Bawazeer · F. Saifuddin
Electrical and Computer Engineering Department, Effat University, Jeddah, Saudi Arabia
e-mail: sqaisar@effatuniversity.edu.sa

M. Saeed
Department of Urology, Sahiwal Teaching Hospital, Sahiwal, Pakistan

© The Author(s), under exclusive license to Springer Nature Switzerland AG 2023
S. Mian Qaisar et al. (eds.), *Advances in Non-Invasive Biomedical Signal Sensing and Processing with Machine Learning*, https://doi.org/10.1007/978-3-031-23239-8_4

4.1   Introduction

The World Health Organization (WHO) estimates that there are over 1 billion impaired persons, 20% of whom experience severe functional challenges on a daily basis [1]. For example, 75 million individuals use wheelchairs every day. This amounts to 1% of the global population. That is equivalent to double Canada's population [2]. Brain-Computer Interface (BCI) technology can significantly improve the lives of this sizable segment of the population.

With the use of the BCI, a person may interact with or control the outside environment without utilizing regular neuromuscular pathways. Hence, supporting people with severe motor impairment, paralysis, or those who lost their limbs by translating their brain activity and intentions into actions allowing them to assist themselves [3]. Such invention helps a big slice of society regain their social lives and become productive again rather than being a burden, thus implying the prosperity of society.

Using BCI, translating brain waves into commands to control assistive devices can be a convoluted process with many parameters to consider. For example, when the brain signals are acquired with the non-invasive method of EEG, the signals are subjected to a lot of noise because the skull and scalp act as barriers between the electrodes and the brain [4]. Therefore, the challenge is to apply appropriate filtering and conditioning to the acquired brain signals to get clear patterns that can be decoded with Artificial Intelligence (AI) algorithms. After all, an accurate start to the interface reduces intent translation errors and ensures more precise robot control at the end.

4.2   The Evolution of BCI

The history of BCI goes back to 1875 when Richard Canton discovered the presence of electrical signals in animals' brains [5]. About a hundred years ago, Canton's discovery inspired Hans Berger, a German neuroscientist, to record in 1924. It was the first ever non-invasive EEG study employing needle electrodes with a clay tip to record electrical activity in the human brain [6]. In a 17-year-old adolescent with a possible case of brain cancer, the electrodes were positioned at the trepanation site and attached to a galvanometer. In 1929, Berger demonstrated that electrical current variations could be recorded with electrodes put on the skin above the skull gap in a paper titled "Über das Elektrenkephalogramm des Menschen" [7].

Then, the University of California, Los Angeles (UCLA) started doing true BCI research in the 1970s with studies on animals to create a new, direct connection between their brains and the world [6]. The phrase "brain-computer interface" was first used in 1973 by UCLA Professor Jacques Vidal, who also outlined the objectives of the research to analyze EEG data via a brain-computer interface. He published a paper titled: "Toward Direct Brain-Computer Communications", and in

1976 UCLA's BCI laboratory demonstrated that a single visual trial elicited potential such that they might be utilized for cursor control in a two-dimensional labyrinth [8].

In 1988, P300 spellers were first introduced by Farwell and Donchin in a paper named "Talking off the top of your head: toward a mental prosthesis utilizing event-related brain potentials" [9]. Based on the detection of a positive deflection in potential 300 msec following a stimulus, the device was named "P300" [9, 10]. The objective of a P300 speller was to display letters selected mentally by the patient. The first trials were when the patient was required to choose a character from a 6×6 or 5×5 matrix in which the rows and columns start flashing for a certain period. This made the brain generate a unique potential value for each letter, hence, detecting the required character [10].

Ten years later, in 1998, researcher Philip Kennedy implanted the first BCI into a human [11]. That person was a locked-in amyotrophic lateral sclerosis (ALS) patient. Despite their being no effort at "typewriter" control, she was able to make binary choice decisions until her death 76 days after implantation [12]. After that, he implanted his second locked-in patient's main cortical region near the hand, where he learnt to control the mouse cursor's 2D location while using a virtual keyboard. He had to visualize particular hand gestures in order to choose the desired letters and activate the imagery cortex. Despite the fact that the patient could only type three letters per minute, this method represented a tremendous advancement in the area of brain mapping [13].

A significant step in the development of BCI systems was made when Matthew Nagle became the first person to have the commercial BCI CyberKinetics BrainGate implanted in him in 2004 [14]. In the same year, a study from the Wadsworth Center of the New York State Department of Health showed how a BCI might be used to operate a computer. Patients participated in the study by donning a cap with electrodes to record EEG signals from the motor cortex, a region of the brain responsible for controlling movement [15].

As a neuroprosthetic technology that aids in hearing restoration, cochlear implants have been put in over 220,000 patients globally by 2010 [16]. A paraplegic 58-year-old lady and a 66-year-old man were implanted with electrodes in their brains in 2012, according to Leigh Hochberg, a neurologist at Massachusetts General Hospital, to operate a robotic arm. They could grasp small objects, reach them, and even use a straw to sip coffee from a bottle. He predicted that someday, BCI technology would allow paralyzed persons to carry out routine tasks [17].

Additionally, in 2016, scientists at the University of California, Berkeley developed "neural dust," the tiniest and most effective wireless implant in the world. In their idea, a cue-based system transformed visual representations of motor activities into instructions for operating an orthosis for the hand or a virtual keyboard [18].

In 2019, University of California, San Francisco (UCSF) researchers presented a BCI that synthesizes speech of patients with speech problems brought on by nervous system illnesses using deep learning techniques. It was the first research to decode brain activity in order to generate whole phrases at a rate similar to normal speech [19].

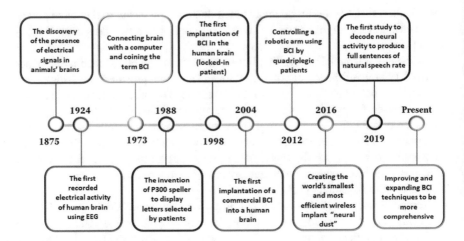

Fig. 4.1 The evolution of BCI systems

Nowadays, researchers are improving and expanding BCI techniques to be more comprehensive. To illustrate the universal applicability of such an innovation, researchers from the University of Washington in the United States investigated extending the design of the p300 speller with English to two additional languages, Spanish and Greek. Such investigations enable extending BCI system accessibility to further individuals, especially in underdeveloped nations [20].

Figure 4.1 below illustrates the evolution of BCI systems over time starting from the discovery of the presence of electrical signals in animals' brains in 1875 until the present.

4.3 Studies on the BCI

In this review, we primarily focus on previous methods that have been done in the field of BCI over the past years. Researchers and pioneers in the world of BCI can benefit from this review in a way that can extend their vision of how BCI should be developed in the future. By highlighting some of the experiments that have been done in the past in the field of BCI, we expect the reader to experience a glimpse of how the pioneers in the world of BCI were thinking, hence, be able to follow a similar approach that contributes in the advancement of BCI systems.

Controlling machines with brains and vice versa is a problem that scientists have been looking at for quite a while. Delgado [21], in his book "Physical Control of the Mind: Toward a psychocivilized society" had the vision to build a psycho-civilized society by controlling the citizens' brains to diminish their aggressive and violent behavior. His vision came after he developed a device called "Stimoceiver" and inserted it into the cortex of several bulls, some were fighting bulls and others were tame bulls. He did that to study the functional differences in the brains of the two breeds so he could discover some clues about their neurological basis of aggression. After the surgical implantation of electrodes, several cerebral points were explored by radio stimulation and motor effects in the bull were evoked, such as head-turning, lifting of one leg, and circling.

In his experiment, when Delgado pushed a button, he electronically manipulated the bull's muscle reflexes and forced the bull to stop the attack (See Fig. 4.2). The same scientist later used non-invasive approaches to control monkeys and other animals' brains. However, Delgado's idea of controlling brains using computers was strongly objected to. Therefore, his funding ran out at the end of the seventies.

Kennedy [12] developed a new electrode in 1998 called the "Neurotrophic Electrode", this technology allowed a patient with locked-in amyotrophic lateral sclerosis (ALS), to restore communication by making binary choices. Using her differential eye movement to indicate yes or no, she was able to control the neural signals in an on/off fashion but with no typewriter attempts (See Fig. 4.3).

After which, he allowed another Locked-in Syndrome (LIS) patient to type words on a 2D virtual keyboard only using his mind [13]. That patient was implanted in the hand area of his primary motor cortex and learned to control the mouse cursor's position by imagining his hand movements. It was possible to capture many signals of various intensities, and each wave shape's spikes were then turned into a pulse train. To simulate a mouse click, the brain signals were transformed into transistor-transistor logic (TTL) pulses with three major pulse outputs. The X and Y voltage input determine the cursor's location on the screen. The cursor is moved by two pulse trains, one in the X direction and the other in the Y direction. The speed at which the firing rate increases impacts how quickly the pointer goes across the screen. The "enter" or "select" command, which is short for "mouse click," is activated by the third pulse (See Fig. 4.4).

Kennedy later went a bit extreme by planting the device in his head for two years recording his brain activity during speech. Nowadays, he is trying to decode the recorded data to build the "silent speech" technology that aims to restore speech for those who have LIS, that is, paralyzed and mute by allowing a computer to speak for them when they speak inside their head [22].

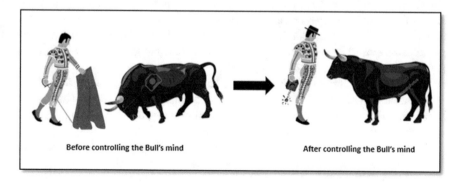

Before controlling the Bull's mind   After controlling the Bull's mind

Fig. 4.2 Delgado's experiment of controlling a bull's mind to stop its violence

Fig. 4.3 Recording brain
activity and analyzing the
brain wave in an ON/OFF
fashion

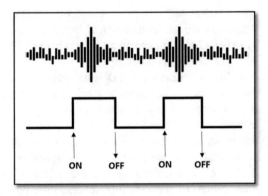

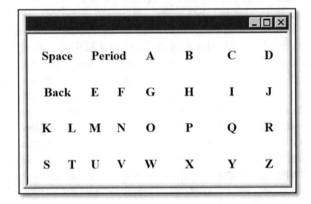

Fig. 4.4 A virtual 2D keyboard where the cursor is moved across the X and Y dimensions

Goebel [23] in his study "exploring the Mind" experimented with Functional
Magnetic Resonance Imaging (fMRI) to record signals, where two participants
played a Ping-Pong game together in real-time using their minds only. In his experiment, BCI converted fMRI signals into racket position on the y axis, the higher the
signal level, the higher the racket position. The first participant imagined dancing
alone or with an increasing number of partners. And the second imagined driving a
racing car with a varying number of other contestants. Goebel explained that the
participants moved rackets on the screen to hit the ball and gain points with "brainpower" instead of a joystick (See Fig. 4.5).

Nicolelis [24] in his study "A Brain-to-Brain Interface for Real-Time Sharing of
Sensorimotor Information" used invasive brain implants in mice to study their
behavior. His team sat up two champers 7000 miles away, the first (Encoder Setup)
in Brazil and the second (Decoder Setup) in the USA.

Each of the champers contained a mouse with a BCI implant that is connected to
the internet, two levers, two LED lights (one over each lever), and a window where
the mouse could receive a sip of water as a reward. Both mice were trained to push
the lever when seeing the LED light flashing up, then go to the window where they

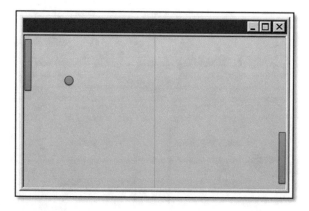

Fig. 4.5 Playing Ping-Pong using "brainpower" by recording (fMRI) signals for two participants

received their reward. The first mouse was the encoder; when he noticed the light, he moved the lever underneath it to obtain his reward. By comparing the encoder's brain signal pattern to a template trial, the decoder was able to capture and transmit the encoder's cerebral activity at the same time (previously built with the firing rate average of a trial sample). The Zscore for the neural ensemble was determined by comparing the number of spikes in each trial to the template trial. The Zscore was then transformed into an ICMS pattern using a sigmoid function that was centered on the mean of the template trial. As a result, the microstimulation patterns changed in real-time, trial by trial, in accordance with the quantity of spikes recorded from the encoder's brain signal.

On the other side, the other mouse or the decoder had the two lights flashing up, so naturally, he did not know which lever to push. Nevertheless, once microstimulation was delivered to the cortex of the decoder mouse, he knew which lever to push to get the reward (See Fig. 4.6). This brain-to-brain communication experiment proved that transferring thoughts was possible with an accuracy of 69%.

In 2013, besides thoughts, Nicolelis proved that transferring sensory inputs was also possible. He experimented with two mice; the first mouse sensed a narrow width aperture with his whiskers. The sensory input of that mouse was sent to the other mouse with a wide aperture but behaved according to the first mouse's sensory input (See Fig. 4.7).

Rezeika et al. [10] in their review "Brain-Computer Interface Spellers" explained that the first P300 speller consisted of a 6x6 matrix of flashing symbols displayed on a monitor, the participant was then asked to select which character he wished to display by only focusing on the desired one and counting how many times it flashes up. This technique depended on the detected positive potential difference that the brain created when stimulated by the flashes, which occurred 300 msec after the stimulus. After processing the EEG signal, the P300 signal was correlated to the order in which the rows and columns flashed. After analyzing these data, we were able to determine the exact row and column which produced the P300 signal, the intersection of which was the selected letter (See Fig. 4.8).

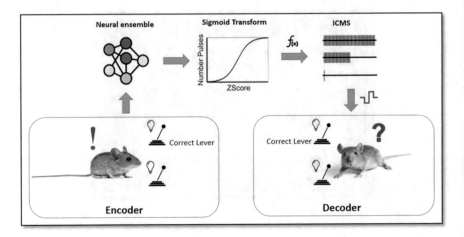

Fig. 4.6 Transferring cortical motor signals through Encoder/Decoder mice experiment with lever and LED lights

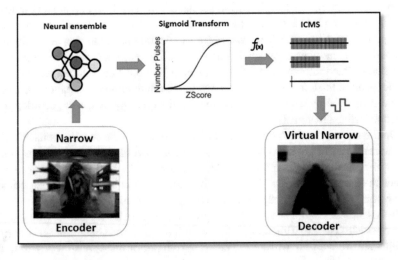

Fig. 4.7 Transferring cortical tactile information through Encoder/Decoder mice experiment with aperture and whiskers

P300 spellers are way more developed nowadays, they predict and display suggested words for the user to select which makes the system way faster and more efficient. More languages are also added to the device so more nations can benefit from such inventions, especially developing countries.

In this section, we shed light on some of the most recent problems and limitations of EEG-based BCI systems. In addition, in each of the papers and letters discussed, we focus on the opportunities and developments these researchers provide

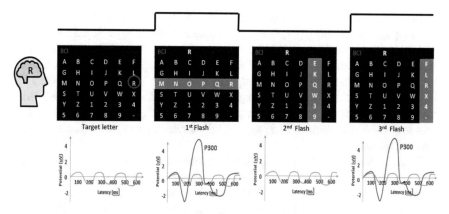

Fig. 4.8 The P300 speller's 6x6 matrix where the patient can select a letter by focusing on it and counting how many times it flashes up

in this field as well as their contribution to the overall future enhancement of BCI systems.

The issue that EEG signals have a limited spatial resolution, with electrodes collecting overlapping signals, is covered in Mishuhina and Jiang's article "Feature Weighting and Regulariza-tion of Common Spatial Patterns in EEG-Based Motor Imagery BCI" [25]. Spatial filtering is frequently used in motor imagery brain-computer interfaces (BCI) to extract discriminative characteristics and reduce over-fitting. However, only a small number of common spatial patterns (CSP) are chosen as features, and the others are disregarded. This applies that discriminating information is lost, hence, BCI performance is restricted. In their paper, they propose a method that includes all CSP features avoiding information loss and enhancing BCI performance. This method is named Feature Weighting and Regularization (FWR) and proves its effectiveness in increasing the classification accuracy compared to other conventional feature selection approaches. Finally, they propose that FWR must be applied in all CSP-based approaches in MI-BCI in the future instead of the conventional FS methods.

Song et al. raise the issue that supervised deep learning methods frequently demand a large-scale annotated dataset, which is very hard to gather in EEG-based applications [26]. They concentrate on how deep learning techniques are essential for EEG analysis to work as expected. Deep learning can enhance EEG categorization, but its potential is constrained by the amount of difficult-to-obtain data required for good classification. They suggest an unique deep learning approach based on the Multi-Task Learning framework (DMTL-BCI) to assist in EEG-based classification tasks in order to resolve this problem. They test their model using the competition IV dataset 2a, which shows that it is beneficial in improving the performance of classification for EEG-based BCI systems with sparse EEG data. It also outperforms the most recent technique by 3%. To enhance the efficacy of EEG-based categorization in the future, they suggest combining semi-supervised learning and making full use of unlabeled data.

Belo et alEEG-based. 's Auditory Attention Detection (ADD) method is the main topic of their study [27]. They talk about how hearing-impaired people who have cochlear implants have poor auditory reception in loud settings because of the limited spectral resolution of these devices. Their findings show that cortical tracking of the envelope of the attended speech is improved as compared to the unattended speech in a multi-speech setting. This opens up the prospect of future hearing aids using both conventional technology and AAD. Finally, they discuss its possible uses in non-clinical passive BCI, such as interactive musical performances or educational settings.

It has always been challenging for BCI systems to deal with data-related issues such as insufficient data and data corruption. However, Fahimi et al. [28] highlight a potential solution utilizing artificial data generation. They discuss the generative adversarial networks (GANs) method among other generative techniques as it proved its effectiveness in image processing over time. In this work, the authors look at how well convolutional GANs do in simulating the temporal, spectral, and spatial properties of genuine EEG. For instance, it aids with data augmentation and the restoration of damaged data. Hence, their approach of artificial data generation helps in the analysis process by eliminating any real EEG data issues. It also opens the door for researchers to investigate more about the future possibilities of such discoveries in the BCI world.

Finally, Abiri et al. [29] in their review of EEG-based BCI paradigms address the issues of reliability of BCI paradigms and platforms. For instance, the signal-to-noise ratio of the data derived from EEG signals is insufficient to control a sophisticated neural system. The time needed to teach the patient to understand the system and how results are severely impacted when the patient is fatigued is another challenge. The study concludes that selecting the most trustworthy, accurate, and practical paradigm is crucial when using a neuro gadget or carrying out a particular neuro-rehabilitation program. They assess the benefits and drawbacks of several EEG-based BCI paradigms for this aim. They contend that because EEG approaches aid in comprehending how the brain behaves and dynamics in many contexts, they have the potential to be marketed for the general population. They also advocate using BCI as neurofeedback to help people better themselves by adjusting brainwaves to improve different elements of cognitive control.

4.4 Methodology

The block diagram below, Fig. 4.9, illustrates the proposed BCI system's architecture in a sequence of following described steps:

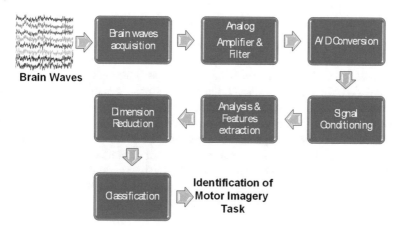

Fig. 4.9 The block diagram of proposed method

4.4.1 Brain Waves Acquisition

The study begins by acquiring the participant's brain waves using a multi channel EEG neuroheadset. The neuroheadset comprises of several electrodes placed symmetrically on selected positions on the cerebral cortex to collect brain waves. These electrodes sense the brain's electrical waves and convert them into analog electrical signals that are wirelessly paired with a computer for further processing. In this study, the participants are asked to imagine moving their right hand and left foot without actually moving them, hence, the data is collected from the imagery cortex.

In this investigation, the BCI competition dataset IVa [30] is utilized. The acquisition of this dataset was made possible by the five healthy volunteers. Each participant under consideration completed 140 trials in each category. There were a total of 280 trials per individual as a result of the two kinds of assignments being assessed. Each trial takes place for 3.5 seconds. The data consists of various-sized training and testing sets for each category.

4.4.2 Analog Amplifier and Filter

The acquired EEG signal, generated by electrodes, are of considerably tiny amplitude and noisy. It is because the scalp and skull act as a barriers between the brain and the electrodes. Moreover, the power line interference and artifacts do impact the content of electrodes generated EEG signals. Therefore, after transduction the brain waves are immediately amplified. It enhances their robustness against noise and improves the signal to noise ratio (SNR). Afterward, the amplified signals are band-pass filtered, to avoid noise and aliasing after analog to digital conversion. In this study, the EEG signals are band limited between [0.15, 200]Hz.

4.4.3 Analog to Digital (A/D) Conversion

After that, the filtered and amplified analog signal is converted to digital to ease the analysis and calculations. To do so, the signal goes through an analog to digital converter (ADC). Within the ADC, the analog signal is sampled, quantized, and encoded to get a digital signal instead of the analog one. Sampling takes certain values of the signal separated by certain time intervals, hence, making the signal discrete in time. After that, quantization gives values of certain levels for each sample by rounding off their values, making the signal discrete in amplitude [31, 32]. Finally, the encoding process maps the quantized values to digital values with length in bits. The result is converting the analog continuous signal into a digital discrete one. In this study the analog filtered signals are sampled at a conversion rate of 1 kHz.

4.4.4 Signal Conditioning

Thence after, the signal is conditioned first by using a discrete-time Finite Impulse Response (FIR) filter, where each value of the output sequence is a weighted sum of the most recent input values. In this study, a low-pass FIR filter, with a cut-off frequency of 50 Hz, is applied on the digitized version of signal. Then the digitally filtered signal is decimated to obtain an effective sampling rate of 100 Hz [33, 34]. Then, to take specific intervals of our signal, windowing using a window function is applied where all the values outside the boundaries selected by us are set to zero. Windowing the signal helps in focusing on the important parts of it, neglecting any unnecessary information.

4.4.5 Features Extraction

Analysis for the windowed signal starts by decomposing the conditioned and windowed signal into four sets or levels (sub-bands) using the Discrete Wavelet Transform (DWT). This transform function down-samples the original signal into several cascaded sets using high- and low-pass filters. It is represented as a dual-tree and named "filter bank". Each set or level in the filter bank is a time series of approximation coefficients describing the time evolution of the signal in the corresponding frequency band. To analyze and decompose our digital signal into sub-bands, we used the DWT. In this study, this transform function down-samples the original signal into several cascaded sets using high- and low-pass filters with a subsampling factor of two. A time series of approximation coefficients that describe the temporal development of the signal in the relevant frequency range makes up each set or level in the filter bank. The signal is first split into low and high frequencies after passing through two filters: a high-pass filter, *h[n]*, and a low-pass filter, *g[n]*. The first high-pass filter produces the first level's coefficients, and the remaining half of the original signal which passes through the low pass filter goes through another similar decomposition to be halved again producing the second level's coefficients. This process repeats four times producing four sub-bands and four levels of approximation coefficients. In this instance, a denoised segment is run through a wavelet decomposition based on the Daubechies technique that uses half-band high-pass and low-pass filters. This makes it possible to calculate the detail, d_m^i, and approximation, a_m^i, coefficients at each level of decomposition (a mi and d mi, respectively).

Following that, each sub-band of the analyzed signal is extracted for features. The feature extraction process reduces the amount of redundant data from a dataset. By implementing several mathematical notations such as the standard deviation, minimum absolute value, maximum absolute value, mean of absolute value, energy, skewness, entropy, and kurtosis. Also, Zero Crossing (ZC), the Root Mean Square (RMS) value of the Instantaneous Amplitude (IA), and Absolute Peak-to-Peak Difference (APPD).

4.4.6 Dimension Reduction

To reduce the number of attributes while keeping as much of the variation in the original dataset a dimension reduction is applied. In our study, the Butterfly Optimization Algorithm (BOA) is used [33]. It is a Swarm-Intelligence based (SI-based) approach of optimization. SI-based algorithms are a subset of bio-inspired, and the latter is a subset of nature-inspired algorithms. The process can be presented as: *SI-based ⊂ bio-inspired ⊂ nature-inspired*.

The food-finding and mating strategies of butterflies serve as the basis for this optimization technique. The five senses that butterflies often employ are smell, sight, taste, touch, and hearing. The butterfly uses each of these senses to perform various functions. For instance, the butterfly uses her sense of smell to obtain nourishment (flower nectar), lay her eggs, and flee from predators. According to scientific research, butterflies have a highly developed ability to identify the source of scent and gauge its potency.

Therefore, in this algorithm, butterflies act as search agents that produce scents of varying strengths and travel arbitrarily from one place to another if they detect no scent, while moving in the direction of the butterfly with the strongest scent otherwise. The initiation phase, the iteration phase, and the final phase are the three phases of this approach. It also depends on the three crucial factors power exponent, stimulus intensity, and sensory modality (a). The BOA is depicted in the flowchart in (Fig. 4.10) below.

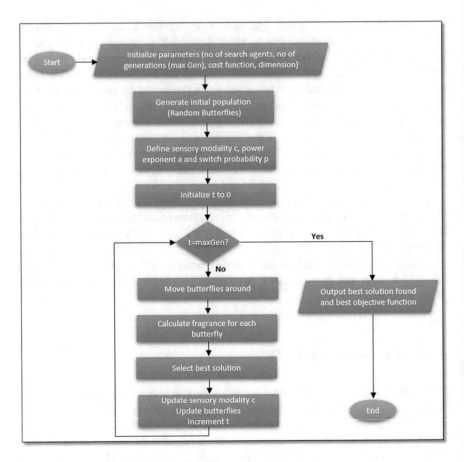

Fig. 4.10 The block diagram of proposed method

4.4.7 Classification

After features extraction and dimension reduction, the data is represented in the form of reduced matrix. The data for the BOA is an 840x33 matrix. Using the MATLAB R2021a classification learner application, several classification (categorization) algorithms based on ML are used to create a model that predicts the value of a target variable. For example, we use the Support Vector Machine classifier (SVM), the k-Nearest Neighbors (k-NN) classifier and the Artificial Neural Network (ANN) classifier to create a model that predicts the value of a target variable. Following is a description of each classifier with some mathematical Equations according to [35].

4.4.7.1   Support Vector Machine Classifier (SVM)

Using the SVM classifier, which is one of the most popular supervised machine learning algorithms for classification can classify not only linear models but also non-linear using the Kernel trick. SVM counts on creating margins to separate the available classes. These margins of separation are gaps that lie between the different categories and they contain the classification threshold. When misclassification is allowed to increase the classification accuracy, the distance between the observations where the threshold is in the middle is called a soft margin. For instance, the support vector classifier is a single point on a one-dimensional number line when the data is one-dimensional.

The support vector classifier looks like a line when the data is two-dimensional and linearly separable. In this instance, the soft margin is calculated using the support vectors (observations on the edge and inside the soft margin), and any new data is classified by determining where it falls on the line. Additionally, the support vector classifier produces a plane rather than a line when the data are three-dimensional (See Fig. 4.11). And we classify new observations by determining which side of the plane they are on. For example, the classification will be under or above the plane, and the new observation will be classified either under or above the plane accordingly.

Therefore, we know that the support vector classifier is a single point (zero-dimensional hyperplane) on a one-dimensional number line for one-dimensional data, and that it is a one-dimensional hyperplane for two-dimensional data (line). Additionally, the support vector classifier is a two-dimensional hyperplane when the data is three-dimensional (plane). Since the support vector classifier has less dimensions than the dimensions of the data, it is a hyperplane. As a result, the support vector classifier is a hyperplane of certain dimensions that are smaller than the dimension of the data when the data is four dimensions or more. In Eq. (4.1), the method of separating the hyperplane is mathematically stated.

$$h(x) = sign\left(\omega.x^T + b\right) \qquad (4.1)$$

Fig. 4.11 Two-dimensional SVM linear classification represented by a line margin separator

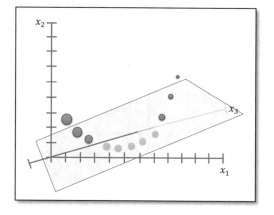

Where x is a sample vector $x = [x_1, x_2 ... x_p]$ with p attributes, $\omega = [\omega_1, \omega_2 ... \omega_p]$ is the weights vector, and b is a scalar bias.

4.4.7.2 k-Nearest Neighbors (k-NN)

The k-NN is another classifier; it is regarded as one of the simplest classifiers. It presumes that there are comparable objects close by.

The k-NN classifier finds the distances between a query and each example in the data, chooses the k instances (or as many as are given) that are closest to the query, and then votes for the label that is most frequently assigned. For example, if $K = 1$, then we will use only the nearest neighbor to define the category that which the sample belongs. In (Fig. 4.12), if $k = 1$, then the unknown dot belongs to the nearest dot, which is blue. Hence, the unknown dot is classified as blue. However, if $k = 15$, then we will take the 15 nearest neighbors and vote. In our example, if $k = 15$, then we have one green, three yellows, and 11 blues. Accordingly, the highest votes go to the blue category and the unknown dot is classified as blue.

Let v_j stand for a sample and $<v_j, l_j>$ stand for a tuple consisting of a training sample and its label, $l_j \epsilon [1, C]$ where C is a set of classes. Equation (4.2) illustrates the mathematical procedure for determining the closest neighbor j given a test sample z.

$$argmin\, dist\left(d_j, t\right) \forall j = 1 ... N \tag{4.2}$$

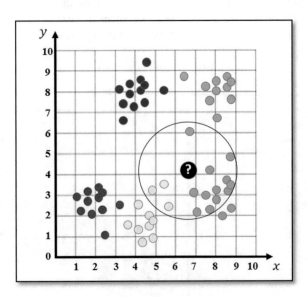

Fig. 4.12 Classifying an unknown sample using the k-NN classifier with k = 15

4.4.7.3 Artificial Neural Network (ANN)

A computational approach for machine learning that uses linked, hierarchical functions is the ANN classifier. ANNs function like a human brain; they rely on the input and then do some complex processing to finally present an output. ANNs consist of nodes and a spider web to connect these nodes. Nodes create layers, the main three layers that form any ANN are the input layer, the output layer, and the hidden layers (all layers lying between the input and output layers) (See Fig. 4.13). Within the hidden layers, activation functions like the Sigmoind, Softplus, or ReLU are used. These activation functions or responsible for constructing a squiggle that can fit the complex existing data and give an indication about the classification of the new samples.

4.4.8 Evaluation Measures

After For the following calculations, the following values from each classifier's confusion matrix are considered (True Positives (TP), False Positives (FP), False Negatives (FN), and True Negatives (TN)).

4.4.8.1 Accuracy

The accuracy value represents the data that has been correctly classified. The mathematical formula to calculate the accuracy is shown in Eq. (4.3). Accuracy has a maximum value of one, the higher the value of accuracy and closer to one, the better the performance of the classifier.

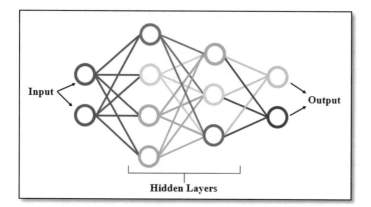

Fig. 4.13 Artificial Neural Network (ANN) classifier layout

$$Accuracy = \frac{TP + TN}{TP + TN + FP + FN} \tag{4.3}$$

4.4.8.2 Precision

To avoid any lack of precision or bias in estimating the classification performance due to the limited dataset, cross-validation with 10 folds is used in this study. Training and testing are applied for all classifiers in each fold for the three datasets. Precision is calculated as seen in Eq. (4.4).

$$Precision = \frac{TP}{TP + FP} \tag{4.4}$$

4.4.8.3 Recall

In a classification issue with two classes, recall (also known as sensitivity) is determined as the ratio of true positives to both true positives and false negatives (See Eq. (4.5)).

$$Recall = \frac{TP}{TP + FN} \tag{4.5}$$

4.4.8.4 Specificity

Specificity (also known as true negative) represents the accuracy of a test that reports the presence or absence of a condition. The total number of true negatives divided by the sum of true negatives and false positives is used to compute it (See Eq. 4.6).

$$Specificity = \frac{TN}{TN + FP}. \tag{4.6}$$

4.4.8.5 F-Measure

The F-measure (F1) gives a relation between the precision and recall values. It is represented mathematically in Eq. (4.7).

$$F = \frac{2 * precision * recall}{precision + recall} \tag{4.7}$$

4.4.8.6 Kappa

The agreement between two clustering findings is determined by the Kappa statistic. Due to the fact that it considers the potential of the agreement occurring by coincidence, it is often greater than accuracy. Equation (4.8) is the mathematical expression of Cohen's kappa measure.

$$kappa = 1 - \frac{1 - p_0}{1 - p_e} \tag{4.8}$$

Where p_e is the fictitious probabilistic probability of such an agreement occurring randomly and p_0 is the percentage of agreement between the anticipated and actual numbers. Eq. (4.9) is used to get the value of p_e.

$$p_e = \frac{(TP + TN)(TP + FN) + (FP)(FP + FN)}{(TP + TN + FP + FN)^2} \tag{4.9}$$

4.5 Results and Discussion

The considered classifiers are modeled, trained and tested by using the MATLAB R2021a classification learner application. The experimentation is conducted while following the cross-validation strategy.

The results obtained for the k-NN classifier are outlined in Table 4.1. It is conspicuous that all the classes showed results with a satisfactory level of the accuracy, with the score of 83.7% for both (C1) and (C2(. The precision of the classifiers also ranged between 83.1% (C1) and 84.3% (C2). The highest value of recall achieved is 84.5% for C1 while the lowest value is 82.8%. The results from specificity ranged from 82.9% (C1) to 84.5% (C2). Furthermore, the highest result achieved through

Table 4.1 Calculated values of the k-NN classifier

Classes	Accuracy	Precision	Recall	Specificity	F1	Kappa
Class-1	0.837%	0.831%	0.845%	0.829%	0.838%	0.674%
Class-2	0.837%	0.843%	0.828%	0.845%	0.836%	0.674%
Average	0.837%	0.837%	0.837%	0.837%	0.837%	0.674%

F1 is 83.8% (C1) and the lowest result is 83.6% (C2). The kappa score for both classes is 67.4%.

The average accuracy score is 83.7%. The average precision and recall scores are also 83.7% for the case of SVM classifier when it is used with the DWT based decomposition and BOA based dimension reduction. The average specificity and F1 scores are also 83.7% and the Kappa index, average for both intended classes, is 67.4%.

The results obtained for the SVM classifier are outlined in Table 4.2. It is conspicuous that all the classes showed results with a satisfactory level of the accuracy, with the score of 81.8% for both (C1) and (C2). The precision of the classifiers also ranged between 81.7% (C1) and 81.8% (C2). The highest value of recall achieved is 81.9% for (C1) while the lowest value is 81.6% for (C2). The results from specificity ranged from 81.6% (C1) to 81.9% (C2). Furthermore, the highest result achieved through F1 is 81.7% (C1) and the lowest result is 81.8% (C2). The kappa score for both classes is 63.6%.

The average accuracy score is 81.7%. The average precision and recall scores are also 81.8% for the case of SVM classifier when it is used with the DWT based decomposition and BOA based dimension reduction. The average specificity and F1 scores are also 81.8% and the Kappa index, average for both intended classes, is 63.6%.

The results obtained for the ANN classifier are outlined in Table 4.3. It is conspicuous that all the classes showed results with an appropriate level of the accuracy, with the score of 74.4% for both (C1) and (C2). The precision of the classifiers also ranged between 77.3% (C2) and 77.4% (C2). The highest value of recall achieved is 77.4% for (C1) while the lowest value is 77.3% for (C2). The results from specificity ranged from 77.3% (C1) to 77.4% (C2). Furthermore, the highest result achieved through F1 is 77.4% (C1) and the lowest result is 77.3% (C2). The kappa score for both classes is 54.8%.

The average accuracy score is 77.4%. The average precision and recall scores are also 77.4% for the case of SVM classifier when it is used with the DWT based decomposition and BOA based dimension reduction. The average specificity and F1 scores are also 77.4% and the Kappa index, average for both intended classes, is 54.8%.

While comparing performance of the SVM, k-NN and ANN classifiers for processing the extracted feature set, by using the suggested combination of the preprocessing, DWT and BOA, it is clear that the k-NN outperforms the SVM and the ANN. The average accuracy score, obtained with the k-NN classifier is respectively 2.0% and 6.3% superior than the average accuracy scores of the SVM and ANN

Table 4.2 Calculated values of the SVM classifier

Classes	Accuracy	Precision	Recall	Specificity	F1	Kappa
Class-1	0.818%	0.8171%	0.819%	0.816%	0.818%	0.636%
Class-2	0.818%	0.818%	0.816%	0.819%	0.817%	0.636%
Average	0.817%	0.818%	0.818%	0.818%	0.818%	0.636%

Table 4.3 Calculated values of the ANN classifier

Classes	Accuracy	Precision	Recall	Specificity	F1	Kappa
Class-1	0.774%	0.774%	0.774%	0.774%	0.774%	0.548%
Class-2	0.774%	0.773%	0.773%	0.773%	0.773%	0.548%
Average	0.774%	0.774%	0.774%	0.774%	0.774%	0.548%

classifiers. It is mainly due to a superior pruning capability of the k-NN, while processing the extracted feature set of the intended dataset, as compared to the SVM and ANN classifiers.

The dataset, used in this study, is publicly available. In future, we shall collect a motor imagery dataset by using the EMOTIV EPOC 14-channel neuroheadset, the idea and processes are similar. The EEG signals will be recorded from the imagery cortex when the participants imagine moving their hand and foot. The study will be enhanced by increasing the number of participants, number of trials recorded, and perhaps focusing on other cortices such as the visual cortex along with the motor imagery. This will result in a more flexible and comprehensive technology that aids those in need to function better in their daily routines.

The addition of event-driven approach can enhance the performance of this system in terms of implementation complexity, processing activity, compression and computation cost effectiveness [36–39]. This axis could be explored in future while achieving an embedded realization of this system.

4.6 Conclusion

To sum up, the BCI allows the brain to control external devices while bypassing the neuromuscular channels. This invention is beneficial in many ways, especially for people with severe motor impairments as it enables them to assist themselves and regain their independence. In this study, the IVa data set (motor imagery, small training sets) provided by the Berlin BCI Group is used. In this data set, five healthy participants imagined moving their hands and foot, hence, the data contains two classes. The EEG signals of these participants were recorded using a non-invasive electrode cap from ECI. Thence after, the data is digitally low-pass filtered to a bandwidth of 50 Hz. The filtered signal is decimated to achieve a final sampling rate of 100 Hz. In next step the decomposition is carried out by using the discrete wavelet transform. The sub-bands are further analyzed for features mining. Afterward, the dimension of extracted feature set is diminished by using the Butterfly Optimization Algorithm. The selected feature set is onward processed by three robust machine learning algorithms for the categorization of considered motor imagery tasks. The considered machine learning algorithms are the k- Nearest Neighbor, Support Vector Machine and Artificial Neural Network. The performance of these algorithms is compared for classification of considered signals, while processing the mined feature set with the devised combination of pre-processing, discrete wavelet transform based decomposition, sub-bands features extraction and Butterfly Optimization based dimension reduction. The results have shown that the k-NN outperforms the SVM and the ANN. The highest average accuracy score of 83.7% is secured by the k-Nearest Neighbor classifier for the studied case. The average accuracy score, obtained with the k-NN classifier is respectively 2.0% and 6.3% superior than the average accuracy scores of the SVM and ANN classifiers. It is mainly due to a superior pruning capability of the k-NN, while processing the extracted feature set of the intended dataset, as compared to the SVM and ANN classifiers.

In future a new motor imagery dataset can be collected and used to study the robustness of the devised solution. The study will be enhanced by increasing the number of participants, number of trials recorded, and perhaps focusing on other cortices such as the visual cortex along with the motor imagery. This will result in a more flexible and comprehensive technology that aids those in need to function better in their daily routines. Moreover, the performance of other optimizers such as the Genetic Algorithm and Ant Colony Algorithm will be compared with the Butterfly Optimization Algorithm for the dimension reduction. Also the performance of other robust machine learning algorithms such as the Naïve Bayes, Decision Trees and Random Forest will be investigated. Additionally, investigating the feasibility of incorporating the ensemble and deep learning algorithms in the proposed solution is another prospect.

4.7 Assignments for Readers

- Describe your thoughts and key findings about the use of EEG signals in brain-computer interface.
- Mention the important processes that are involved in the pre-processing and EEG data collection stages.
- Describe how the performance of post feature extraction and classification stages is affected by the signal conditioning process.
- Identify your thoughts and key points about the EEG categorization techniques used in this chapter.
- Identify your thoughts and key points on the dimension reduction technique used in this chapter.

References

1. V. Schiariti, The human rights of children with disabilities during health emergencies: The challenge of COVID-19. Dev. Med. Child Neurol. **62**(6), 661 (2020)
2. G.L. Krahn, WHO world report on disability: A review. Disabil. Health J. **4**(3), 141–142 (2011)

3. N. Veena, N. Anitha, A review of non-invasive BCI devices. Int. J. Biomed. Eng. Technol. **34**(3), 205–233 (2020)
4. T. Choy, E. Baker, K. Stavropoulos, Systemic racism in EEG research: Considerations and potential solutions. Affect. Sci. **3**, 1–7 (2021)
5. X. Wan et al., A review on electroencephalogram based brain computer interface for elderly disabled. IEEE Access **7**, 36380–36387 (2019)
6. A. Kübler, The history of BCI: From a vision for the future to real support for personhood in people with locked-in syndrome. Neuroethics **13**(2), 163–180 (2020)
7. H. Berger, Über das elektroenkephalogramm des menschen. Arch. Für Psychiatr. Nervenkrankh. **87**(1), 527–570 (1929)
8. I. Arafat, Brain-computer interface: Past, present & future. Int. Islam. Univ. Chittagong IIUC Chittagong Bangladesh, 1–6 (2013)
9. L.A. Farwell, E. Donchin, Talking off the top of your head: Toward a mental prosthesis utilizing event-related brain potentials. Electroencephalogr. Clin. Neurophysiol. **70**(6), 510–523 (1988)
10. A. Rezeika, M. Benda, P. Stawicki, F. Gembler, A. Saboor, I. Volosyak, Brain–computer interface spellers: A review. Brain Sci. **8**(4), 57 (2018)
11. Y. Zhang, Invasive BCI and noninvasive BCI with VR/AR technology, 12153, 186–192 (2021)
12. P.R. Kennedy, R.A. Bakay, Restoration of neural output from a paralyzed patient by a direct brain connection. Neuroreport **9**(8), 1707–1711 (1998)
13. P.R. Kennedy, R.A. Bakay, M.M. Moore, K. Adams, J. Goldwaithe, Direct control of a computer from the human central nervous system. IEEE Trans. Rehabil. Eng. **8**(2), 198–202 (2000)
14. M. Korr, RI physician traces tragedy, triumphs in'Man with bionic brain'. R I Med. J. **96**(2), 47 (2013)
15. G.E. Fabiani, D.J. McFarland, J.R. Wolpaw, G. Pfurtscheller, Conversion of EEG activity into cursor movement by a brain-computer interface (BCI). IEEE Trans. Neural Syst. Rehabil. Eng. **12**(3), 331–338 (2004)
16. T. Fujikado, Brain machine-interfaces for sensory systems, in *Cognitive Neuroscience Robotics B*, (Springer, 2016), pp. 209–225
17. L.R. Hochberg et al., Reach and grasp by people with tetraplegia using a neurally controlled robotic arm. Nature **485**(7398), 372–375 (2012)
18. D. Seo et al., Wireless recording in the peripheral nervous system with ultrasonic neural dust. Neuron **91**(3), 529–539 (2016)
19. G.K. Anumanchipalli, J. Chartier, E.F. Chang, Speech synthesis from neural decoding of spoken sentences. Nature **568**(7753), 493–498 (2019)
20. P. Loizidou et al., Extending brain-computer interface access with a multilingual language model in the P300 speller. Brain Comput. Interf., 1–13 (2021)
21. J.M.R. Delgado, *Physical Control of the Mind: Toward a Psychocivilized Society*, vol 41 (World Bank Publications, 1969)
22. P. Kennedy, A. Ganesh, A. Cervantes, Slow Firing Single Units Are Essential for Optimal Decoding of Silent Speech (2022)
23. G. Zu Putlitz et al., Exploring the Mind
24. M. Pais-Vieira, M. Lebedev, C. Kunicki, J. Wang, M.A. Nicolelis, A brain-to-brain interface for real-time sharing of sensorimotor information. Sci. Rep. **3**(1), 1–10 (2013)
25. V. Mishuhina, X. Jiang, Feature weighting and regularization of common spatial patterns in EEG-based motor imagery BCI. IEEE Signal Process. Lett. **25**(6), 783–787 (2018)
26. Y. Song, D. Wang, K. Yue, N. Zheng, Z.-J. M. Shen. EEG-based motor imagery classification with deep multi-task learning, 1–8 (2019)
27. J. Belo, M. Clerc, D. Schön, "EEG-based auditory attention detection and its possible future applications for passive BCI," Brain-Comput. Interf. Non-Clin. Home Sports Art Entertain. Educ. Well- Appl. (2022)
28. F. Fahimi, Z. Zhang, W. B. Goh, K. K. Ang, C. Guan. Towards EEG generation using GANs for BCI application, 1–4 (2019)

29. R. Abiri, S. Borhani, E.W. Sellers, Y. Jiang, X. Zhao, A comprehensive review of EEG-based brain–computer interface paradigms. J. Neural Eng. **16**(1), 011001 (2019)
30. B. Blankertz et al., The BCI competition III: Validating alternative approaches to actual BCI problems. IEEE Trans. Neural Syst. Rehabil. Eng. **14**(2), 153–159 (2006)
31. S.M. Qaisar, A custom 70-channel mixed signal ASIC for the brain-PET detectors signal readout and selection. Biomed. Phys. Eng. Express **5**(4), 045018 (2019)
32. S. Mian Qaisar, Isolated speech recognition and its transformation in visual signs. J. Electr. Eng. Technol. **14**(2), 955–964 (2019)
33. S. M. Qaisar, S. I. Khan, K. Srinivasan, and M. Krichen. Arrhythmia classification using multirate processing metaheuristic optimization and variational mode decomposition. J. King Saud Univ. Comput. Inf. Sci. (2022)
34. S.M. Qaisar, A. Mihoub, M. Krichen, H. Nisar, Multirate processing with selective subbands and machine learning for efficient arrhythmia classification. Sensors **21**(4), 1511 (2021)
35. H. Fatayerji, R. Al Talib, A. Alqurashi, S. M. Qaisar. sEMG signal features extraction and machine learning based gesture recognition for prosthesis hand, 166–171 (2022)
36. S. Mian Qaisar, F. Alsharif, Signal piloted processing of the smart meter data for effective appliances recognition. J. Electr. Eng. Technol **15**(5), 2279–2285 (2020)
37. S. Mian Qaisar, Signal-piloted processing and machine learning based efficient power quality disturbances recognition. PLoS One **16**(5), e0252104 (2021)
38. S. Mian Qaisar, A proficient Li-ion battery state of charge estimation based on event-driven processing. J. Electr. Eng. Technol. **15**(4), 1871–1877 (2020)
39. S.M. Qaisar, Efficient mobile systems based on adaptive rate signal processing. Comput. Electr. Eng. **79**, 106462 (2019)

Chapter 5
Advances in the Analysis of Electrocardiogram in Context of Mass Screening: Technological Trends and Application of AI Anomaly Detection

Illya Chaikovsky and Anton Popov

Abstract Electrocardiography is still the most wide-spread method of functional diagnosis. The chapter has been targeted towards the debate on evolution and current attitude on the heart failure screening electrocardiography, reviewing the clinical practices of applying remote electrocardiogram (ECG) recording gadgets, the quantity and origin of data possible to be collected with ECG gadgets having various number of sensors using different modern methods of mathematical transformation of ECG signal, i.e. fourth generation ECG analysis. Accent has been made towards the application of the modern machine learning method – anomaly detection to heart activity analysis. Anomaly detection is one of the machine learning methods which identifies the data samples who deviate from some concept of normality. Such samples represent novelty, or outliers in the dataset, and often carry important information. As an example of application of anomaly detection in biomedical signal analysis, the problem of identifying the subtle deviations from the population norm based on the ECG is presented. The time-magnitude features derived from six leads of Signal Averaged ECG are used in the Isolation Forest anomaly (IFA) detector to quantify the distance of the single ECG from the cluster of normal controls. Input data to the IFA technique consists of diverse tree amounts as well as several pollution factors. For comparison, five different groups were examined: patients with proven coronary artery diseases, military personnel with mine-explosive injuries, COVID-19 survivors, and two subgroups involving participants of widespread-screening in one of the countryside areas in Ukraine.

I. Chaikovsky (✉)
Glushkov Institute of Cybernetics of National Academy of Science of Ukraine, Kyiv, Ukraine

A. Popov
Electronic Engineering Department, Igor Sikorsky Kyiv Polytechnic Institute, Kyiv, Ukraine

Faculty of Applied Sciences, Ukrainian Catholic University, Lviv, Ukraine

© The Author(s), under exclusive license to Springer Nature Switzerland AG 2023
S. Mian Qaisar et al. (eds.), *Advances in Non-Invasive Biomedical Signal Sensing and Processing with Machine Learning*, https://doi.org/10.1007/978-3-031-23239-8_5

5.1   Introduction

Increasingly engaging patient participation into diagnosis and treatment decision-making (patient empowerment) is one of the main trends in modern medicine [1], supported, among other things, at the level of legislative initiatives in the healthcare system. Modern information technologies are a prerequisite for the implementation of this trend. An important part of these technologies is the increasing distribution of aesthetic hand-size gadgets for electrocardiography tests, which users may apply to some extent themselves only, without their doctor's supervision. It is more correct to call these devices as combined software - hardware systems, because. How they all have the appropriate software. The progress of microelectronics and the development of the Internet, especially "cloud" services, make these devices affordable for any user and determine their annual sales of hundreds of thousands (possibly millions) of pieces, and the devices of most manufacturers are available globally, in any country, including number in Ukraine. The analysts at Global Industry Analyst Inc. report the US portable electrocardiograph market alone being around $1.1 billion. The annual growth of this market is at least 6% [2]. Thus, the individual use of portable electrocardiographic devices is becoming a significant social phenomenon. It can be said that with the help of such devices spontaneous screening of heart diseases occurs, far exceeding in scale any screening programs using classical 12-lead electrocardiography.

I must say that in addition to the obvious advantages, this trend also carries a certain danger. The possibilities of partial lead electrocardiography are, of course, significantly limited compared to classical electrocardiography, which is often not recognized by users who do not have professional medical knowledge. This certainly applies to screening opportunities for various heart conditions. It is also important to note that the value of even routine 12-lead electrocardiography in screening for heart diseases, primarily coronary artery disease, i.e. its ability to increase predictive accuracy over traditional risk factors is currently under intense debate. Special attention in this context is paid to the use of artificial intelligence (AI) for the analysis of the electrocardiogram (ECG). One of the main driving elements of AI in medical imaging is an aim for higher effectiveness of healthcare. The amount of medical data grows at a disproportionately high rate compared to the number of physicians available. Innovations in portable and wearable medical devices don't only bring a certain amount of useful data, but at the same time provide new opportunities for screening of certain diseases, as they can increase the number of monitoring timeframes. In this context it is extremely important to analyze slight ECG changes that are not obvious by applying common visual and/or automatic electrocardiogram interpretation as well as to develop metrics which are valid not only for 12-leads ECG but also for ECG with limited number of leads [3]. The electrocardiogram (ECG) has proved a valuable data source for AI studies [4]. Current chapter focuses on contemporary electrocardiography role opinions analysis in heart disease screening, to present portable electrocardiographic gadgets operation experience, to discuss data quantity and entity to be collected applying electrocardiography gadgets having varying lead numbers.

In addition, the results of our own research are presented, the approach based on AI method is proposed in order to define the subtle deviations of the ECG from the population norm to use in diagnosis and prognostic systems.

5.2 Evolution of Views on the Role of the Electrocardiogram in Assessing the Risk of Major Adverse Cardiovascular Events

There is no doubt that assessing an individual's risk for serious cardiovascular events is extremely important.

Many different models have been developed to assess the overall risk of developing coronary artery disease and other cardiovascular diseases. Probably the first of them was the Framingham risk scale, which includes 7 parameters [5]. The SCORE (Systematic Coronary Risk Evaluation) scale, developed on the basis of European Institutions studies results [6], is widely known.

Currently, these scales are a reliable tool for determining the likelihood of developing cardiovascular events in the next 5–10 years in patients with existing CVD and in individuals without clinical manifestations of cardiovascular pathology. At the same time, an individual profile of risk factors and concomitant cardiovascular conditions is measured in order to determine the need, tactics and intensity of clinical intervention.

However, despite all the obvious advantages, these scales, which are widely used and included in clinical guidelines, also have a number of limitations. A reflection of this fact is the emergence in recent years of new scales such as JBS3 risk score and MESA risk score, which include 15 and 12 parameters, respectively.

The most obvious problem is the practical implementation of certain interventions in people without clinical symptoms of cardiovascular diseases. How much cost will this entail? Is it possible to follow the recommendations even with a highly developed healthcare system?

According to S. Shalnova and O. Vikhireva [7], if we apply the SCORE scale to the adult population of Norway, the country with the highest life expectancy, it turns out that among 40-year-old Norwegians, every fifth woman and most men have a high risk of cardiovascular disease. Vascular diseases. At the age of 50, these figures increase to 39.5% and 88.7%, respectively. For age 65, 84.0% of women and 91.6% of men fall into the high-risk category. From a practical point of view, the strict implementation of the European recommendations seems to be very difficult even for such a prosperous country as Norway, especially in countries with a much less developed system of insurance medicine, such as Ukraine.

Individual risk is determined based on the results of extrapolation of cohort observations. It is clear that the probability of matches with a small set of features included in the risk scales for specific individuals may be low.

Naturally, risk scale estimation has no reason to be personalized, i.e. to add the conventional venture factors to personal physiologically crucial parameters obtained with equipped techniques.

Variety of all instrumental techniques makes electrocardiography undoubtedly outstanding. 12-lead electrocardiography has been used in epidemiological studies since the late 40s of the last century, in fact, from the very first steps in the epidemiology of non-communicable diseases. Especially for epidemiological studies, a method was created for measuring the elements of the electrocardiogram and describing its changes, called the Minnesota code, which makes the analysis of the electrocardiogram unified, and therefore suitable for analyzing a large amount of data. Subsequently, this classification system has been improved more than once, and related systems have appeared, such as Novacode, MEANS and some others. In accordance with these analysis systems, all ECG changes are classified into a certain number of diagnostic classes, each change can be recognized as small (minor) or large (major).

Since the late 1970s, articles based on large sample analyzes and long-term (usually 10 to 30 years) follow-up periods have been regularly published in the most reputable journals, demonstrating the value of both large and small ECG changes (in according to the Minnesota code or similar classifier) as separate warning items of lethal and non-lethal cardiovascular accidents [8–13]. There was no doubt that the use of electrocardiographic predictors increased the predictive accuracy of SCORE and other risk scales.

However, in 2011, a team of authors [14] published a systematic review commissioned by the US Commission on Preventive Services Tasks (USPSTF), which analyzed 62 studies, including almost 174,000 participants with a follow-up period from 3 to 56 years.

The key questions addressed by the authors of these guidelines are: Does electrocardiographic screening in asymptomatic individuals lead to a more accurate classification into groups having heightened, moderate, or neglectable coronary artery disease risks compared with traditional (Framingham) risk factors, what are the benefits of screening with compared to not doing it in terms of CHD outcome, whether doing screening is harmful.

The authors did not find convincing evidence that analysis of the 12-lead electrocardiogram improves the accuracy of classification into risk groups, nor evidence that the implementation of electrocardiographic screening positively affects the outcome of coronary heart disease or the appointment of a risk-reducing drug vascular treatment events (statins, aspirin). On the other hand, there are no studies demonstrating direct or indirect harm caused by electrocardiographic screening. There are only works containing general arguments about the undesirability of coronary angiography or other functional tests associated with visualization of the myocardium, when there are no sufficient grounds for this. This review formed the basis of the USPSTF recommendations [15]. The general conclusion of these recommendations is that annual routine electrocardiographic examination should not be performed in asymptomatic individuals who are at low risk on the basis of traditional risk scales. With regard to individuals belonging to groups of medium or high risk, the authors were unable to draw a definite conclusion about the balance of benefits and potential harm in the implementation of ECG screening. This strategy is also consistent with the findings of other recommendations and extensive studies published in recent years [16–18]. It must be said that these recommendations and studies have the highest evidentiary power according to modern systems for assessing the quality of recommendations for diagnostic tests, such as GRADE [19], because they are based on a meta-analysis of a large amount of data and rely on an assessment of how much a diagnostic test improves the outcome of a disease or predicts the onset of that disease.

It is interesting to note that the latest European Society of Cardiology guidelines in a field of cardiovascular disease prevention [20] advise treating individuals with a low risk of cardiovascular events, as defined by SCORE, but with evidence of LV hypertrophy on ECG, as individuals at medium risk. For other ECG syndromes, this recommendation is not given.

Separately, electrocardiographic screening should be considered in people of older age groups, and vice versa, in young people, in the latter case, in order to detect structural heart diseases and prevent sudden cardiac death, especially in people experiencing great physical and psychological overload, such as athletes and staff power structures. As for the elderly, the study by R. Auer et al. is very informative [21]., which was published after the publication of the mentioned USPSTF recommendations. In this work, on significant material (more than two thousand participants, follow-up period of 8 years), it was shown that in people aged 70–80 years, electrocardiographic signs, compared with traditional risk factors, significantly increase the predictive accuracy of screening, compared with screening only applying conventional venture factors. The most complete and context-relevant are the recommendations of the American Heart Association (AHA) published in 2014. The AHA supports such screening in principle but is not pushing for it to be mandatory. It is emphasized that significant resources are needed to conduct mandatory annual screening of all competing athletes, so the decision on the need for such screening is delegated to the local level. This view is broadly shared by the US National Institutes of Health and the European Society of Cardiology Sports Cardiology Working Group. At the same time, the International Olympic Committee more specifically recommends an electrocardiographic examination of all competitive athletes at least every two years.

Regarding law enforcement personnel, national programs of mandatory electrocardiographic screening are carried out mainly in military aviation, especially in relation to candidates for entry into the ranks of the air force (USA, Israel, Italy, etc.). For military personnel of other military branches, electrocardiographic screening is usually required only after 40 years. In younger military personnel, it is carried out only if there is evidence, for example, a burdened family history. In Ukraine, in accordance with the orders of the heads of law enforcement agencies, an electrocardiographic examination is a mandatory part of the annual medical examination, regardless of age.

In addition to electrocardiographic screening, carried out based on such long-established systems for analyzing 12-channel electrocardiograms as the Minnesota code and its derivatives (Novacode, MEANS), works have recently appeared that describe screening using new tools for analyzing electrocardiograms. Such efforts have, in our opinion, sufficient grounds. At one time, the ECG indicators included in the above classifiers of electrocardiographic signs were selected not because of their special clinical significance or exceptional physiological nature, but due to the existence at that time of extensive studies of clinical and electrocardiographic relationships in relation to these parameters. Therefore, nothing prevents other electrocardiographic signs from being investigated in the context of their value for electrocardiographic screening.

These works can be divided into two categories: one is represented by studies in which routine amplitude-time indicators are calculated, but their unusual combinations are used. An example of such works are, for example, studies of the Froelicher group [22]. In our opinion, the work of E. Gorodeski et al. [23] is of considerable interest, which shows the ability of a decision rule that includes 6 demographic and 14 electrocardiographic amplitude-time parameters selected from more than four hundred indicators to forecast the all-round reasons for women's mortality in post-menopausal period. It is important to note that in accordance with the Minnesota code, the electrocardiogram in 12 leads in all examined (more than 33 thousand observations) was normal. The follow-up period in this work was 8 years.

Another category includes works that use characteristics that are relatively complex compared to the usual amplitude-time indicators and parameters that require signal conversion using computer technology.

Such methods are currently known as the fourth generation of electrocardiography, where the first generation of electrocardiography used to be a quasi-manual assessment of the time-vs-amplitude ECG data including the eye-related analysis of plotted electrocardiographic curves, the second one included the automatically-processed measurement of the time-vs-amplitude ECG data and, similar to prior generation, graphs optical analysis. Third descent uses both automated measurement and electrocardiographic diagnostics which is followed by stating a syndromic electrocardiographic summary.

Having this said, it is obvious that the automated tools taken from both the second and the third ECG generations just copy and ease the functions of a person - a doctor of functional diagnostics. The crucial contribution of the fourth generation is the software-related assessment of the information given by these analysis methods going beyond the visual data analysis.

An example of such work is a multicenter study by T. Shlegel et al. [24], which demonstrated the advantages of a multi-parameter scale that, in addition to routine amplitude-time parameters, includes technologies such as high-frequency analysis of the QRS complex, analysis of T-wave morphology, and some others, in screening for coronary heart disease, hypertrophy left ventricle, left ventricular systolic dysfunction.

It must be said that studies belonging to the latter category have a rather weak evidentiary value in accordance with the already mentioned GRADE scale, since they provide only diagnostic accuracy (sensitivity, specificity) and no data on a clinically important outcome of the disease. It has been clear that a long-term follow-up stage is necessary in evaluating the outcome.

Let us separately discuss the ethnic difference in the parameters of a normal electrocardiogram. The ethnic and even more so racial difference in the quantitative indicators of the electrocardiogram of a healthy person has long attracted the attention of researchers. Knowing the exact limits of the ranges of normal values in different ethnic groups is necessary in order to decide which electrocardiogram is abnormal and to what extent. Ethnic and racial differences in several main amplitude-time parameters of the electrocardiogram, as well as criteria based on the assessment of the amplitudes of left ventricular hypertrophy, were studied in detail [25, 26]. There are papers describing the influence of racial differences on the effectiveness of electrocardiographic decision rules based on artificial intelligence [27]. However, multilateral, universal electrocardiogram analysis systems such as Minnesota coding, to the best of our knowledge, have not been investigated in terms of ethnic and racial variability. In addition, the problem of the influence of ethnic and racial differences on the prognostic value of certain electrocardiographic parameters is still waiting for its researcher.

5.3 The Systems of Electrocardiographic Leads, Electrocardiogram with Limited Number of Leads for Heart Disease Screening

This section briefly looks back to the development stages of the currently widespread accepted scheme for recording and analyzing the 12-lead ECG. It has been known that those 3 leads having a bipolar limb design have been exploited in clinically-performed electrocardiography, shaping the Einthoven triangle in the frontal plane, for several decades. These leads today are called standard. In 1942, Goldberger proposed enhanced unipolar limb leads that supplement the three standard leads from the point of view of areal heart electrical activity analysis, despite they are also located at the frontal plain and not equationally independent from the standard leads. Before that, in the 1930s, F. Wilson suggested 6 chest unipolar leads, which entered the practice with varied success by the end of the 1940s. The clinical contribution of the invention was broken down by Wilson himself in an iconic 1948 article [28]. These leads' value is proven by their unique feature to detect and differentiate the QRST complex pathological changes, as it was reported by the group of modern cardiography inventors. They often diagnose pathology when the limb leads remain unchanged or uninformative". The special significance of these leads in the diagnosis of ischemia in the anterior septal region of the left ventricle is emphasized. Thus, the Wilson-invented leads, which came into practice, we repeat, from the end of the 1940s of the last century, increased the sensitivity of the electro-cardiography method to local changes in the myocardium and, especially, in relation to changes in the anterior wall. For time being, the standard was the ECG in 3, and later in 6 leads from the limbs.

This information is provided here to re-emphasize the importance of clearly articulating the scope and limitations of portable electrocardiographs having a certain quantity of leads.

The development of miniaturized miniaturized aesthetic hand-size gadgets for electrocardiography tests, which users may apply to some extent themselves only, without their doctor's supervision is a part of a broader tendency, given the name of POST (point-of-care testing), that among the patients briefly stands for a medical test carried out directly anywhere, not attending the doctors'.

The pioneers at this home-available gadgets area were, actually, the household automatic measurers of the blood pressure, which worldwide production was started by OMRON in 1988, having had their distribution begun 20–25 years ago.

Later, in the 90's, the personal blood testers also became available, primarily glucose level detectors. Pluggable electrocardiographs with just several electrocardiographic leads represent the next POST-tools wave that has been produced since the very beginning of the twenty-first century.

The first such devices for mass use were apparently CheckMyHeart electrocardiographs (Great Britain).

There are currently dozens of different types of portable electrocardiograph devices on the market for individual use. Basically, they represent a sole-channel electrocardiographs having finger contacts. We list some of them, namely those that are most often mentioned in the relevant reviews: AfibAlert (USA), AliveCor/Kardia (USA), DiCare (China), ECG Check (USA), HeartCheck Pen (Canada), InstantCheck (Taiwan), MD100E (China), PC-80 (China). REKA E 100 (Singapore), Zenicor (Sweden), Omron Heart Scan (Japan), MDK (The Netherlands).

All listed devices have one or more international technical certificates (ISO, CE, FDA) and are registered as electrocardiographic devices. AliveCor/Kardia and ECG Check devices are structurally integrated with smartphones, other devices are specialized electrocardiographic attachments for mobile devices (smartphone, tablet, laptop) capable of registering an ECG signal and transmitting it over a distance without distortion. Most devices are available on the open market without restrictions, manufacturers of some models (REKA E 100, ECG Check) declare that they are intended primarily for distribution by prescription. In this case, their purchase (or temporary use) is usually covered by health insurance. Many devices (for example, Zenicor) have a Web service that allows you to immediately bring the registered electrocardiogram in one lead to the doctor. Without exception, all single-channel devices have extensive and categorical disclaimers (i.e. disclaimers) explaining that for any, even the most minor, symptoms of heart disease, you should immediately consult a doctor, not relying only on the results of automatic ECG analysis in one lead.

The leading area of these gadgets' clinical use is the arrhythmic phenomenon registration, as it has been stated by the producing entities, primarily atrial fibrillation. In this regard, the experience of AliveCor/Kardia is very interesting. The company was founded in 2011. A year later, the company received the first certificate from the US Food and Drug Administration. The wording of the intended use of the certified product includes recording, displaying, storing, and transmitting a single-lead electrocardiogram using an iPhone-integrated device. In 2013, AliveCor/Kardia received a second FDA certification confirming that the electrocardiogram obtained with its device is fully equivalent to a single lead electrocardiogram recorded by a standard commercial electrocardiograph. These certificates have given the right to professional cardiologists to prescribe the AliveCor/Kardia device, combined with the iPhone. patients. In 2014, the company received permission from the FDA to freely sell its devices without intermediaries to anyone. At this stage, the device was still used only for recording, visualization and wireless transmission of the electrocardiogram, without the function of its automatic analysis. However, a few months later, an FDA certificate was obtained for the algorithm for automatic diagnosis of atrial fibrillation, which was implemented in the software. From that moment on, the user of the technology began to receive immediate feedback on the presence or absence of this type of arrhythmia. Finally, the latest FDA approval the company has received is a certification for the so-called Normal Detector, an algorithm that tells the user if their electrocardiogram is normal or abnormal, not only in relation to atrial fibrillation, but in relation to rhythm regularity in general.

Thus, modern miniature electrocardiographic software and hardware systems are developing in the direction of complicating the built-in algorithms for analyzing and interpreting an electrocardiogram - from devices designed only for recording a single-channel electrocardiogram and transmitting it to a specialist, to peculiar communicators that immediately and directly provide the user with more or less significant information about the state of his heart.

The detection of previously undiagnosed arrhythmias is one of the most natural areas for widespread use of miniature electrocardiographic devices.

Among these arrhythmias, atrial fibrillation seems to take the first place, due to its prevalence, social significance, and the relative reliability of automatic algorithms for diagnosing atrial fibrillation on a single ECG lead.

The already mentioned company AliveCor/Kardia has apparently conducted the most extensive screening studies on this topic.

Also, large-scale screening was carried out using a single-channel portable cardiograph MDK. The results of these and other similar studies convincingly prove the clinical and cost-effectiveness of atrial fibrillation screening using specialized electrocardiographic attachments for mobile devices. It is important that there is no need to organize special events for such screening. Screening is carried out during a routine visit, for example, to a family doctor, or even simply at home, if each screening participant is provided with a mobile device with an electrocardiographic attachment during the study.

Other types of screening (detection of structural heart diseases or risk factors for their occurrence), carried out using electrocardiographic gadgets having a certain lead quantity, are hardly mentioned in known studies. We can only recall the already old work [29], which shows the predictive value of T-wave flattening in the first lead in relation to myocardial infarction in young and middle-aged men. However, the sample and follow-up period presented in this paper are small and have not been confirmed in later and larger studies.

For a number of years, Ukraine's NAS Glushkov Institute of Cybernetics has been developing original electrocardiographic devices. The" philosophy" of these devices software relies on subtle ECG alterations analysis, non-obvious to the classical visual and/or automatic electrocardiogram representation, that are invisible based on conventional optical and/or automated electrocardiogram reading. The proprietary metric is developed, which allows to define the "distance" from each current electrocardiogram to the gender and age benchmark. We interpret this distance as an additional risk factor for MACE as well as a qualifier for distant future events.

Hierarchical classification of miniature electrocardiographic devices has been suggested according to two criteria – the ability of ECG signal acquisition and software capabilities (Table 5.1).

Obviously, the class of any electrocardiographic device can be defined as the sum of the scores on both of the above criteria.

The role of routine 12-lead electrocardiography in classical epidemiological studies in cardiology is being intensively discussed by the scientific community. However, the increasing use of miniature electrocardiographic devices without the participation of medical personnel will remain one of the main technological trends in the coming years. An inevitable, perhaps most important, part of this trend is the screening component, ie. identification of various, including non-trivial, electrocardiographic signs that will be interpreted by users (mostly clinically healthy people) as signs of a heart disease or indicators of an increased risk of such a disease in the future. As shown above, there is indeed a need for new, individualized indicators of increased cardiovascular complaints chances, taken from physiological response

Table 5.1 Classification of miniature electrocardiographic devices

Level	
	According to the possibilities of ECG signal acquisition
1	Only the 1st standard ECG lead
2	3 standard ECG leads (consecutive)
3	3 standard leads (parallel
4	All 6 leads from the extremities
	According to the capabilities of the software
1	Only ECG visualization, measurement of some of the simplest amplitude - time parameters of ECG and parameters of heart rate variability (HRV)
2	Ability to immediately assess the functional state and its trends based on the analysis of subtle changes in the shape, magnitude and duration of waves and intervals of ECG signal
3	Ability to immediately assess the functional state based on the formation of a multilateral integrated indicator. Elements of ECG analysis of the fourth generation

Table source: Ilya Chaikovsky

analysis of a particular person, in addition to traditional risk scales. Methods for analyzing the value of periodically emerging new risk factors for cardiovascular diseases were recently summarized by M.A. Hlatky et al. [30]. As with the GRADE scale, the main criterion is the predictive value for a clinically important outcome of the disease. It is interesting that considerable attention is paid to complex indicators, consisting of several particular ones.

However, long-term follow-up studies are only the final phase of investigating the value of a new risk marker. The conclusions of such studies become available only after many years of the "life" of a new indicator. For quite a long time, it can (and, due to the technological trend described above, will) be used without strict scientific evidence of its value. Therefore, when creating such new indicators, it is necessary to strive to make them as multilateral and complex as possible. So, with regard to new electrocardiographic markers that can be obtained using portable devices for individual use, this means using the maximum possible number of electrocardiographic leads in portable devices and a prognostic conclusion based not on any particular indicator, but on a combination of several indicators.

5.4 The Generations of ECG Analysis, some Modern Approaches Based on Mathematical Transformation of ECG Signal

As it was mentioned above, we propose to divide the methods of electrocardiogram analysis into 4 generations.

Methods of the fourth generation, in turn, can be divided into 2 groups. The first group consists of approaches that are based only on improved methods of data analysis, more informative criteria and biomarkers, electrocardiogram registration is carried out in the usual way. These 2-nd group of methods includes new technical means of signal recording.

All these methods have a common pathophysiological basis: all of them are aimed at assessing the electrical homogeneity of the myocardium by various means. In this case, the greater the heterogeneity of the myocardium from an electrical point of view, in other words, the greater the dispersion of the generated transmembrane action potentials in amplitude and length, the greater the likelihood of serious cardiovascular events.

It should be noted that one of the main areas of application of fourth generation technologies is the screening of cardiac diseases.

The feasibility of electrocardiographic screening for the most common heart diseases, especially coronary heart disease, in terms of price / effect ratio is intensively discussed. Early detection of myocardial ischemia by resting electrocardiography or ambulatory electrocardiography in individuals over 40 years without symptoms of coronary heart disease, with atypical chest pain, or with stable low-grade angina reduces the risk of severe cardiovascular events. However, the cost of a mass survey is very significant [31]. Thus, to increase the effectiveness of electrocardiographic screening, it is necessary to solve two tasks: on the one hand to reduce the cost and simplify the procedure of examination and interpretation of results, on the other hand to increase the sensitivity of the test.

fourth generation electrocardiography is aimed at solving both problems.

The most famous of the methods of the first group of fourth-generation electro-cardiography technologies is the so-called "signal-averaged electrocardiogram". From the semantics point of view, a signal – averaged electrocardiogram is an elec-trocardiogram obtained by averaging several electrocardiographic complexes in order to improve signal quality. The averaging procedure is used in many modern methods of electrocardiogram analysis, but in the scientific literature, unfortunately, the narrow meaning of the term signal-averaged electrocardiogram (synonymous with high-resolution ECG) has taken root. This is usually called the analysis of late potentials, i.e. time and spectral study of low-amplitude and high-frequency signals in the final part of the QRS complex and the initial part of the ST segment. This method is widely used, there are consensus documents of various cardiological societies (such as the American College of Cardiology) [32]. The value of the analy-sis of late potentials to determine the risk of ventricular tachycardia in patients with myocardial infarction has been proven. Less strong, but still sufficient evidence suggests that this method is also useful for determining the risk of ventricular tachy-cardia in patients with non-coronary cardiomyopathy [33]. An improvement of this method is the analysis of the late potentials of P-wave, which is used to assess the risk of paroxysms of atrial fibrillation [34].

However, it can be said that recent analysis of late potentials has been replaced by newer and more modern methods of electrocardiogram analysis, which have not yet been tested as widely as late potential analysis but are even more promising in terms of their value in determining cardiovascular events.

We consider the morphology (shape) analysis of the electrocardiogram T-wave as potentially interesting and electrophysiologically reasonable. Mathematically, this method is the decomposition of the electrocardiographic signal by values at special (singular) points with the analysis of the main components [35]. In the framework of this method, the so-called coefficient of complexity of the T-wave is calculated.

This coefficient indicates the extent to which the electrocardiogram T-wave shape can be described by a simple dipole model of the electrocardiogram source and, accordingly, the contribution of more complex sources. The higher this coeffi-cient, the more heterogeneous the myocardium in electrical terms.This T-wave mor-phology consideration has proved to be a good predictor of the risk of cardiovascular events in the general population [36], among young athletes [37] and for myocardial infarction patients. Other, simpler approaches to the consideration of the electrocar-diogram T-wave shape, also exist. Thus here, it is necessary to mention the ECG analysis in the phase space. If the system is described by two variables, then the phase space has two dimensions, and each variable corresponds to one dimension. In this case, the phase space is a phase plane, i.e. a rectangular coordinate system, along the axes of which the values of the two variables are being plotted. Having said that, the technology nature states that at each point of the initial electrocardiographic response in the time domain, its first derivative is estimated by quantitative methods, and all further processing is carried out on the phase plane. This approach to ECG analysis has been used for a long time, at least since the late 70's of last century [38]. The Cybernetic Center of the National Academy of Sciences of Ukraine has been developing a different approach to ECG phase analysis for several years. This treatment involves dividing the phase trajectory into separate cardiac cycles, selecting trajectories with the same morphology, trajectories being averaged in phase space with subsequent "reference cycle" assessment on the average phase trajectory.

Thus, it is the indicators of the shape of the average phase trajectory that are evaluated, and the trajectories of ectopic cardiocomplexes are not considered, while in the other above-mentioned works on ECG phase analysis, on the contrary, they are the subject of analysis. We have proposed a number of quantitative indicators for the analysis of the shape of the average phase trajectory, the most sensitive of which was the symmetry index, i.e. the ratio of the maximum velocity at the rising segment of the T-wave to the maximum velocity at the descending segment of T-wave (at positive T) or the ratio of the maximum velocity on the descending segment of the T-wave to the maximum speed on the ascending segment of the T-wave (with negative T).

The diagnostic value of this approach to ECG analysis in many clinical situations has been demonstrated, including the analysis of only first electrocardiographic lead [39].

Also, a certain reserve of increasing diagnostic informativeness in the assessment of repolarization patterns may be linked to the evolution of mathematical description models of the ST-segment and T-wave by several approximation functions [40].

Another promising approach is the so-called high-frequency analysis of the QRS complex. It consists in calculating the signal power in the band 150–250 Hz in the middle of the QRS complex part of ECG. It has been shown that a decrease in this indicator is a reliable predictor of myocardial ischemia, both in acute coronary syndrome and in chronic asymptomatic ischemia [41].

It is reasonable to mention a simple and clear approach based on the calculation of the spatial angle between the vertices of the QRS complex and the T wave of the electrocardiogram. This parameter is essentially an improved ventricular gradient of Wilson, known since 1934. In recent years, large-scale studies have shown that this simple indicator is a strong predictor of cardiovascular events and mortality in the general population, and especially among women [42].

At the end of the last and the beginning of our century, such an electrocardiographic indicator of myocardial electrical homogeneity was widely used as the spatial variance of the QT interval, i.e. the difference between the longest and shortest QT interval in 12 leads. Recently, this indicator has been criticized, but certainly has not yet exhausted its usefulness [43].

The approach developed by L. Titomir [44], called dipole electrocardiotopography (DECARTO), is interesting and well-founded. This is a method of visual display and analysis of information obtained using 3 orthogonal leads. It is a quasi-mapping of the electrical process in the ventricles of the heart based on orthogonal ECG, based on the use of a model of ventricular depolarization wave, which is reflected by the electrical vector of the heart. The components of this vector are proportional to the corresponding signals of orthogonal leads. At each point in time, the depolarization front is projected onto a spherical quasipericardium (a sphere centered in the geometric center of the ventricles that covers the heart) in the form of a spherical segment. The main area of application of this method is acute coronary syndrome, the prognosis of short-term and long-term results of treatment of acute myocardial infarction.

Finally, a separate subgroup should include methods based not on the analysis of indirect electrocardiographic signals, but rather the variability of certain characteristics of individual cardio-complexes over a period of time. It is necessary to distinguish these methods from the analysis of heart rate variability, when analyzing not the parameters of your own cardiocycle, but only R-R intervals.

There are many methods and estimates of variability of certain elements of the cardiac signal from complex to complex. This is an analysis of the variability of the amplitude of the T-wave at the microvolt level, and some others. The most common of these is the analysis of the duration of the variability of the QT interval (QTV). This indicator is also used to assess the risk of life-threatening ventricular arrhythmias in patients diagnosed with heart diseases [45].

This review is far from being complete. There are other modern methods of electrocardiogram analysis, the authors of which insist on their high efficiency. In all this diversity, the clinician can easily "drown". Therefore, information technologies should be developed that summarize the data obtained with several modern computerized methods of electrocardiogram analysis and offer the doctor an integral coefficient that shows the probability of a heart disease or cardiovascular event. In this regard, it should be noted the results obtained by the Laboratory of Functional Diagnostics of the US National Aerospace Administration (NASA) in Houston.

In recent years, much attention of researchers is attracted by electrocardiogram analysis using artificial intelligence methods. As a matter of fact, ECG pays benefits for AI applications deep learning. The ECG is highly accessible and provides iterable unprocessed data which is available for digital storing and transferring. Another feature is totally automated ECG representation, when the accurate study applications use huge ECG data banks and sets of clinical data, cooperated with cutting-edge computer abilities, are demonstrating the usefulness of the AI-engaged ECG, the detection apparatus of ECG signs and structures unseen to the man's eye. These structures are able to spot the cardiac disease, such as left ventricular (LV) systolic dysfunction, silent atrial fibrillation (AF) and hypertrophic cardiomyopathy (HCM), but might also reflect systemic physiology, such as a person's age and sex or their serum potassium levels etc. [46] Of course, the use of AI for ECG analysis in the context of predicting various heart diseases is of particular interest. In the work [47] it is shown that the ECG-AI model based solely on information extracted from ECG independently predicts HF with accuracy comparable to existing FHS and ARIC risk calculators. There are several other high-quality works on this topic.

Also, we would especially like to emphasize the work in which it is demonstrated that the difference between individual biological age, defined by AI ECG, and chronological age is an independent predictor of all-cause and cardiovascular mortality. Discrepancies between these possibly reflect disease independent biological aging [48].

It should be noted that the further development of fourth generation electrocardiography is impossible without mathematical and computer modeling. However, models of heart electrical activity which are set with high levels of the object spatial distribution have considerable gaps with empirical models mostly used to define the links of electrophysiological phenomena in a heart at the visceral level with ECG changes. The latter primarily involves the task of understanding the ECG pathology changes mechanisms in myocardial ischemia due to the rise in its electrical inhomogeneity and gradually its unsteadiness. Given the inconsistency of a few sets of testing volumes, this context complicates the new algorithm evolution for diagnosing ischemia in its early stages, as well as methods for quantifying some manifestations of ECG disorders ofheart muscle activation and repolarization applying the only model.

The development of computer technology and information technology has given a new impetus to electrocardiography. The electrocardiographic signal, which is easily recorded and digitized, allegedly "provokes" doctors and mathematicians to cooperate under the motto of Galileo Galilei: "Measure everything that can be measured, make measurable everything that has not been measured before." The result of this collaboration is the creation of new effective methods of electrocardiographic diagnosis, which over time will find a place in every clinic and doctor's office and may replace traditional electrocardiography.

5.5 Anomaly Detection in ECG Using Machine Learning Approach

Many devices can provide ECG in clinical controlled conditions, as well as during exercise and in 24/7 regime during everyday life activities. Comparatively wide availability of the ECG recordings, both clinically and from wearable devices supports its usage as a basis of the online diagnosis tool. Performing ECG anomaly detection tries to serve as the prediction and prevention tool for dangerous health conditions associated with heart malfunctioning.

In ECG the anomalous behavior may be represented as the irregular heart rhythms or heartbeats with unusual time-magnitude parameters. Despite many deviations from the conditional normal ECG have been described in the literature, their combination, or the tiny changes at the beginning of the disease development, may not be obvious, be rare events, or be hidden. Therefore, application of rule-based anomaly detection may be less effective than use of the data-driven machine learning approach.

Anomaly detection is one of the fundamental tasks in data mining and consists of identifying the objects which considerably deviate from some concept of normality in each dataset [49]. Depending on the context, such objects can be irregular, unexpected, rare, or simply "strange". Due to the fuzzy and application-dependent definitions for "deviation" and "normality", there exist a lot of anomaly detection algorithms. The algorithms of anomaly detection may be roughly subdivided into two major classes: unsupervised and supervised, depending on the availability of the labeled data. Excellent description of the anomaly detection techniques can be found in [50].

Unsupervised methods do not use the information about the labels of the data (normal or anomalous) in the training set. This group of methods contains model-based methods (relying on the description of the data generation model) and proximity-based methods (which use the distances between data points in the feature space). In supervised anomaly detection, the prior information about the labels in the training dataset is available. In this case, many general-purpose classification methods can potentially be used. But in case of application to anomaly vs. normal object classification, this is less used than unsupervised, because the number of anomalies is usually limited, and often the anomalies are not available beforehand.

Many methods of anomaly detection have been applied to the ECG analysis, focusing on the different types of animal characteristics. In [51], the review of most widely used approaches is presented. Authors of [52] applied Support Vector Machine classifier after wavelet-based extraction of heart rate variability features to of arrhythmic beat classification. Multilinear principal component analysis is used to process ECG for extracting disease-altered patterns, followed by anomaly detection using deep support vector data description in [53]. The proposed framework achieves superior performance in detecting abnormal ECG patterns, such as atrial fibrillation, right bundle branch block, and ST-depression. Recently, deep learning networks training is getting more attention for ECG anomaly detection development. In [54] a novel hybrid architecture consisting of Long Short Term Memory cells and Multi-Layer Perceptrons. Simultaneous training pushes the overall network to learn descriptive features complementing each other for making decisions, which led to the average classification accuracy of 97% across several records in the ECG database.

5.6 Isolation Forest Anomaly Detection for Quantifying the Deviation of Signal Averaged ECG from Population Norm

5.6.1 Isolation Forest Unsupervised Anomaly Detection

Isolation Forest (IF) [55] is one of the most popular methods for anomaly detection [56]. To define if the vector of features representing the ECG under analysis is an anomaly or not in the group of vectors, unsupervised learning is used for isolating the anomalies. The idea is that the anomalies are easier to separate from the cluster than non-anomalous vectors because they lie on the outskirts of the cluster. To isolate a vector in space, the IF algorithm recursively selects the axis in a feature space, and then randomly splits this axis by selecting the value between the minimum and maximum of the corresponding feature values. After several partitions, the coordinate of the single vector appears to be separated. The number of partitions required to isolate each vector is used to compute the score of anomalies of that vector. If the vector is located far from the rest of the vectors, the number of partitions required to isolate it is quite small, since the coordinates of the vector deviate substantially from the coordinates of other vectors. This method is applied to the identification of tiny changes in ECG from several groups of subjects.

5.6.2 Subjects Data

Five different groups were examined [57]: healthy subjects with no reported cardiovascular problems (Normal Controls, NC), subjects with proven coronary artery diseases (CID), subjects recovered from COVID-19, military personnel with mine-explosive injuries (Combatants), and two subgroups of participants of mass-screening in one of the rural region of Ukraine. Subgroup 1 consisted of persons, who died during five- years follow-up (all-cause mortality), subgroup 2 - persons, who didn't die during this period.

Signal averaged ECG (SAECG) considering a group of 181 people (males, aged from 18 to 28) is used in this study. Originally the data contained ECGs recorded in six ECG leads (I, II, III, aVR, aVL, aVF). From each of six SAECG leads, 34 features were extracted:

- Durations of P, Q, R, S peaks, and QRS complex,
- Durations of PR, QR, TR intervals,
- Duration of JT segment, duration from J to the top of T peak, duration from the top to the end of T peak,
- Amplitudes of P, Q, R, S, T peaks, and J wave,
- Mean magnitude over the ST segment, the magnitude at the end of ST-segment,
- Area under P peak, area under the QRS complex,

- Areas under the T peak from the beginning to the top, and from the top to the end,
- Ultimate derivative values are at ascending/descending parts of T peak.

In total, 204 features from each lead are calculated to characterize multichannel SAECG.

5.6.3 Quantification of the Distance to the Norm

After SAECG features are extracted, each ECG can be presented as a vector in the 204-dimensional feature space. The value of every feature is the coordinate of the particular ECG in that space with respect to the corresponding axes. In the case of having the group of ECG with similar characteristics, the corresponding feature vectors will form in the cluster in the space. If the particular ECG is located far from the cluster, this might indicate that their features are distinct from those of the cluster members. The vector of ECG which is similar to the group of ECGs forming the cluster will be located within the cluster.

In this work, the concept of outlier/inlier is proposed to be used for detecting the deviations of the ECG from the group of other ECGs. To define whether the particular ECG is an outlier or not, the Isolation Forest anomaly detector is used.

The procedure to use IF in defining the deviation of the current ECG from the group of the norm is as follows:

1. For the group of normal ECGs, SAECG is obtained, and the features of SAECGs are extracted.
2. Train the IF anomaly detector using the group of normal ECGs.
3. For the new ECG under analysis, pass it through the IF and obtain the anomaly score.

The negative values of the anomaly score indicate that the ECG is an anomaly; this is interpreted as the substantial deviation of the ECG from the norm. Additionally, the absolute value of the anomaly score can be used as a degree of deviation from the normal group. The bigger the absolute value is, the more distant the SAECG is located from the population norm, and therefore the difference between the current ECG and the normal group is more significant.

5.6.4 Experiment Results

In Fig. 5.1 the distribution of subjects from NC, CID, and COVID groups are presented. As vertical axes, the projection on the main eigenvector from PCA decomposition of the feature matrix is provided for reference, to construct the 2D plot. Table 5.2 contains mean and standard deviation values of the distance from the centers of the cluster for different groups.

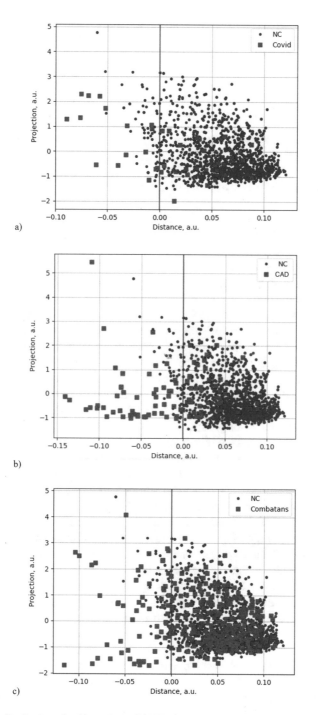

Fig. 5.1 The distribution of subjects from COVID group (**a**), CAD group (**b**), and Combatants group (**c**) with respect to NC subjects. (Image source: Illya Chaikovsky, Anton Popov)

Table 5.2 Mean and standard deviation of the anomaly score

Group name	Mean ± std. of the anomaly score
Healthy volunteers	0.0583 ± 0.0318
CAD	−0.0129 ± 0.0522
Wounded combatants	0.0389 ± 0.0431
COVID patients	0.0157 ± 0.0481
Subjects, died within 5 years of follow-ups (all-cause mortality)	−0.0102 ± 0.0601
Subjects, didn't die within 5 years of follow-ups	0.0204 ± 0.0498

Table source: Illya Chaikovsky, Anton Popov

As one can see, the distribution of distances and relative amount of outliers differs for the different groups, suggesting the receptiveness of the proposed method to the characteristics of the original SAECG. In case of COVID subjects, the positions are distributed quite equally, and points representing the COVID patients have both positive and negative distance values. This suggests that ECG of COVID subjects does not contain subtle deviations from the NC group. In contrast, many of CAD subjects have a negative distance from the NC group, which suggests the difference between the SAECG characteristics due to the changes of heart activity.

When estimating distance between the studied groups and normal controls it was found that the largest distance takes place between healthy volunteers' group and CAD patients group and group of subjects who died within 5 years of follow-ups (all-cause mortality). This may suggest further development of the mortality predictive score based on the outlier detection. The minimal distance from NC was detected in the Combatants group.

As already mentioned, the role of artificial intelligence methods in ECG analysis is increasing significantly. Of course, the disadvantages of this method should not be underestimated [58, 59]. Among these shortcomings, the need to analyze a large amount of data is usually noted, which requires a high qualification of the researchers. Often there is a need to update the used models during the study or after deployment due to the shift in the data. Another important problem is overfitting, i.e. a situation where the algorithm over-adjusts to the training sample, reaching maximum accuracy in it, but its performance is much worse on other populations. Solving this problem requires "fine tuning" of the training process.

However, the biggest problem hindering the widespread implementation of AI methods in the practice of cardiologists seems to be the "black box nature" of the findings obtained using AI. This means that clinicians have a poor understanding of the logical chain of inferences that lead to certain results, and therefore do not trust them. To solve this problem, in recent years, a special line has been developing in the theory and practice of machine learning methods, which is called explainable machine learning [60]. Of course, this approach also has its limitations.

The above limitations, especially the "black box nature", probably lead, among other things, to the fact that AI-assisted ECG analysis methods are used mainly for solving more specific problems, and are rarely used to determine the global risk of death from all causes. Only a few works on this topic are known. In the work of A.A. Mahayni and co-authors [61] used AI to predict long-term mortality after cardiac surgery. They used preoperative ECGs from subjects with detected left ventricular ejection fraction to train convolutional neural network for binary classification, and demonstrated increased prognostic value in the prediction of long-term mortality in patients undergoing cardiac surgical procedures. Another work [62] used a massive amount of the 12-lead resting-state ECGs to train deep neural network and predict the 1-year mortality with high efficacy. It was demonstrated that even the ECG, which is interpreted as normal by a qualified electrocardiologist, may provide important prognostic information to the AI algorithm and help to build correct predictions.

We, within the framework of our metric, interpret the distance from each current electrocardiogram to the threshold as a risk factor for long-term outcomes .

The novelty of our approach is the ability to specify the groups of SAECGs, from which we want to find the deviations. This enables adjustment of the risk analysis to the cohorts of people who inherently have specific characteristics of heart electrical activity, such as sportsmen, children, etc. We demonstrated that the same framework could be used to catch the tiny deviations from the group norm, and quantify its value, which may be used as a prognostic feature of the risk. The advantages of the employed Isolation Forest anomaly detector is its ability to work with smaller sample sizes, which is useful for the case of having relatively small groups to compare the ECG with. At the same time, IF can scale to handle the extremely large data volume and is robust to the presence of the irrelevant features. Together with its ability to directly isolate the anomalies in the dataset and provide a quantified score of the distance from the cluster, it is best suitable for the detection of subtle changes in the SAECGs with respect to the group norm.

5.7 Teaching Assignment

1. Describe the evolution and current opinion regarding the role of the electrocardiogram in assessing the venture for major adverse cardiovascular accidents.
2. Describe the basic characteristics and classification of the miniature electrocardiographic devices.
3. Highlight the generations of ECG analysis, describe the basic characteristics of each.
4. Describe your reflection of the adjustments of the risk factors to different groups of subjects, proposed in this chapter.
5. Describe the main idea of the interpretation of the distance from the group of feature vectors, proposed in this chapter.

5.8   Conclusion

In the nearest time there will certainly be more cases for delegating the patients with rights to test their heart state. Electrocardiographic tools with mobile phone size and simple access to analyzing cloud servers are becoming crucial for giving the patients personalized medicine approach.

Electrocardiograms analysis cloud platforms with few leads are going to develop gradually from oversimplified processing of just several rhythm disturbances to more sophisticated analysis, services, and diagnosis. The decision-making developments involving artificial intelligence as their base will give estimations for everyone. Their goals are severe cardiovascular risks both in the general population and, especially in certain cohorts, such as those with diabetes, pre-diabetes, and heart failure patients. The attempts are to be made to cope with the most powerful barrier to the engagement of machine learning logics – their black-box character, i.e., the difficulty, especially for clinicians, to perceive and moreover trust the representation of data leading to the diagnosis. Based on electrocardiogram and heart rate variability analysis, individualized recommendations will be made regarding frequency, duration, intensity, type, and total amount of physical activity, as well as detailed dietary recommendations.

On the other hand, the classic 12-lead electrocardiogram will remain the most frequently used technology in clinical cardiology for the long time. The progress in biomedical computing and signal processing, and the available computational power offer fascinating new options for electrocardiogram analysis relevant to all fields of cardiology. Successful implementation of artificial intelligence technologies for the analysis of routine 12-channel electrocardiogram is a critical step to further increase the power of electrocardiography. In this respect, the huge amount of digitized electrocardiogram recordings from affordable and widespread devices enables the growth of artificial intelligence data-driven machine learning approaches. The sophisticated algorithms requiring the training data will be more available both on the devices and as the cloud-based services, providing the automated diagnosis, prediction, and prevention of cardiovascular diseases and supporting human well-being.

References

1. J. Calvillo, I. Román, L.M. Roa, How technology is empowering patients. A literature review. 2013. Available: https://citeseerx.ist.psu.edu/viewdoc/download?doi=10.1.1.893.3296&rep=rep1&type=pdf
2. Single lead ECG equipment market size. [cited 16 Feb 2021]. Available: https://www.grandviewresearch.com/industry-analysis/single-lead-ecg-equipment-market
3. I. Chaikovsky, Electrocardiogram scoring beyond the routine analysis: Subtle changes matters. Expert Rev. Med. Devices 17(5), 379–382 (2020)
4. Z.I. Attia, D.M. Harmon, E.R. Behr, P.A. Friedman, Application of artificial intelligence to the electrocardiogram. Eur. Heart J. 42(46), 4717–4730 (2021)

5. K.M. Anderson, P.W. Wilson, P.M. Odell, W.B. Kannel, An updated coronary risk profile. A statement for health professionals. Circulation **83**, 356–362 (1991)
6. R.M. Conroy, K. Pyörälä, A.P. Fitzgerald, S. Sans, A. Menotti, G. De Backer, D. De Bacquer, P. Ducimetière, P. Jousilahti, U. Keil, I. Njølstad, R.G. Oganov, T. Thomsen, H. Tunstall-Pedoe, A. Tverdal, H. Wedel, P. Whincup, L. Wilhelmsen, Graham IM; SCORE project group. Estimation of ten-year risk of fatal cardiovascular disease in Europe: The SCORE project. Eur. Heart J. **24**(11), 987–1003 (2003)
7. S.A. Shal'nova, O.V. Vikhireva, Otsenkasummarnogoriskaserdechno-sosudistykhzabolevaniy. Ratsional'nayafarmakoterapiya v kardiologii. 2005; 1. Available: https://cyberleninka.ru/article/n/7138553
8. Pooling Project Research Group. Relationship of blood pressure, serum cholesterol, smoking habit, relative weight and ECG abnormalities to incidence of major coronary events: Final Report of the Pooling Project.. American Heart Association; 1978
9. W.B. Kannel, K. Anderson, D.L. McGee, L.S. Degatano, M.J. Stampfer, Nonspecific electrocardiographic abnormality as a predictor of coronary heart disease: The Framingham study. Am. Heart J. **113**, 370–376 (1987)
10. D. De Bacquer, G. De Backer, M. Kornitzer, H. Blackburn, Prognostic value of ECG findings for total, cardiovascular disease, and coronary heart disease death in men and women. Heart **80**, 570–577 (1998)
11. M.L. Daviglus, Y. Liao, P. Greenland, A.R. Dyer, K. Liu, X. Xie, C.F. Huang, R.J. Prineas, J. Stamler, Association of nonspecific minor ST-T abnormalities with cardiovascular mortality: The Chicago Western Electric Study. JAMA **281**(6), 530–536 (1999)
12. P. Greenland, X. Xie, K. Liu, L. Colangelo, Y. Liao, M.L. Daviglus, A.N. Agulnek, J. Stamler, Impact of minor electrocardiographic ST-segment and/or T-wave abnormalities on cardiovascular mortality during long-term follow-up. Am. J. Cardiol. **91**(9), 1068–1074 (2003)
13. P. Denes, J.C. Larson, D.M. Lloyd-Jones, R.J. Prineas, P. Greenland, Major and minor ECG abnormalities in asymptomatic women and risk of cardiovascular events and mortality. JAMA **297**, 978–985 (2007)
14. Chou R, Arora B, Dana T, Fu R, Walker M, Humphrey L. Screening asymptomatic adults with resting or exercise electrocardiography: a review of the evidence for the U.S. preventive services task force. Centre for Reviews and Dissemination (UK); 2011
15. Moyer VA. Screening for Coronary Heart Disease With Electrocardiography: U.S. Preventive Services Task Force Recommendation Statement. Annals of Internal Medicine. 2012
16. AAFP recommendations for preventive services guideline. In: AAFP [Internet]. [cited 28 Feb 2020]. Available: https://www.aafp.org/online/etc/medialib/aafp_org/documents/clinical/CPS/rcps08-2005.Par.0001.File.tmp/October2012SCPS.pdf
17. P. Greenland, J.S. Alpert, G.A. Beller, E.J. Benjamin, M.J. Budoff, Z.A. Fayad, E. Foster, M.A. Hlatky, J.M. Hodgson, F.G. Kushner, M.S. Lauer, L.J. Shaw, S.C. Smith Jr., A.J. Taylor, W.S. Weintraub, N.K. Wenger, A.K. Jacobs, S.C. Smith Jr., J.L. Anderson, N. Albert, C.E. Buller, M.A. Creager, S.M. Ettinger, R.A. Guyton, J.L. Halperin, J.S. Hochman, F.G. Kushner, R. Nishimura, E.M. Ohman, R.L. Page, W.G. Stevenson, L.G. Tarkington, C.W. Yancy, American College of Cardiology Foundation; American Heart Association, 2010 ACCF/AHA guideline for assessment of cardiovascular risk in asymptomatic adults: A report of the American College of Cardiology Foundation/American Heart Association task force on practice guidelines. J. Am. Coll. Cardiol. **56**(25), e50–e103 (2010)
18. A. Groot, M.L. Bots, F.H. Rutten, H.M. den Ruijter, M.E. Numans, I. Vaartjes, Measurement of ECG abnormalities and cardiovascular risk classification: A cohort study of primary care patients in the Netherlands. Br. J. Gen. Pract. **65**, e1–e8 (2015)
19. British Medical Journal Publishing Group, GRADE: grading quality of evidence and strength of recommendations for diagnostic tests and strategies. BMJ **336**, 1106 (2008). https://doi.org/10.1136/bmj.a139
20. Committee for Practice Guidelines ESC. European Guidelines on cardiovascular disease prevention in clinical practice (version 2012) The Fifth Joint Task Force of the European Society

of Cardiology and American Heart Association. Eur. Heart J. 2012. Available: https://academic.oup.com/eurheartj/article-abstract/33/13/1635/488083

21. R. Auer, D.C. Bauer, P. Marques-Vidal, J. Butler, L.J. Min, J. Cornuz, S. Satterfield, A.B. Newman, E. Vittinghoff, N. Rodondi, Health ABC Study, Association of major and minor ECG abnormalities with coronary heart disease events. JAMA **307**(14), 1497–1505 (2012)

22. S.Y. Tan, G.W. Sungar, J. Myers, M. Sandri, V. Froelicher, A simplified clinical electrocardiogram score for the prediction of cardiovascular mortality. Clin. Cardiol. **32**, 82–86 (2009)

23. E.Z. Gorodeski, H. Ishwaran, U.B. Kogalur, E.H. Blackstone, E. Hsich, Z.M. Zhang, M.Z. Vitolins, J.E. Manson, J.D. Curb, L.W. Martin, R.J. Prineas, M.S. Lauer, Use of hundreds of electrocardiographic biomarkers for prediction of mortality in postmenopausal women: The Women's Health Initiative. Circ. Cardiovasc. Qual. Outcomes **4**(5), 521–532 (2011)

24. T.T. Schlegel, W.B. Kulecz, A.H. Feiveson, E.C. Greco, J.L. DePalma, V. Starc, B. Vrtovec, M.A. Rahman, M.W. Bungo, M.J. Hayat, T. Bauch, R. Delgado, S.G. Warren, T. Núñez-Medina, R. Medina, D. Jugo, H. Arheden, O. Pahlm, Accuracy of advanced versus strictly conventional 12-lead ECG for detection and screening of coronary artery disease, left ventricular hypertrophy and left ventricular systolic dysfunction. BMC Cardiovasc. Disord. **10**, 28 (2010)

25. A.L. Arnold, K.A. Milner, V. Vaccarino, Sex and race differences in electrocardiogram use (the National Hospital Ambulatory Medical Care Survey). Am. J. Cardiol. **88**, 1037–1040 (2001)

26. P.M. Okin, J.T. Wright, M.S. Nieminen, S. Jern, A.L. Taylor, R. Phillips, V. Papademetriou, L.T. Clark, E.O. Ofili, O.S. Randall, L. Oikarinen, M. Viitasalo, L. Toivonen, S. Julius, B. Dahlöf, R.B. Devereux, Ethnic differences in electrocardiographic criteria for left ventricular hypertrophy: The LIFE study. Losartan intervention for endpoint. Am. J. Hypertens. **15**(8), 663–671 (2002)

27. P.A. Noseworthy, Z.I. Attia, L.C. Brewer, S.N. Hayes, X. Yao, S. Kapa, P.A. Friedman, F. Lopez-Jimenez, Assessing and mitigating bias in medical artificial intelligence: The effects of race and ethnicity on a deep learning model for ECG analysis. Circ. Arrhythm. Electrophysiol. **13**(3), e007988 (2020)

28. F.N. Wilson, The clinical value of chest leads. Br. Heart J. **10**(2), 88–91 (1948)

29. M.L. Løchen, K. Rasmussen, P.W. Macfarlane, E. Arnesen, Can single-lead computerized electrocardiography predict myocardial infarction in young and middle-aged men? J. Cardiovasc. Risk **6**(4), 273–278 (1999)

30. M.A. Hlatky, P. Greenland, D.K. Arnett, C.M. Ballantyne, M.H. Criqui, M.S. Elkind, A.S. Go, F.E. Harrell Jr., Y. Hong, B.V. Howard, V.J. Howard, P.Y. Hsue, C.M. Kramer, M.C. JP, S.L. Normand, C.J. O'Donnell, S.C. Smith Jr., P.W. Wilson, American Heart Association Expert Panel on Subclinical Atherosclerotic Diseases and Emerging Risk Factors and the Stroke Council, Criteria for evaluation of novel markers of cardiovascular risk: a scientific statement from the American Heart Association. Circulation **119**(17), 2408–2416 (2009)

31. W. Stanford, Screening of coronary artery disease: Is there a cost-effective way to do it? Am. J. Cardiol Imaging **10**(3), 180–186 (1996)

32. ACC Consensus Document on Signal-Averaged Electrocardiography. JACC **27**(1), 238–249 (1996)

33. J.F. Robillon, J.L. Sadoul, D. Jullien, P. Morand, P. Freychet, Abnormalities suggestive of cardiomyopathy in patients with type 2 diabetes of relatively short duration. Diabete Metab. **20**(5), 473–480 (1994)

34. F. Cecchi, A. Montereggi, I. Olivotto, P. Marconi, A. Dolara, B.J. Maron, Risk for atrial fibrillation in patients with hypertrophic cardiomyopathy assessed by signal averaged P wave duration. Heart **78**(1), 44–49 (1997)

35. F. Extramiana, A. Haggui, P. Maison-Blanche, R. Dubois, S. Takatsuki, P. Beaufils, A. Leenhardt, T-wave morphology parameters based on principal component analysis reproducibility and dependence on T-offset position. Ann. Noninvasive Electrocardiol. **12**(4), 354–363 (2007)

36. P.M. Okin, R.B. Devereux, R.R. Fabsitz, E.T. Lee, J.M. Galloway, B.V. Howard, Principal component analysis of the T wave and prediction of cardiovascular mortality in American Indians: The strong heart study. Circulation **105**(6), 714–719 (2002)
37. A. Pelliccia, F.M. Di Paolo, F.M. Quattrini, C. Basso, F. Culasso, G. Popoli, R. De Luca, A. Spataro, A. Biffi, G. Thiene, B.J. Maron, Outcomes in athletes with marked ECG repolarization abnormalities. N. Engl. J. Med. **358**(2), 152–161 (2008)
38. C.N. Mead, S.M. Moore, K.W. Clark, B.F. Spenner, L.J. Thomas Jr., A detection algorithm for multiform premature ventricular contractions. Med. Instrum. **12**(6), 337–339 (1978)
39. I.A. Chaikovsky, L.S. Fainzilberg, *Medical aspects of the use of the FASAGRAPH device in clinical practice and at home* (Kyiv, IRT Center ITIS, 2009), p. 74
40. O.V. Baum, I.A. Chaĭkovskiĭ, L.A. Popov, V.I. Voloshin, L.S. Faĭnzil'berg, M.M. Budnik, Electrocardiographic image of myocardial ischemia: Real measurements and biophysical models. Biofizika **55**(5), 925–936 (2010)
41. T.T. Schlegel, W.B. Kulecz, J.L. DePalma, A.H. Feiveson, J.S. Wilson, M.A. Rahman, M.W. Bungo, Real-time 12-lead high-frequency QRS electrocardiography for enhanced detection of myocardial ischemia and coronary artery disease. Mayo Clin. Proc. **79**(3), 339–350 (2004)
42. P. Rautaharju, C. Kooperberg, J. Larson, A. LaCroix, Electrocardiographic abnormalities that predict coronary heart disease events and mortality in postmenopausal women. Circulation **113**, 473–480 (2006)
43. M. Malik, V.N. Batchvarov, Measurement, interpretation and clinical potential of QT dispersion. J. Am. Coll. Cardiol. **36**(6), 1749–1766 (2000)
44. L.I. Titomir, N.E. Barinova, *Electrocardiographic mapping* (Methodological Guide, Moscow, 2006) 51 p
45. W.L. Atiga, H. Calkins, J.H. Lawrence, G.F. Tomaselli, J.M. Smith, R.D. Berger, Beat-to-beat repolarization lability identifies patients at risk for sudden cardiac death. J. Cardiovasc. Electrophysiol. **9**(9), 899–908 (1998)
46. K.C. Siontis, P.A. Noseworthy, Z.I. Attia, P.A. Friedman, Artificial intelligence-enhanced electrocardiography in cardiovascular disease management. Nat. Rev. Cardiol. **18**(7), 465–478 (2021)
47. O. Akbilgic, L. Butler, I. Karabayir, P.P. Chang, D.W. Kitzman, A. Alonso, L.Y. Chen, E.Z. Soliman, ECG-AI: Electrocardiographic artificial intelligence model for prediction of heart failure. Eur. Heart J. Digit. Health **2**(4), 626–634 (2021)
48. A.O. Ladejobi, J.R. Medina-Inojosa, M. Shelly Cohen, Z.I. Attia, C.G. Scott, N.K. Le Brasseur, B.J. Gersh, P.A. Noseworthy, P.A. Friedman, S. Kapa, F. Lopez-Jimenez, The 12-lead electrocardiogram as a biomarker of biological age. Eur. Heart J. Digit. Health **2**(3), 379–389 (2021)
49. L. Ruff, J.R. Kauffmann, R.A. Vandermeulen, G. Montavon, W. Samek, M. Kloft, T.G. Dietterich, K.R. Müller. A unifying review of deep and shallow anomaly detection. Proceedings of the IEEE. 2021 Feb 4
50. C.C. Aggarwal, *Outlier analysis* (Springer, Cham, 2017), p. 466
51. H. Li, P. Boulanger, A survey of heart anomaly detection using ambulatory electrocardiogram (ECG). Sensors **20**(5), 1461 (2020)
52. C. Venkatesan, P. Karthigaikumar, P. Anand, S. Satheeskumaran, R. Kumar, ECG signal preprocessing and SVM classifier-based abnormality detection in remote healthcare applications. IEEE Access **6**, 9767–9773 (2018)
53. H. Zhou, C. Kan, Tensor-based ECG anomaly detection toward cardiac monitoring in the internet of health things. Sensors **21**(12), 4173 (2021)
54. G. Sivapalan, K.K. Nundy, S. Dev, B. Cardiff, D. John, ANNet: a lightweight neural network for ECG anomaly detection in IoT edge sensors. IEEE Trans. Biomed. Circuits Syst. **16**(1), 24–35 (2022)
55. F. T. Liu, K. M. Ting and Z. Zhou, "Isolation Forest," 2008 Eighth IEEE International Conference on Data Mining, 2008, pp. 413–422. https://doi.org/10.1109/ICDM.2008.17

56. F.T. Liu, K.M. Ting, Z.-H. Zhou, Isolation-based anomaly detection. ACM Trans. Knowl. Discov. Data (TKDD) **6**(1), 1–39 (2012)
57. I. Chaikovsky, A. Popov, D. Fogel, A. Kazmirchyk, Development of AI-based method to detect the subtle ECG deviations from the population ECG norm. Eur. J. Prev. Cardiol. **28**(Supplement_1), zwab061–zwab229 (2021)
58. T. Reichlin, R. Abächerli, R. Twerenbold, M. Kühne, B. Schaer, C. Müller, C. Sticherling, S. Osswald, Advanced ECG in 2016: Is there more than just a tracing? Swiss Med. Wkly. **146**, w14303 (2016)
59. R. Cuocolo, T. Perillo, E. De Rosa, L. Ugga, M. Petretta, Current applications of big data and machine learning in cardiology. J. Geriatr. Cardiol. **16**(8), 601–607 (2019)
60. J. Petch, S. Di, W. Nelson, Opening the black box: The promise and limitations of explainable machine learning in cardiology. Can. J. Cardiol. **38**(2), 204–213 (2022)
61. A.A. Mahayni, Z.I. Attia, J.R. Medina-Inojosa, M.F.A. Elsisy, P.A. Noseworthy, F. Lopez-Jimenez, S. Kapa, S.J. Asirvatham, P.A. Friedman, J.A. Crestenallo, M. Alkhouli, Electrocardiography-based artificial intelligence algorithm aids in prediction of long-term mortality after cardiac surgery. Mayo Clin. Proc. **96**(12), 3062–3070 (2021)
62. S. Raghunath, A.E. Ulloa Cerna, L. Jing, D.P. VanMaanen, J. Stough, D.N. Hartzel, B.K. Fornwalt, Prediction of mortality from 12-lead electrocardiogram voltage data using a deep neural network. Nat. Med. **26**(6), 886–891 (2020)

Chapter 6
Application of Wavelet Decomposition and Ma-Chine Learning for the sEMG Signal Based Ges-Ture Recognition

Hala Rabih Fatayerji, Majed Saeed, Saeed Mian Qaisar, Asmaa Alqurashi, and Rabab Al Talib

Abstract The amputees throughout the world have limited access to the high-quality intelligent prostheses. The correct recognition of gestures is one of the most difficult tasks in the context of surface electromyography (sEMG) based prostheses development. This chapter shows a comparative examination of the several machine learning-based algorithms for the hand gestures identification. The first step in the process is the data extraction from the sEMG device, followed by the features extraction. Then, the two robust machine learning algorithms are applied to the extracted feature set to compare their prediction accuracy. The medium Gaussian Support Vector Machine (SVM) performs better under all conditions as compared to the K-nearest neighbor. Different parameters are used for the performance comparison which include F1 score, accuracy, precision and Kappa index. The proposed method of hand gesture recognition, based on sEMG, is thoroughly investigated and the results have shown a promising performance. In any case, the miscalculation during feature extraction can reduce the recognition precision. The profound learning technique are used to achieve a high precision. Therefore, the proposed design takes into account all aspects while processing the sEMG signal. The system secures a highest classification accuracy of 92.2% for the case of Gaussian SVM algorithm.

H. R. Fatayerji · S. Mian Qaisar (✉) · A. Alqurashi · R. Al Talib
Electrical and Computer Engineering Department, Effat University, Jeddah, Saudi Arabia
e-mail: sqaisar@effatuniversity.edu.sa

M. Saeed
Department of Urology, Sahiwal Teaching Hospital, Sahiwal, Pakistan

© The Author(s), under exclusive license to Springer Nature Switzerland AG 2023
S. Mian Qaisar et al. (eds.), *Advances in Non-Invasive Biomedical Signal Sensing and Processing with Machine Learning*, https://doi.org/10.1007/978-3-031-23239-8_6

6.1 Introduction

The hands are the most versatile and dexterous component of the human body, capable of interacting with the world through a wide range of motion techniques such as touch, grasp, manipulation, and so on. Amputees all throughout the world are currently struggling to achieve anything more than the bare minimum with their prosthetics. In fact, according to the World Health Organization (WHO), only 1 in 10 individuals who need assistive devices, such as prostheses, have access to them currently due to the costly expense of the items as well as a lack of knowledge, availability, trained staff, policy, and funding [1]. Furthermore, in the varying circumstances, the system, and signal acquisition and detection should be effective. Therefore, the proposed system design identifies hand gestures by processing surface electromyography (sEMG) signals in order to contribute to the development of prosthetic hands.

The myoelectric signal (MES), also known as an electromyography (EMG) signal, obtained from the forearm skin surface gives vital information regarding neuromuscular processes. The complexity, non-linearity, and a considerable variance characterize the signals generated by EMG, which makes the signals difficult to interpret. Hence, before the usage of EMG signals to build a classification system for hand motions (pattern recognition and classification), there should be an identification process of the signals' attributes (features). In this situation, the pattern is represented by the temporal signal in an EMG signal. In most circumstances, the acquired signal may be defined in terms of its amplitude, frequency, and phase, all of which are time-variant. Electrical currents are formed in the muscle during a muscle contraction, showing neuromuscular activity, because muscle contraction and relaxation are constantly under the control of the neurological system. The nervous system and anatomical and physiological features of muscles interact to generate a complex EMG signal. While passing through various tissues, the EMG signal picks up noise. Moreover, if the EMG detector is placed near the skin's surface, it might gather signals from many motor organs at the same time, resulting in signal interference.

Clinical diagnosis and biological applications are the primary drivers of interest in EMG signal analysis, and evidently one of the key application areas is the treatment and rehabilitation of people with motor disabilities. EMG signals including MUAPs (Motor Unit Action Potentials) contain valuable information for the identification of diseases of the neuromuscular system. An understanding of EMG signals may be gained if the relevant algorithms and methods for their analysis are easily accessible. As a consequence, hardware implementations for different EMG signal-related applications can advance and be applied to invigorate the field's stagnation, but the high unpredictability of sEMG and the scarcity of available data restrict the deployment of gesture recognition technology [2].

The necessity for another generation of upper appendage prostheses prompted the development of a cost-effective prosthetic hand with an easy-to-use control interface. Advanced signal processing apparatuses and a programmed control calculation have been incorporated into the myoelectric hand to enable the replacement of costly, precise actuators and sensors with less expensive components and to reduce the difficulty associated with the gadget's activation and navigation. High-level control is used to discern the client's goal to impel the hand model, which was meticulously created and built for this duty. Correspondingly, low-level control naturally plays out the problem of gaining a hold on it. Low-level input provides the control with both power and joint position data, whilst a vibrotactile feedback framework (undeniable level input) provides the client with a circuitous experience of touch [3]. When a prosthetic device is limited by electromyography signals produced by the muscles of the remaining of the amputated limb, six key perspectives must be considered to provide successful control:

(a) To comprehend the characteristics of sEMG signals and how they are acquired.
(b) To describe in detail the numerous advances produced.
(c) To become acquainted with the various machine learning algorithms and their workings by evaluating how well they function.
(d) Client control ought to be intuitive and need little mental effort.
(e) There shouldn't be any discernible postponement in the reaction time of the framework.
(f) To put into practice a paradigm that will benefit amputees from all societal strata.

6.2 Literature Review

6.2.1 Background

After centuries of many American Civil War losses, there was a large increase in demand for prosthetic limbs. Due to the limited functionality of the available limbs, many veterans began creating their own prostheses. One of the first amputees of the war, James Hanger, invented the "Hanger Limb." Samuel Decker was a pioneer in the development of modular limbs and also created his own mechanical arms. Decker's design has a spoon that is hooked to his artificial arms in recognition of the requirement for him to be able to carry out daily tasks with his prosthesis. Designs now needed to restore some of the amputees' prior abilities in addition to replacing the lost limb. A generation of young men was finally be able to live independent lives with artificial limbs. Specialized artificial limbs were a notion that the forerunners of prosthetic design had started to explore and around the 1900s, limb design grew more specialized and focused on purposes other than decoration [4]. Slowly, the fundamental idea behind surface EMG-based human-machine interfaces developed to be the use of machine learning techniques to transform sEMG data into controlled signals. The implementation of prosthetic hand control and high dependability of the human-machine interface have been made possible by the accuracy and adaptability of the information processing and classification algorithms.

The deep learning has lately drawn more interest of academicians for studying the detection of sEMG based patterns. By bypassing the tedious feature extraction and optimization procedures, it can automatically learn features of various abstract levels from a variety of input samples to achieve an end-to-end sEMG based gesture recognition [2]. The wavelet transform is the most commonly acknowledged approach for dissecting the EMG in the time-recurrence space. The organizing stage entails selecting the class to which the element vector retrieved from an EMG belongs. Support vector machines and neural networks are the most commonly used continuous models for characterization. A mix of decision trees, k-means clustering, and hidden Markov models is employed. In this case, a mix of support vector machines (SVMs) and hidden Markov models (HMMs) is applied. Signal acknowledgement frameworks have had to work constantly for a long time. The precision of these frameworks should be comparable to that of disconnected frameworks. A motion acknowledgment framework must be able to detect a move in less than 300 milliseconds in order to function constantly. This is equivalent to at least three motions per second. Furthermore, these frameworks are typically executed with limited computational resources. These requirements impose a requirement on the complexity of an acknowledgment model. As a result, the test is to design a continuous signal acknowledgment framework with a cheap computational expense and excellent performance. Although other machine learning techniques have been discussed in earlier research, the k-Nearest Neighbor (k-NN), SVM, and Artificial Neural Networks (ANNs) are the three classifiers that produce the best classification results [5].

6.2.2   Preprocessing for sEMG Based Gesture Recognition

The sEMG-based hand motion recognition technique is divided into several steps. The initial step is to acquire the raw signals. The number and location of electrodes must be determined based on the type of motion done in the experiment. Because each action is dependent on multiple muscles, most observations about motion identification for whole-hand movements have been recorded from four or more channels on the entire arm. However, in hand-posture research, the utilized muscles are primarily in the forearm, and thus the number of channels can be decreased. Although this may affect the accuracy quality, it can be improved by integrating feature data from multiple channels appropriately. The major sEMG processing blocks are shown in Fig. 6.1. A description of different blocks is provided in the following.

Active segment signals and information from inactive segment are both included in the continual process of collecting sEMG signals. Non-active segment information must be removed in order to increase the recognition model's precision and speed [6]. The sEMG signal is considered a noisy one, which indicates that the sEMG's probability distribution varies with time. The non-stationarity signal of sEMG can be reduced by filtering. Filtering is used to remove the noise and obtain

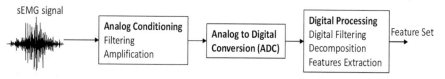

Fig. 6.1 The signal acquisition and preprocessing stages

Fig. 6.2 The analog band-pass filter

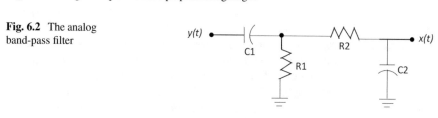

the most important information. Because roughly 95% of the sEMG signal strength is concentrated at 400–500 Hz, the sensor's lowest sample frequency must be more than double the sEMG's maximum frequency, according to the Nyquist–Shannon sampling theorem. In the meanwhile, the filter uses a low-pass filtering approach, or a moving average method, which might be considered a special low-pass filter. Some characteristics (such as MAV, ARV, or RMS) are computed using the moving average technique by windowing the signals and then averaging the features of all channels, or by computing the features of the average of all channels directly (Fig. 6.2).

Signal conditioning is the process of altering an analog signal such that it complies with the demands of the following step of further processing. Anti-aliasing filtering and voltage or current limiting are examples of signal conditioning used in analog-to-digital converter applications. The voltage and current, frequency, and electric charge are all acceptable input formats. Devices for signal conditioning can use a variety of outputs including voltage, current and frequency. Amplification, filtering, range matching, isolation, and other procedures are used in signal conditioning to prepare sensor output for further processing.

Analog signals are converted into digital signals by a device called an analog-to-digital converter (ADC). It converts a signal with continuous time and amplitude to one with discrete time and amplitude. The first step is band-pass filtering between the frequency range of [0.5; 150] Hz, given by Eq. (6.1) and shown in Fig. 6.1. In Eq. (6.1), $x(t)$ is the filtered version of signal $y(t)$ and $h(t)$ is the impulse response of this filter. In second step, the sampling is carried out, given by Eq. (6.2) and shown in Fig. 6.3. In Eq. (6.2), $x_s(t)$ is the sampled version of $x(t)$ and $s(t)$ is the sampling function. Onward, the input is quantized throughout the quantization process. We employed 500 Hz sampling rate and 12-bit resolution quantizer during the A/D conversion. The process of quantization involves condensing an infinite set of continuous values into a more manageable set of discrete values. It involves estimating the real-world values with a digital representation that restricts the precision and range of a value in the context of simulation and embedded computing. Rounding mistakes, underflow or overflow, and computational noise are all introduced by

Fig. 6.3 The sampling process

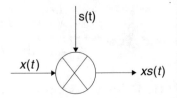

quantization. The behavior of an ideal system and estimated numerical behavior, thus, differ numerically. When choosing suitable data types for capturing real-world signals, one must take into account the precision, range, and scaling of the data type used to encode the signal as well as the non-linear cumulative effects of quantization on the numerical behavior of your algorithm. When mechanisms such as feedback loops are present, the cumulative influence of quantization is increased.

In embedded systems, the quantization is an essential step in accelerating inference while reducing memory and power usage. As a result, it may be installed on hardware with a reduced memory footprint, which frees up more RAM for control logic and extra algorithms. For a particular hardware architecture, examples of quantization features include integer processing, employing hardware accelerators, and fusing layers [7, 8]. The quantization process is given by Eq. (6.3). In Eq. (6.3), $x[n]$ is the digitized version of $x_s[n]$ and $Qe[n]$ is its corresponding quantization error. The upper bound on the $Qe[n]$ is posed by the quantum q and the relation ship is given by Eq. (6.4) [9, 10].

$$x(t) = y(t) * h(t).$$
(6.1)

$$x_s(t) = x(t) \times s(t).$$
(6.2)

$$x[n] = x_s[n] + Qe[n].$$
(6.3)

$$Q_e[n] \leq \pm \frac{q}{2}.$$
(6.4)

Each prolonged sEMG signal was divided into 6-second segments comprising 3000 samples to increase information size and the rectangular window approach was used to complete the division, with the windowing process is given by Eqs. (6.5) and (6.6) [11–13].

$$zw_n = x_n \times w_n.$$
(6.5)

$$zw_n = \sum_{\frac{-T}{2}}^{\frac{T}{2}} z_n.$$
(6.6)

Where, the digitized version of the sEMG band limited signal acquired from the examined dataset is denoted by x_n. Its segmented form is zw_n. w_n represents the vector of window function coefficients. It has a period of 6-seconds and 3000 magnitude 1 coefficients. The windowing method breaks up the longer sEMG signal into reduced chunks. Each segment is treated as a distinct instance. A total of 180 cases are examined, with 30 from each class.

The basic principle behind wavelets is to interpret data based on scale. The size with which we examine data is important in wavelet analysis. Wavelet algorithms operate on data at various sizes or resolutions. Gross characteristics can be seen if the signal is seen via a big "window." Similarly, minor characteristics would be seen if the signal was viewed via a narrow "window." Wavelet analysis produces the ability to view both the forest and the trees. Approximating functions that are cleanly confined in finite domains can be employed with wavelet analysis. Wavelets are ideal for estimating data with severe discontinuities. A wavelet function, known as an analyzing wavelet or mother wavelet is used in the wavelet analysis. If the best wavelets are not selected for the intended data or if the coefficients resolution is decreased below a certain threshold, then the data will not be correctly represented [7, 14]. The Eq. (6.7) can be used to express wavelet mathematically. Where s denotes the scaling operator and u is the translation operator.

$$\Psi(t) = \frac{1}{\sqrt{S}} \Psi\left((t-u)/s\right). \tag{6.7}$$

$$W_x(u,s) = \frac{1}{\sqrt{S}} \int_{-\infty}^{+\infty} x(t)\Psi *\left((t-u)/s\right)dt. \tag{6.8}$$

The Eq. (6.8) demonstrates how to use the wavelet transform to break down a signal $x(t)$. When it comes to the decomposition of signals in terms of a base set of functions, the Discrete Wavelet Transform (DWT) is similar to the Fourier transform. A single parameter is used in Fourier transformations, and the basis set is made up of sines and cosines, whereas the expansion has only one parameter. A single "mother" wavelet is used to create the functions (wavelets) in the wavelet transform, with dilation and offsets matching to the two variables of the expansion being used to construct the functions.

The Discrete Time Wavelet Packet Decomposition (DWPD) is a wavelet transform that applies additional filters to the signal than the DWT. Wavelet packets are one-of-a-kind linear wavelet combinations. Many of the orthogonality, smoothness, and localization characteristics of their parent wavelets are retained in the bases they produce. The DWPD is a wavelet transform that applies additional filters to the signal than the DWT. Wavelet packets are one-of-a-kind linear wavelet combinations. Many of the orthogonality, smoothness, and localization characteristics of the parent wavelets are retained in the bases they produce. Each freshly created wavelet packet coefficient sequence serves as the root of its own analysis tree as the coefficients in the linear combinations are computed recursively. The WPD decomposes both the detail and approximation coefficients. The WPD creates 2^n separate sets of coefficients (or nodes) for n degrees of decomposition, whereas the DWT produces (n + 1) sets. However, because of the down sampling process, the total number of coefficients remains constant and there is no redundancy [15]. The process of computing the approximation an detailed coefficients is respectively given by Eqs. (6.9) and (6.10).

$$a_m = \sum_{k=1}^{K_g} xd_n \cdot g_{2n-k} \cdot \qquad (6.9)$$

$$d_m = \sum_{k=1}^{K_g} xd_n \cdot h_{2n-k} \cdot \qquad (6.10)$$

The wavelet decomposition, utilized to produce the sub-bands of the sEMG signal is shown in Fig. 6.4. The wavelet decomposition approach has been shown to lower the empirical risk in certain circumstances. Results from sEMG signal time series show that our method makes sense [16].

6.2.3 Feature Selection Techniques for sEMG Based Gesture Recognition

A feature is a functional requirement of a system. In general, the phrase feature includes both functional and non-functional criteria. The feature is an observable behavior of the system that the user might activate in this research. One of the most difficult aspects of programming is comprehending how a certain feature works. One must first locate the feature's implementation in the code before they can fully understand it. In many cases, systems are composed of many modules, each of which contains tens or hundreds of lines of code. Most of the time, it's difficult to tell wherein the source code a specific functionality is implemented. Original architects of the system may not be available, or their perspective may be skewed due to alterations made by others since the documentation's creation (if any). Maintaining

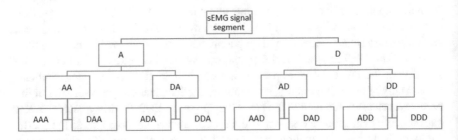

Fig. 6.4 The Wavelet Decomposition

a system introduces illogical modifications that weaken its overall structure. Every time something is altered in the system, it becomes more difficult to understand. One alternative is to reverse engineer the system from the ground up to get out of this rut, identifying all of its components and assigning functions to them. An incremental semiautomatic procedure uses established automatic ways for retrieving component data and validating them by hand before using them. Exhaustive procedures, on the other hand, are not economically viable. Fortunately, understanding the components that implement a certain set of functionalities is often sufficient [17].

For a system to be understood in its implementation of a specific feature, it must first be identified as to which computing units within the system are responsible for that characteristic. There are many instances where mapping features to source code is not well documented. The intended behavior of a system is described in abstract terms by its features. While concentrating solely on the implementation details and static structure of a system, reverse engineering methodologies neglect the dynamic relationships between the many pieces that only show when the system is in operation. By developing a model in which characteristics are tied to structural entities, we want to enhance the static and dynamic analyses that have already been performed. When it comes to dynamic analysis, there is a multitude of information available; nevertheless, this amount of knowledge creates a challenge in the analysis. In order to cope with it, we used Latent Semantic Indexing, an information retrieval technique that works with both documents and keywords. The objectives were to find linked features, as well as associated classes that participate in features in order to complete the task. For the text corpus, they used function calls from the traces; for the document corpus, they employed two mappings to documents: classes as documents as well as traces as documents.

The reduction of duplicate data in a data source is made possible through feature extraction. Data reduction expedites the learning and generalization stages of the machine learning process while also assisting the computer in building the model with less manual labor. Standard deviation, absolute minimum of nth level approximation coefficients, highest absolute value of nth level detail coefficients, mean of average absolute of all sub-bands, ratios of the mean of average absolute of succeeding sub-bands, root-mean-square value of time series, skewness & kurtosis of subband coefficients, absolute peak-to-peak difference of sub-band coefficients, and energies are all mined for each considered sub-band [18].

6.2.4 Machine Learning and Deep Learning Techniques for sEMG Based Gesture Recognition

In order to manage complicated activities autonomously or with little to no human participation, artificial intelligence (AI) is generally defined as any approach that allows computers to imitate or surpass human decision-making and mimic human behavior. As a result, it has connections to a wide range of tools and approaches and is concerned with a broad range of important issues, such as knowledge representation, reasoning, learning, planning, perception, and communication. A computer might then use logical inference techniques to reason about hard-coded positions in formal languages, which were the main focus of early AI research. The knowledge base technique is another name for this. However, the paradigm has significant disadvantages since individuals fail to articulate all of their tacit knowledge necessary to do difficult tasks. Such constraints exist.

Artificial intelligence is divided into several subfields, including deep learning, machine learning, and neural networks. Deep learning, a type of machine learning, is divided into neural networks. Both deep learning and machine learning use distinctive learning techniques. The majority of the feature extraction process is automated using deep learning, eliminating the requirement for some manual human interaction and enabling the usage of larger data sets. Traditional, or "non-deep," machine learning is taught by humans. Human experts create a collection of traits to recognize differences in data inputs, which frequently require the use of additional organized data to understand. Although they are not necessary, labeled datasets or supervised learning can help "deep" machine learning algorithms. Unstructured data may be ingested in its raw form, and it can automatically recognize the properties that set distinct data types apart. Data analysis, in contrast to machine learning, does not need human contact, allowing us to scale machine learning in more intriguing ways. Speech recognition, natural language processing, and computer vision have all advanced more quickly as a result of deep learning. Deep learning is a term used to describe the number of layers in a neural network. More than three layers of inputs and outputs make up a deep learning algorithm, sometimes referred to as a deep neural network. There are just two or three layers in a simple neural network [19].

According to ML, a computer program's performance generally increases over time in relation to a range of tasks and performance indicators. It attempts to automate the process of developing analytical models in order to carry out cognitive tasks like object identification and language translation. This is accomplished by employing algorithms that continually learn from training data specific to the task at hand, giving computers the ability to identify intricate patterns and hidden insights without being explicitly trained. For high-dimensional data operations like classification, regression, and grouping, machine learning is incredibly helpful. It can assist in obtaining reliable and repeatable findings by learning from earlier calculations and seeing patterns in huge databases. Machine learning algorithms have succeeded in a number of fields as a result, including fraud detection, credit scoring, analysis of the next-best offer, audio and image identification, and natural language processing (NLP). On the basis of the problem and the data provided, three types of ML may be identified:

(a) Supervised learning,
(b) Unsupervised learning
(c) Reinforcement learning

Using labeled datasets, supervised learning is the process of creating algorithms that can accurately categorize data or forecast outcomes. When new input data is added, the model's weights are changed until it is well fitted. To make sure the model is not overfitting or underfitting, this is done as part of the cross validation stage. Organizations may solve a variety of complex real-world problems with the help of supervised learning, such as separating spam from email. In supervised learning, classification and regression techniques including Naive Bayes, Neural Networks, Linear Regression, Logistic Regression, Random Forest, Support Vector Machine (SVM), and others are utilized. The user trains the algorithm to provide a response based on a collection of known and labeled data.

Unsupervised machine learning analyzes and sorts unlabeled data sets using machine learning techniques; these algorithms find hidden patterns or data groupings. Because of its capacity to identify similarities and differences in data, it is the ideal choice for exploratory data analysis, cross-selling tactics, consumer segmentation, and picture and pattern recognition. Additionally, it is used in the dimensionality reduction process to reduce the number of features in a model; principal component analysis (PCA) and singular value decomposition are two typical techniques for this (SVD). There are several unsupervised learning techniques and clustering algorithms available, including neural networks, k-means clustering, probabilistic clustering, and others. The algorithms create answers from unlabeled and unknown data. Data scientists frequently employ unsupervised approaches to uncover patterns in fresh data sets, and they may build machine learning algorithms utilizing a variety of technologies and languages, as well as pre-built machine learning frameworks, to speed up the process [19, 20].

Deep learning is a subcategory of machine learning that employs both supervised and unsupervised learning techniques. It is based on the representation learning subfield of machine learning theory (or feature learning). Artificial neural networks (ANN), also known as deep learning neural networks, mimic the workings of the human brain by using data inputs, weights, and bias. Together, these elements describe, categorize, and identify data items. Each layer of deep neural networks, which are made up of several interconnected ones, improves and fine-tunes categorization or prediction. A network's transmission of calculations is referred to as forward propagation. The layers of a deep neural network that are visible are the input and output layers. The layers of a deep neural network that are visible are the input and output layers. Before producing the final prediction or classification in the output layer, the deep learning model processes data in the input layer.

Deep learning models provide results quicker than traditional machine learning approaches because they employ a hierarchical learning process to extract high-level, complicated abstractions as data representations. In other words, rather of requiring the data scientist to select the important attributes manually, a deep learning model will learn them Backpropagation is a different approach that uses methods like gradient descent to produce prediction errors before altering the weights and biases of the function by repeatedly going back through the layers to train the model. Forward and back-propagation function in tandem to allow a neural network to foresee and correct for errors. Deep learning models provide results quicker than traditional machine learning approaches because they employ a hierarchical learning process to extract high-level, complicated abstractions as data representations.

In other words, rather of requiring the data scientist to select the important attributes manually, a deep learning model will learn them. Backpropagation is a different approach that uses tools like gradient descent to produce prediction errors before changing the function's weights and biases by repeatedly going back through the layers to train the model. Forward and back-propagation function in tandem to allow a neural network to foresee and correct for errors. The algorithm's accuracy improves with time, and the "deep" in deep learning refers to the several layers used in deep learning models:

The completion of tasks like object detection and identification is made possible by convolutional neural networks (CNNs), which are extensively employed in computer vision and image classification applications. CNNs are able to recognize patterns and discriminate between properties in an image. CNN can be made up of numerous layers of models, each accepting input from the previous layer, processing it, and then passing it on to the next layer in a daisy-chain pattern. Recurrent neural networks (RNNs), on the other hand, are often utilized in natural language and speech recognition applications because they utilize sequential or time series data [20, 21].

6.3 Methodology

Figure 6.5 displays the designed system block diagram. The following describes several processing phases with materials and methods.

6.3.1 Dataset

The dataset came from a research that involves frequently and freely grasping of different items [22]. The individuals were given complete control over the speed and force of grasping. The six motions, shown in Fig. 6.6, were asked to be repeated by five healthy volunteers between the ages of 20 and 22. Figure 6.7 displays the surface plots of feature sets that were retrieved from examples of various categories. For each fundamental movement, the experiment was repeated 30 times with the subject performing each one for 6 seconds. 180 sEMG signals were therefore acquired for each subject.

In addition to being non-invasive, repeating patterns, and capable of categorizing signals in real time, sEMG has a wide range of applications, including gesture recognition, prosthesis development, and human-computer interfaces. The sEMG signals in this dataset can also be used to enhance other datasets for more accurate categorization of similar signals. There are 16 recorded EMG signals, each lasting 70 seconds, in the sEMG database of objects gripping activities. The signals were gathered from a healthy person. Six tasks were offered to the participant: spherical, palmar, tiny tools, lateral, cylindrical and hook gestures (cf. Figure 6.6) [22, 23].

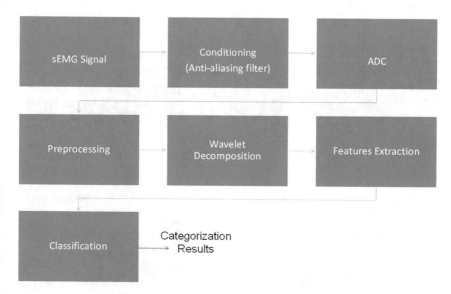

Fig. 6.5 The proposed system block diagram

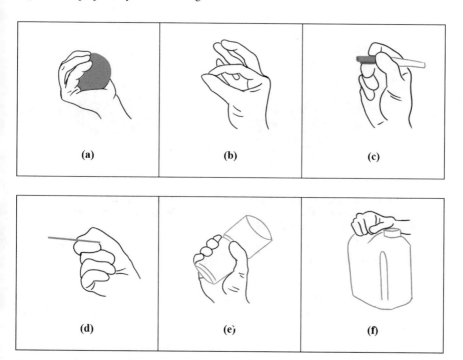

Fig. 6.6 (a) Spherical Gesture, (b) Tiny Tools Gesture, (c) Palmar (Grip) Gesture, (d) Lateral Gesture, (e) Cylindrical Gesture, and (f) Hook Gesture

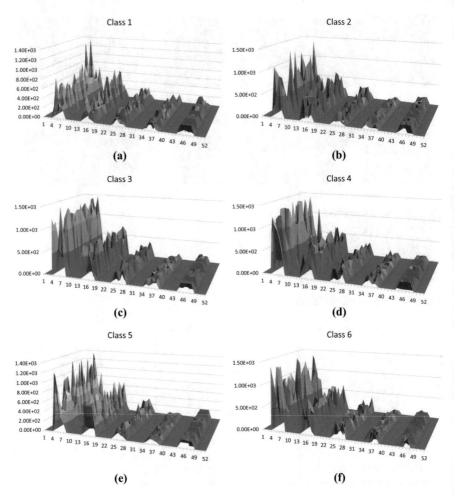

Fig. 6.7 (**a**) Class 1: Spherical, (**b**) Class 2: Tip, (**c**) Class 3: Cylindrical, (**d**) Class 4: Palmar, (**e**) Class 5: Lateral, (**e**) Class-6: Hook. The x-axis is presenting the number of attributes and y-axis is presenting their corresponding magnitudes

6.3.2 Machine Learning Algorithms

The classifier is an algorithm for performing the categorization tasks. It learns from the labeled dataset and onward the trained classifier may then be used to classify unknown documents or nodes based on the samples that were passed through the classifier to learn what makes a specific class where some parameters are set to better understand the status of the signal. Optimizer options are hyper-parameter options deactivated and all features used in the model before PCA are set to the default of "Gaussian Naive Bayes" in Model Type Preset. Gaussian is the distribution name for numerical predictors. Multivariate multinomial distribution is the name of the distribution used for categorical predictors (MVMN). The default choice for the feature selection and cost matrix is MVMN. Fine KNN, Euclidean distance metric, weight equality, and standardize data are all true. Hyper-parameter options are deactivated in the optimizer settings, and feature selection is enabled for the model type preset. PCA is disabled and the Misclassification Cost Matrix is set as the default for all features in the model prior to PCA. Our method considers K of these data points, which is the predefined number. Therefore, the distance metric and K value of the KNN algorithm are crucial elements to take into consideration. As far as distance measurements go, there's no better option than using Euclidean distance. In addition to this, you have the option of using the Hamming, Manhattan, or even the Minkowski distance. The training dataset's data points are all taken into account when predicting the class or continuous value of a new data point. Use feature space, class labels, or continuous values to find the "K" Nearest Neighbors of new data points. In Discriminant Linear All features used in the model prior to PCA are selected, and PCA is deactivated. The Misclassification Costs Matrix is set to Default. The Model Type Preset is Linear Discriminant, and the Covariance Structure is full. In the SVM Model Type Preset, the Gaussian Kernel Function, the 7.2-scale kernel, the one-level box constraint, and the One-vs-One (OvO) multiclass method are all set to the default values of medium. Settings for hyper-parameters are disabled; All features used in the model before to PCA are referred to as feature selection; The Misclassification Cost Matrix has a True default value since PCA is deactivated. There are 30 learner types and 26 subspace dimensions in Ensemble Classifiers' model type pre-sets, and hyper-parameter choices have been deactivated in the optimizer settings. There are no PCA or misclassification cost matrices since the model uses all characteristics before PCA.

6.3.2.1   Support Vector Machine Classifier (SVM)

A sparse kernel decision machine, the SVM approach builds its learning model without taking posterior probabilities into account. SVM provides a systematic solution to machine learning problems because to its mathematical foundation in statistical learning theory. Frequently used for classification, regression, novelty detection, and feature reduction problems, SVM develops a solution by using a subset of the training input.

When a program is executing, it generates new parameter values. Preventative maintenance can save a lot of money in the long run if the engine begins to show signs of failure early on. In order to solve the problem that the diagnostic model's generalization ability decreases due to the motor's variable operating circumstances, this research proposed a rolling application bearing cross-domain defect detection strategy based on a medium Gaussian SVM. End-to-end diagnostics is made possible using only the original signal as an input. To evaluate a model, this approach requires prior knowledge of the label for the target domain in order to achieve supervised domain adaptation.

The SVM approach creates its learning model without taking posterior probabilities into account. It is a sparse kernel decision machine. Due to its mathematical

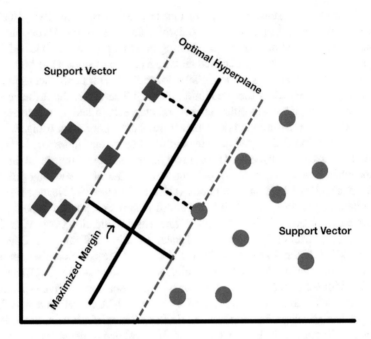

Fig. 6.8 Support vector machine

basis in statistical learning theory, SVM provides a systematic solution to machine learning problems. SVM is often used for classification, regression, novelty detection, and feature reduction problems and provides a solution by using a subset of the training input. These are their two main advantages (in the thou-sands). This method is perfect for problems involving text classification when a dataset of a few thousand tagged samples is the norm (Fig. 6.8).

6.3.2.2 K-Nearest Neighbor (KNN)

Using no previous knowledge of the original dataset, the KNN is a nonparametric classification technique. It is renowned for both its efficiency and ease of usage. The class of the unlabeled data can be predicted because the data points in a labelled training dataset are divided into multiple classes. Although this classifier is straightforward, the 'K' value is crucial for identifying unlabeled data. The term "k nearest neighbor" refers to the ability to repeatedly run the classifier with various values to determine which one produces the best results.

Automated model parameter estimation and manual setting of model hyper parameters are used to estimate model parameters. As the components of machine learning that need to be manually set and tweaked, model hyper parameters are sometimes referred to as "parameters." The K Nearest Neighbors operates in this manner. The nearest neighbors of our new data point are the data points that are

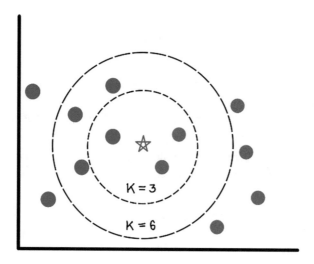

Fig. 6.9 K-nearest neighbor

separated from it by the least feature space. Our approach considers K of these data points, which is a fixed quantity. The distance metric and K value of the KNN algorithm are therefore important parameters. The Euclidean distance is the distance unit that is used the most frequently. There are also the Minkowski and Hamming distances, as well as the Manhattan and Manhattan distances. When determining the class or continuous value of a new data point, the training dataset's whole collection of data points is considered. Finds the K nearest neighbors of new data points by searching feature space, class labels, or continuous values (Fig. 6.9).

6.3.3   Evaluation Measures

6.3.3.1   Accuracy

According to [24], the disarray framework concept is used to evaluate the classifier's demonstration. The total number of predictions made to determine classification accuracy divides the total number of accurate predictions given a dataset. Accuracy is insufficient as a performance metric for imbalanced classification problems. This is mostly due to the fact that the dominant class(es) will exceed the minority class(es), which implies that even untrained models can get accuracy scores of 90% or 999%, depending on how severe the class imbalance is. There are four categories for each administered class. Focusing on the classes of lateral and hook gestures, we are defining:

Lateral and hook gestures

- True Positive (TP): How frequently does the characterization computation predict "lateral" even when "lateral" is the true class?
- False Positive (FP): How frequently does the categorization computation predict "lateral" even when the real class is "hook"? Also known as a "Type I Error".
- False Negative (FN): How often does the order computation predict, "hook" when the real class is "lateral"? Also known as a "Type II Error"
- How often does the arrangement computation predict "hook" when the true class is "palmar"? [24].

The accuracy is the range of real orders that can range from 0 to 1, with 1 representing the best accuracy result as given in Eq. (6.11).

$$Accuracy = \frac{T_P + T_N}{T_P + T_N + F_P + F_N} \times 100\%. \tag{6.11}$$

6.3.3.2   Precision

Another statistical measure is called precision. It counts the number of accurate positive forecasts. Precision calculates the accuracy for the minority class as a result. It is determined by dividing the total expected number of positive occurrences by the number of accurately predicted positive cases. When the TNs and TPs classifications are appropriate, Eq. (6.12) may be used to quantitatively describe this measure. Findings from categorization that are FPs or FNs are wrong.

$$Precision = \frac{TP}{(TP + FP)}. \tag{6.12}$$

6.3.3.3   Specificity

As indicated in Eq. (6.13), the percentage of accurately detected adverse events is known as specificity.

$$Specificity = \frac{TN}{(TN + FP)}. \tag{6.13}$$

6.3.3.4   Recall

The recall, as it is described in Eq. (6.14), is a measure that counts the actual positive predictions that were made as opposed to all possible positive predictions. Recall takes into account all positive predictions, as opposed to accuracy, which only takes into account the right positive predictions among all positive predictions. Recall in this method indicates the coverage of the positive class [24].

$$Recall = \frac{TP}{(TP + FN)}.$$ (6.14)

6.3.3.5 F-Score

The F-score evaluates the precision of a model on a certain dataset. It is used to assess algorithms that categorize occurrences as either "positive" or "negative," or in between. A statistic for assessing information retrieval systems is the F-score. It is possible to adjust the F-score to emphasize accuracy over recall or the opposite. Equation represents the harmonic mean of accuracy and recall, which is the classic F1 score Eq. (6.15) [25].

$$F = \frac{2 * precision * recall}{precision + recall}.$$ (6.15)

6.3.3.6 Kappa Statistics

Cohen's K-coefficient, which measures inter-rater agreement, measures the degree of agreement between two variables; hence, kappa most frequently deals with data that is the result of a judgment rather than a measurement. The likelihood of agreement is compared by Kappa to what may be expected if the ratings were independent. Kappa is another means of conveying the classifier's accuracy [26]. Conditions, Eqs. (6.16) to (6.18), can be used to calculate Kappa.

$$kappa = 1 - \frac{1 - p_0}{1 - p_e}.$$ (6.16)

$$p_o = \frac{(TP + TN)}{(TP + TN + FP + FN)}.$$ (6.17)

$$p_e = \frac{(TP + TN)(TP + FN) + (FP + TN)(FP + FN)}{(TP + TN + FP + FN)^2}.$$ (6.18)

6.4   Results and Discussion

T The performance of the created method is assessed using the six hand-gesture characteristics. Each gesture was made by the participants 30 times for a total of six seconds each gesture. The recordings were made with a conversion resolution of 12 bits and a sample rate of 500 Hz. The proposed windowing method is used to segment the ADC output. The maximum segment length is three seconds. To provide the qualities of each instance, features from each segment are extracted and combined. The extracted feature set is then processed using ML-based classifiers. The 10-CV approach is used to evaluate performance. Tables - describe the findings obtained for SVM and KNN, respectively.

The confusion matrices, obtained for the case of each hand gesture are outlined in the following Tables 6.1, 6.2, 6.3, 6.4, 6.5, and 6.6.

The evaluation measures for the case of SVM classifier are outlined in Table 6.7.

In Table 6.7, the spherical gesture (C1) shows the highest values of evaluation indices and the best AUC graph in the prediction parameters of all classes of gestures. When the SVM classification technique is used, it is the simplest to discriminate between maneuvers and the rest of the movements. All six classifiers evaluated had an average recall of 92.2% and an average AUC value of 99.0%, with the Medium Gaussian SVM coming out on top (Fig. 6.10)

The evaluation measures for the case of KNN classifier are outlined in Table 6.8.

In Table 6.8, the measures for the Fine KNN algorithm show the lowest outcome in overall accuracy (70.71%). Based on a confusion matrix and a prediction graph, it has the lowest prediction outcomes. Compared to other algorithms, the Weighted KNN method achieved 94.1 percent accuracy and took just 0.97885 Sec. to run. On the other hand, the classification accuracy of Cosine KNN was the lowest at 81.3%. Cubic KNN, on the other hand, took the longest to train at 30.441 seconds. According to the selection of two attributes, the prediction model presents the predicted with accurate and wrong predictions in the X and Y axis. The Euclidian distance measure, equal distance weight, and a default number of neighbors of 10 are all part of the Medium KNN. With the default parameters, this method has a 91.6% accuracy.

Table 6.1 Class 1 Dataset Records

Gesture	Input (Dataset)
	Spherical gesture 30 times for the duration of 6 seconds.
Result	
Fine KNN	Medium Gaussian SVM
TPs: 3	TPs: 29
FPs: 7	FPs: 0
FNs: 0	FNs: 1
TNs: 110	TNs: 137

Table 6.2 Class 2 Dataset Records

Gesture	Input (Dataset)
	Tiny tools gesture 30 times for the duration of 6 seconds.

Result	
Fine KNN	Medium Gaussian SVM
TPs: 28	TPs: 30
FPs: 0	FPs: 1
FNs: 2	FNs: 0
TNs: 112	TNs: 136

Table 6.3 Class 3 Dataset Records

Gesture	Input (Dataset)
	Palmar gesture 30 times for the duration of 6 seconds.

Result	
Fine KNN	Medium Gaussian SVM
TPs: 19	TPs: 22
FPs: 7	FPs: 3
FNs: 11	FNs: 8
TNs: 121	TNs: 144

It employs the Euclidian distance metric, equal weight of the distance, and a default of 100 neighbors as its default settings for coarse KNN. Based on the default parameters, this algorithm's Accuracy is 92.3 percent. In its computation, the cosine KNN uses a cosine distance metric, equal distance weight, and a de-fault number of neighbors of 10. The accuracy of this method is 81.3% with the default parameters. The Cubic KNN method makes use of an initial set of 10 neighbors and an equal distance weight. This algorithm's accuracy with default parameters is 93.5%. WKNN employs Euclidean distance metrics, the square of squared inverse distance weighted by 10 neighbors, and a default number of neighbors. This algorithm is accurate only 81.1% of the time (Fig. 6.11).

The accuracy is 77.8%, total misclassification costs are 40, prediction speed is ~3800 obs/sec, and training time is 0.8864 seconds in the results of the KNN simulation. Model type is acceptable, KNN number of neighbors is one, distance metric is Euclidean, distance weight is equal, standardize data is true, hyper-parameter options are disabled in the optimizer options, all features used in the model are selected, PCA is disabled before misclassification cost analysis, and the default

Table 6.4 Class 4 Dataset Records

Gesture	Input (Dataset)
	Lateral gesture 30 times for the duration of 6 seconds.

Result	
Fine KNN	Medium Gaussian SVM
TPs: 23	TPs: 29
FPs: 9	FPs: 0
FNs: 7	FNs: 1
TNs: 117	TNs: 137

Table 6.5 Class 5 Dataset Records

Gesture	Input (Dataset)
	Cylindrical gesture 30 times for the duration of 6 seconds.

Result	
Fine KNN	Medium Gaussian SVM
TPs: 24	TPs: 29
FPs: 3	FPs: 2
FNs: 6	FNs: 1
TNs: 116	TNs: 137

misclassification cost matrix is used. On the other hand, the SVM's accuracy is 92.2%, the cost of misclassification as a whole is 14, the prediction speed is ~3400 obs/sec, the training time is 0.77719 sec, the model type is Medium Gaussian SVM, the Kernel Function is Gaussian, the Kernel Scale is 7.2, and the Box Constraint Level is 1. One-to-one standardized data is utilized in the multiclass method, hyper parameter choices in the optimizer are deactivated, all features used in the model are selected, PCA is turned off before PCA, and the default misclassification cost matrix is used.

The event-driven tools are beneficial in terms of the computational effectiveness, processing activity and power consumption reduction and real-time compression [27–29]. The feasibility of incorporating these tools in the suggested method can be investigated in future.

Table 6.6 Class 6 Dataset Records

Gesture	Input (Dataset)
	Hook gesture 30 times for the duration of 6 seconds.

Result	
Fine KNN	Medium Gaussian SVM
TPs: 16	TPs: 27
FPs: 14	FPs: 8
FNs: 14	FNs: 3
TNs: 124	TNs:139

Table 6.7 Prediction evaluations of SVM

RF	Accuracy	Precision	Recall	Specificity	F1	Kappa	AUC
C1	0.994	1.000	0.967	1.000	0.983	0.993	1.00
C2	0.994	0.967	1.000	0.992	0.983	0.993	1.00
C3	0.937	0.880	0.733	0.979	0.80	0.921	0.97
C4	0.994	1.000	0.967	1.000	0.983	0.993	1.00
C5	0.982	0.935	0.967	0.985	0.950	0.978	1.00
C6	0.937	0.771	0.900	0.945	0.830	0.921	0.97
Avg	0.973	0.925	0.922	0.983	0.921	0.966	0.99

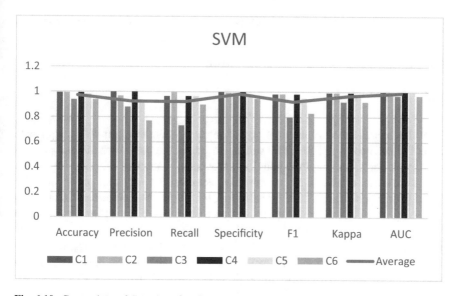

Fig. 6.10 Comparison of Gaussian SVM Prediction Parameters

Table 6.8 Prediction evaluations of KNN

RF	Accuracy	Precision	Recall	Specificity	F1	Kappa	AUC
C1	0.952	0.811	1.000	0.940	0.895	0.938	0.98
C2	0.986	1.000	0.933	1.000	0.965	0.982	0.97
C3	0.886	0.731	0.633	0.945	0.678	0.846	0.79
C4	0.897	0.719	0.767	0.928	0.742	0.862	0.85
C5	0.939	0.889	0.800	0.975	0.842	0.921	0.89
C6	0.833	0.533	0.533	0.899	0.533	0.767	0.72
Avg	0.916	0.780	0.778	0.948	0.776	0.886	0.87

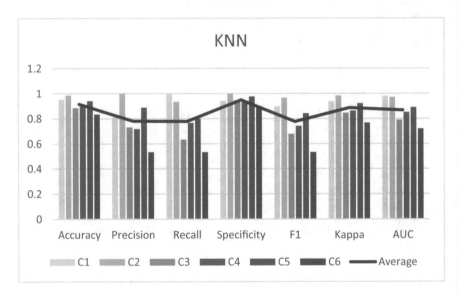

Fig. 6.11 Comparison of KNN Prediction Parameters

6.5 Conclusion

This chapter describes a contemporary automated system that uses sEMG signals to identify hand gestures. The sEMG signals are one of the most often utilized biological signals for predicting the upper limb movement intentions. Turning the sEMG signals to useful control signals frequently necessitates a large amount of computational power and sophisticated techniques. This chapter compares the performance of k-Nearest Neighbor and Support Vector Machine techniques for hand gesture detection based on the processing of sEMG signals. The first stage in this method is to capture the signal from the skin's surface, followed by conditioning, segmentation, and feature extraction. The feature extraction highlights the needed characteristics from the da-ta to recognize the gesture. Following that, the k-Nearest Neighbor and Support Vector Machine techniques were applied on the mined feature set. The training and testing is carried out while following the cross-validation strategy. The prediction of accuracy, AUC, F1 score, precision and Kappa are among the measures utilized in the comparison. The comparison confirms that SVM produces superior results and is best suited, among the studied methods, for the needed application of gesture recognition.

In the conducted study, while processing the sEMG signals with the proposed hybridization of segmentation, discrete wavelet transform, sub-bands feature extraction, and KNN classifiers the tip gesture had the highest accuracy of 98.5%. The accuracy score for the tip gesture is even higher for the case of SVM classifier and it is 99.4%. The average accuracy score of 91.6% and 97.3% is respectively secured by the KNN and SVM classifiers for the 6-intended hand gestures of a mono-subject.

These results are encouraging and the effectiveness of the developed solution will be evaluated in the future for multiple individuals datasets. The Naive bias and other classifiers such as the Artificial Neural Networks, Decision Trees and Random Forests will also be used for categorization. The deep learning and ensemble learning methods will also be investigated.

6.6 Assignments for Readers

- Describe your thoughts and key findings about the use of sEMG signals in prosthetics.
- Mention the important processes that are involved in the pre-processing and sEMG data collection stages.
- Describe how the performance of post feature extraction and classification stages is affected by the sEMG signal conditioning process.
- Identify your thoughts and key points about the sEMG classification techniques used in this chapter.
- Identify your thoughts and key points on the feature s technique used in this chapter.

References

1. WHO standards for prosthetics and orthotics. https://www.who.int/publications-detail-redirect/9789241512480 (Accessed Sep. 01, 2022)
2. A. Chaiyaroj, P. Sri-Iesaranusorn, C. Buekban, S. Dumnin, C. Thanawatta-no, D. Surangsrirat, Deep neural network approach for Hand, wrist, grasping and functional movements classification using low-cost sEMG sensors, in *2019 IEEE International Conference on Bioinformatics and Biomedicine (BIBM)*, (2019), pp. 1443–1448. https://doi.org/10.1109/BIBM47256.2019.8983049
3. A.U. Alahakone, S.M.N. Senanayake, *Vibrotactile feedback sys-tems: Current trends in rehabilitation, sports and information display* (2009), pp. 1148–1153. https://doi.org/10.1109/AIM.2009.5229741
4. W. Park, "The geniuses who invented prosthetic limbs." https://www.bbc.com/future/article/20151030-the-geniuses-who-invented-prosthetic-limbs (accessed Sep. 03, 2022)
5. R. Zhang, X. Zhang, D. He, R. Wang, Y. Guo, sEMG signals characterization and identification of hand movements by machine learning considering sex differences. Appl. Sci. **12**(6), 2962 (2022). https://doi.org/10.3390/app12062962

6. Z. Yang et al., Dynamic gesture recognition using surface EMG signals based on multi-stream residual network. Front. Bioeng. Biotechnol. **9** (2021) Accessed: Sep. 03, 2022. [Online]. Avail-able: https://www.frontiersin.org/articles/10.3389/fbioe.2021.779353

7. What Is Quantization?|How It Works & Applications. https://www.mathworks.com/discovery/quantization.html (Accessed Sep. 03, 2022)

8. S.M. Qaisar, A custom 70-channel mixed signal ASIC for the brain-PET detectors signal read-out and selection. Biomed. Phy. Eng. Express **5**(4), 045018 (2019)

9. A.A. Abualsaud, S. Qaisar, S.H. Ba-Abdullah, Z.M. Al-Sheikh, M. Akbar, *Design and Implementation of a 5-Bit Flash ADC for Education* (2016), pp. 1–4

10. S.M. Qaisar, A. Mihoub, M. Krichen, H. Nisar, Multirate processing with selective subbands and machine learning for efficient arrhythmia classification. Sensors **21**(4), 1511 (2021)

11. S. Kalmegh, Analysis of WEKA Data Mining Algorithm REPTree. Sim-ple Cart and RandomTree for Classification of Indian News **2**(2), 9

12. N. Salankar, S.M. Qaisar, EEG based stress classification by using difference plots of varia-tional modes and machine learning. J. Ambient Intellig. Humanized Comput., 1–14 (2022)

13. S. Mian Qaisar, Baseline wander and power-line interference elimination of ECG signals using efficient signal-piloted filtering. Healthcare Technol. Letters **7**(4), 114–118 (2020)

14. S. Mian Qaisar, N. Hammad, R. Khan, A combination of DWT CLAHE and wiener filter for effective scene to text conversion and pronunciation. J. Electrical Eng. Technol. **15**(4), 1829–1836 (2020)

15. V. Krishnan, B. Anto, Features of wavelet packet decomposition and discrete wavelet trans-form for malayalam speech recognition. **1** (2009)

16. Wavelet Decomposition - an overview | ScienceDirect Topics. https://www.sciencedirect.com/topics/engineering/wavelet-decomposition (Accessed May 09, 2022)

17. What is Feature Extraction? Feature Extraction in Image Processing. https://www.mygreatlearning.com/blog/feature-extraction-in-image-processing/ (Accessed Dec. 13, 2021)

18. 1.3.5.11. Measures of Skewness and Kurtosis. https://www.itl.nist.gov/div898/handbook/eda/section3/eda35b.htm (Accessed Sep. 03, 2022)

19. What is Machine Learning?, Jul. 02, 2021. https://www.ibm.com/sa-en/cloud/learn/machine-learning (Accessed Sep. 03, 2022)

20. H.D. Wehle, Machine Learning, Deep Learning, and AI: What's the Dif-Ference?. (Jul. 2017)

21. What is Deep Learning?. https://www.ibm.com/cloud/learn/deep-learning (accessed Sep. 03, 2022)

22. S.M. Qaisar, A. López, D. Dallet, F.J. Ferrero, *sEMG Signal based Hand Gesture Recognition by using Selective Subbands Coefficients and Machine Learning* (2022), pp. 1–6

23. H. Fatayerji, R. Al Talib, A. Alqurashi, S.M. Qaisar, *sEMG Signal Features Extraction and Machine Learning Based Gesture Recognition for Prosthesis Hand* (2022), pp. 166–171

24. J. Brownlee, How to calculate precision, recall, and F-measure for Im-balanced classification. Machine Learning Mastery, Jan. 02 (2020) https://machinelearningmastery.com/precision-recall-and-f-measure-for-imbalanced-classification/ (Accessed Sep. 04, 2022)

25. F-Score. DeepAI. (2019). https://deepai.org/machine-learning-glossary-and-terms/f-score (Accessed Sep. 04, 2022)

26. Kappa Statistics - an overview | ScienceDirect Topics. https://www.sciencedirect.com/topics/medicine-and-dentistry/kappa-statistics (Accessed Sep. 04, 2022)

27. S. Mian Qaisar, F. Alsharif, Signal piloted processing of the smart meter data for effective appliances recognition. J. Electrical Eng. Technol. **15**(5), 2279–2285 (2020)

28. S.M. Qaisar, S.I. Khan, D. Dallet, R. Tadeusiewicz, P. Pławiak, Sig-nal-piloted processing metaheuristic optimization and wavelet decomposi-tion based elucidation of arrhythmia for mobile healthcare. Biocybernet. Biomed. Eng. **42**(2), 681–694 (2022)

29. S.M. Qaisar, Efficient mobile systems based on adaptive rate signal pro-cessing. Comput. Elect. Eng. **79**, 106462 (2019)

Chapter 7
Review of EEG Signals Classification Using Machine Learning and Deep-Learning Techniques

Fatima Hassan and Syed Fawad Hussain

Abstract Electroencephalography (EEG) signals have been widely used for the prognosis and diagnosis of several disorders, such as epilepsy, schizophrenia, Parkinson's disease etc. EEG signals have been shown to work with machine learning techniques in the literature. However, they require manual extraction of features beforehand which may change from dataset to dataset or depending on the disease application. Deep learning, on the other hand, have the ability to process the raw signals and classify data without requiring any domain knowledge or manually extracted features but lacks a good understanding and interpretability. This chapter will discuss different techniques of machine learning including features extraction and selection methods from filtered signals and classification of these selected features for clinical applications. We have also discussed two case studies i.e., epilepsy and schizophrenia detection. These case studies use an architecture which combines deep learning with traditional ML techniques and compare their results. Using this hybrid model, an accuracy of 94.9% is obtained based on EEG signals obtained from epileptic and normal subjects, while an accuracy of 98% accuracy is achieved in schizophrenia detection using only three EEG channels. The latter result is significant as it is comparable to other state of art techniques while requiring less data and computational power.

F. Hassan
Faculty of Computer Science and Engineering, GIK Institute, Topi, Pakistan
e-mail: gce2044@giki.edu.pk

S. F. Hussain (✉)
Faculty of Computer Science and Engineering, GIK Institute, Topi, Pakistan

School of Computer Science, University of Birmingham, Birmingham, UK
e-mail: s.f.hussain@bham.ac.uk

© The Author(s), under exclusive license to Springer Nature Switzerland AG 2023
S. Mian Qaisar et al. (eds.), *Advances in Non-Invasive Biomedical Signal Sensing and Processing with Machine Learning*, https://doi.org/10.1007/978-3-031-23239-8_7

7.1 Introduction

Biomedical signals carry useful information regarding the physiological activities of the human which might not be directly observed. Significant research has been conducted to extract meaningful information from these signals. This information can be useful in developing automated real-time detection of different disorders using machine learning algorithms. EEG is a neuroimaging technique which records the electrical activity generated by population of neurons inside the human brain. It allows the non-invasive monitoring of patients' health and diagnose different brain disorders such as Epilepsy, Alzheimer, Parkinson's, and other brain disorders. These diseases often cause abnormalities in EEG readings. Generally, clinicians and physicians analyze these signals visually which is laborious, time-consuming and may result in inefficient results.

Brain computer interface (BCI) is another multidisciplinary area which has recently piqued attention due to its potential to provide communication and control to patients with severe movement disorders. It allows a physically disabled person to control an external device such as prosthetics using EEG signals rather than muscle activity. The majority of BCI applications, including wheelchair control, emotion recognition, prosthetic arms, etc., use EEG signals. BCI implementation requires an effective strategy for processing these complex EEG signals. These challenges inspired researchers to develop different signal processing, feature extraction, feature selection algorithms in combination with machine and deep learning. The human brain is divided into two hemispheres, left and right, and four lobes, i.e., Temporal, Frontal, Occipital, Parietal and Central lobe. Each lobe has its own specialized functions, and when performing them, it releases different rhythmic waves. The EEG signals are recorded by means of non-invasive electrodes placed at different positions on the scalp. There are two modes for positioning of electrodes which are unipolar and bipolar. In the first mode, each electrode measures the voltage difference compared to a reference electrode and each electrode-reference pair forms a channel. The voltage difference between two specified electrodes are recorded in bipolar mode and each pair creates a channel [1]. One to 256 channels can be found in a standard EEG system. The EEG waveforms recorded are categorized into five bands based on their frequency ranges. Most of the important information of human brain activity lie in these five bands. These frequency bands along with their frequency ranges are listed in Table 7.1. The *Delta band* consists of slowest waves with highest amplitude. These rhythms occur in deep sleep. *Theta waves* are observed in a state of meditation. *Alpha waves* are normally seen when the subject under observation is awake but is in a state of deep relaxation with eyes closed. When the brain is in a state of active concentration or engaged in activities such as thinking, decision making etc., *Beta waves* are generated. Lastly, *Gamma* waves occur when the subject is intensely focused.

The sensorimotor rhythm which reflects human movement is also a component of the alpha and beta frequency bands. Akbulut et al. [3] extracted features from these bands for the classification of hand movements. Similarly, Jatupaiboon et al.

Table 7.1 Frequency ranges Corresponding to each EEG Band [2]

EEG bands	Frequency range
Delta	< 4 Hz
Theta	4 – 8 Hz
Alpha	8 – 13 Hz
Beta	13 – 30 Hz
Gamma	> 30 Hz

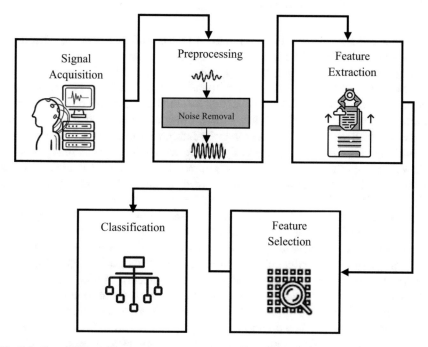

Fig. 7.1 General Block Diagram of AI-based Classifiers for EEG Signals [2]

[4] performed the frequency band analysis and channel-based analysis of EEG signals for emotion classification.

This chapter covers different signal processing techniques and feature extraction methods to extract the relevant and dominant features which are then sent to machine learning models for classification. Figure 7.1 shows the basic block diagram of an artificial intelligence (AI) based classification of EEG signals.

There are five common steps in all AI-based classification algorithms. The first step is signal acquisition which is already discussed above. The next step is signal pre-processing which involves noise and artifacts removal. Researchers have proposed different signal processing techniques depending upon the problem and the type of artifacts. For multi-channel data, some researchers have used channel selection techniques also where only a subset of the channels are selected rather than the entire data. The third step is feature extraction which aims to find the most informative set of features from the raw signals. Among them, the most discriminative features are then selected using feature selection algorithms which discards the irrelevant features. This reduction in features in turn decreases the processing time and improves the accuracy. Finally, the last step is the classification of these features for which different architectures have been proposed.

7.2　Signal Pre-Processing

Although EEG has shown to be a powerful tool in different domains, it still has some limitations that make it difficult to analyze or process. The EEG signals are susceptible to noise and artefacts which can affect the quality of a signal. Artefacts are the unwanted signals due to external and internal interferences, experimental errors and environmental noise, power and line interferences, eye blinking, muscle movements and heartbeat etc. These artefacts may imitate cognitive or pathogenic activity which can affect the neurologist's interpretation and lead to misleading results. Cutting the entire segment of data affected by the artefacts might result in the loss of important information. For real-time processing, manual artefact extraction would be almost impossible. These artifacts should be removed from EEG signals for further processing. There should be some automated technique for artefact separation. Different methods have been used for noise removal and signal filtration. Some of them are discussed briefly here.

EEG signals are regarded as non-stationary due to the presence of high and low frequency noises. The effect of these noises and artifacts can be reduced by basic filters, such as low-pass, band-pass, high-pass, etc. Selection of filters depends upon the frequency range of the artifacts. Low-pass filter attenuates the frequencies which are higher than the certain level. On the other hand, high-pass filter removes the frequencies below a certain threshold. Low-frequency noises in EEG signals can be removed by passing them through low-pass filters. Similarly, noise due to muscle movements is a high frequency noise and therefore can be reduced through high-pass filter [5]. In most of the BCI applications, high pass filters are employed to eliminate the very low frequency noises, such as those of breathing [6]. Moreover, low pass filters that have a cut-off frequency of 40–70 Hz are used to reduce or eliminate high-frequency noise [7].

In case of band-pass filters, only frequencies within a specific range can pass through them. The signals below and upper the limit of this range are discarded. Band-stop filter is the reverse of band-pass filter. The signals below the lower and upper limit of the range remain undistorted and all the signals within this range are discarded. The power line introduces 50 Hz or 60 Hz electromagnetic waves and is the source of the most substantial noise. The value of power line noise is from 10 mV to 1 V whereas the EEG signals without artifacts have a value from 0 to 70μV [8]. It can corrupt the data of a few or even all electrodes. Therefore, Maiorana et al. [9] applied band-stop filter on the signals to eliminate power line noise. It discards the signals within a narrow frequency range. Band-pass filters allow you to focus your study on specific frequency bands that are relevant to your application [9, 10]. Another commonly used filter is a notch filter [11, 12]. Notch filter with a central frequency of 50 or 60 Hz is used to minimize power line interference. It allows all frequencies to pass through except the interfering frequencies [12–15]. used Butterworth filter for noise removal. Adaptive filters are also used for signal denoising. They have the ability to modify themselves according to the properties of signal being analyzed [16].

Some research studies have used Blind Source Separation (BSS) techniques for signal pre-processing. The BSS [17] separates the source signals from mixed signals with little or no knowledge about the source signals or the mixing process. Independent Component Analysis (ICA) is an example of a BSS technique. It decomposes a complex mixed signal into independent components. Some of these components represent original data sources whereas others represent the artifacts. If these artifactual components are used in training machine learning models, they can affect the classification accuracy. Therefore, the features extracted from these artifactual components should be removed. Artifacts such as eye movement, EEG, electrocardiogram (ECG), and electrical grounding noise are all generated by statistically independent signal sources [18]. The ICA method can separate them and extract relevant information from EEG signals. This approach has been reported to detect artefacts in certain papers [19–21]. It also improves the signal quality in multichannel EEG data. This has been proven in numerous studies including various numbers of channels, ranging from 16 to many more [21, 22].

ICA is computationally efficient but requires more computations to decompose a signal into components [18]. Its performance depends upon the volume and length of the data segment. Higher the volume of data, higher will be the performance of ICA in terms of artifact removal. Sai et al. [23] applied ICA along with wavelet multiresolution analysis on EEG signals to filter out artifactual components with minimal distortion to the signals of interest. The EEG signal from each channel is then decomposed to 8 levels using Debauchies (db8) mother wavelet. Among these 8 levels, D1, D2 and A8 were discarded as they contain high frequency noise and artifacts. Then, ICA is applied on remaining levels containing frequencies of interest.

One commonly used BSS technique is the Principal Component Analysis (PCA). PCA works by reducing the dimensionality which is useful for artifact removal and noise reduction [24, 25]. PCA decomposes the EEG signal into linearly unrelated vectors known as principal components which are then split into two groups: one related to brain activity and the other associated to artefacts. The components related to brain activity are then used to reconstruct the clean and filtered EEG signal. However, in real recorded signals, the assumption of orthogonality in PCA is not always met which affects the performance significantly. Some studies employed Empirical Mode Decomposition (EMD) [26, 27]. Patel et al. [28] applied PCA with Ensemble EMD on EEG signals to suppress the effects of eye blink artefacts.

Wavelet transforms (WT) is a proven technique for analyzing non-stationary signals due to their ability to accurately capture transient events [29]. They provide multi-scale analysis of EEG signals in both time and frequency domain [30]. To suppress the effect of noise, different operations such as thresholding are applied in spatial domain [31]. Salis et al. [32] applied discrete wavelet transform (DWT) to eliminate artifacts applied at each scale. Then these wavelet coefficients are transformed back to construct the signal. Zhao et al. [33] also employed wavelet packet transforms (WPT) for artifact removal.

7.3   Features Extraction

Machine Learning algorithms require features for classification. Feature is an identifiable measurement, or a distinguishing attribute which is extracted from data segment of a pattern. These features are required to reduce the computational complexity, number of resources and lower the cost of data processing. The most critical step in any classification model is the extraction of relevant features as it directly affects the classifier's performance [34]. For correct interpretation, it is necessary to extract the most informative statistical features from the EEG signal. Feature extraction involves conversion of raw data into numerical features while preserving the original data's information. Different feature extraction algorithms have been used by the researchers which are discussed here in detail.

7.3.1   Fast Fourier Transform (FFT)

FFT transform the signal from a time to the frequency domain. By doing so, hidden features become more apparent. Suppose $f(t)$ is a continuous-time signal, then a Fourier transform $F(\omega)$ is given by the following mathematical equation:

$$F(\omega) = \int_{-\infty}^{\infty} f(t) e^{j\omega t} dt$$

$$(7.1)$$

Here, ω is the frequency. Delimayanti et al. [35] extracted features using FFT for sleep stage classification. They segmented EEG signals into equal time intervals termed as epochs. These epochs were then subjected to frequency analysis using FFT. Rashid et al. [36] extracted standard deviation, average spectral density, energy entropy and spectral centroid from alpha and beta bands of EEG signals. Average spectral density is computed using FFT. All these features were then fed to a classifier. A study in [37] also used FFT for classification of depressive subjects from the normal ones. FFT has a limitation that it focusses only on spectral information but does not provide any time-domain information.

7.3.2 Short-Time Fourier Transform (STFT)

To cover the limitations of FFT, STFT is proposed which analyses the EEG signals in a time-frequency domain. It divides the signal of interest into short segments using a windowing technique. These short segments are then analyzed using the standard Fourier transform. The mathematical equation of STFT is written as:

$$F(\tau,\omega) = \int_{-\infty}^{\infty} f(t)\omega(t-\tau)e^{-i\omega t}dt$$

$$(7.2)$$

where represents the window function, $f(t)$ is the input signals and $F(\tau\ \omega)$ is the Fourier transform representing the signal over time and frequency. STFT is also used for extracting features from spectrograms. Spectrogram is a 3D representation of a signal amplitude with respect to time and frequency. There are different parameters which should be selected appropriately as they effect the resolution of a spectrogram such as window length, window type, number of FFT points, etc. [10]. Zabidi et al. [10] used Hamming window of width 0.1–0.8 s to compute STFT. Ramos-Aguilar et al. [38] also computed STFT or spectrogram and then extracted features from them to detect epileptic seizures. Although STFT provides both time and frequency information but it has a fixed-time resolution [38].

7.3.3 Continuous Wavelet Transform

It is another feature extraction technique used to extract event related time-frequency features from EEG signals. CWT convolves the scaled and translated wavelet functions $\varphi(t)$ with the input data sequence and generate a two-dimensional time-frequency scalograms. The mathematical equation of CWT is:

$$CWT(n,s) = \frac{1}{\sqrt{s}} \int_{-\infty}^{+\infty} x(t).\varphi^*\left(\frac{t-n}{s}\right)dt$$

$$(7.3)$$

Here, $\varphi\varphi(t)$ is a mother wavelet function, $x(t)$ represents input signal, n and s are scaling and translation parameters. Upadhyay et al. [39] computed statistical features from the CWT coefficients and used them for alcoholism diagnosis. Zhao et al. [40] generated scalograms by applying CWT on the raw EEG signals. The features extracted using CWT are then passed as an input for training classifiers. But CWT based feature extraction is computationally intensive.

7.3.4   Discrete Wavelet Transform

DWT is a common feature extractor for the analysis of time-series data. DWT decomposes the time-series data into different components having different frequencies at different scales using a set of basis function. This function is formed by compression and dilation of a mother wavelet. Let a and b represent the scaling parameter and translation parameter. For an input signal $f(t)$, the DWT would be:

$$DWT(a,b) = \frac{1}{\sqrt{b}} \sum_{m=0}^{p-1} f(t_m).\varphi^* \left(\frac{t_m - a}{b} \right) dt$$

$$(7.4)$$

Here, $\varphi\varphi(t)$ is a mother wavelet function. The input signal is passed through a multiple high and low pass filters and generate detailed coefficient and the approximated coefficients. The approximated coefficients are then further passed through the series of filters. There are seven different wavelets which are commonly used. These are Haar, Symlets, Discrete Meyer, Reverse Biorthogonal, Biorthogonal, Daubechies and Coiflets. Figure 7.2 shows the decomposition of EEG signal ($F[t_m]$) into five sub-bands D_1, D_2, D_3, D_4 and A_4 using the Debauchies wavelet.

Db4 is the most commonly employed mother wavelet for interpretation of EEG signals. Numerous studies [30, 41–43] have employed DWT based feature extraction. Djemal et al. [30] decomposed the pre-processed EEG segment into five frequency bands using level 4 DWT. Different Statistical features and several entropy values (log energy, Renyi entropy, threshold entropy and Shannon entropy) are computed from these wavelet coefficients, i.e., D1, D2, D3, D4, and A4. Research study in [42] extracted Expected Activity Management (EAM), Higuchi fractal dimension (HFD) and sample entropy from the sub-bands. Another study in [44] extracted fourteen statistical features from DWT coefficients and selected the different combinations of these features for training. Among these 14 features, they found out that energy, entropy and variance provided the best classification accuracy. Qaiser et al. [41] also computed statistical features such as signal power spectrum, skewness, mean absolute value, entropy, kurtosis, standard deviation, mean ratio, zero crossings, peak positive value etc. from the approximate and detailed coefficients.

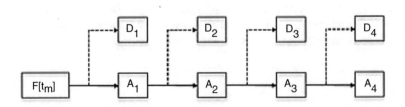

Fig. 7.2 Detailed and Approximate coefficients using Db4 mother wavelet [41]

7.3.5   *Wavelet Packet Decomposition (WPD)*

It is the extended form of DWT which performs multilevel decomposition of EEG signals and used for signal transformation from time domain to frequency domain. In contrast to WT, WPD splits both sub-bands i.e., the low and high frequency band but the frequency bins are of equal width. In wavelet analysis, a signal is divided into approximate and a detail coefficient. The complete binary tree is constructed by decomposing these coefficients. Figure 7.3 shows the block diagram of a 4-level WPD. Studies in [45, 46] extracted features using WPD.

7.4   Features Selection

Some of the features are redundant or are of less importance. These redundant or irrelevant features tend to affect the accuracy. Training the model with the best set of features is a crucial task since selecting the best set of features from any dataset is a difficult process. Using feature selection methods, we can choose the most relevant features and discard the irrelevant ones. The aim of feature selection is to reduce the dimensionality of the features which speeds up the learning and reduce the cost of a learning algorithm. Feature selection methods can be divided into two main types which are discussed below.

Wrapper based feature selection techniques follow a greedy search approach by searching the feature space and testing all the possible feature combinations. The effectiveness of the chosen feature subset is then assessed using the prediction accuracy of the classifiers. Recursive Feature Elimination (RFE) [47] is a wrapper-based method. The method involves fitting the model to the entire dataset initially, then removing the weakest features one at a time until the desired number of features is obtained. There is no specific criterion for elimination of features. The features are recursively eliminated based on the classifier's accuracy. Ting et al. [46] used RFE combined with Support Vector Machine (SVM) classifier. All the features in a

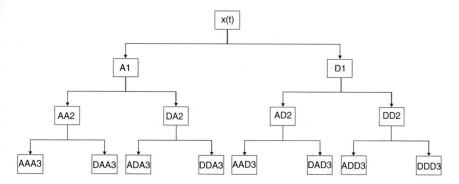

Fig. 7.3   3-Level Wavelet Packet decomposition

feature vector are assigned with a weight value. These weight values are learned by kernel function of SVM. Then, RFE eliminates the features with lowest weight values recursively.

Roy et al. [48] used two strategies to pick the fewest number of features. The first one is PCA, which compresses a dataset into a lower-dimensional feature subspace in such a way that majority of the important information is preserved. Then, RFE technique is used which assigns a score to each feature and choose the ones with the highest score. As, the wrapper-based methods are optimized according to the learning algorithm therefore, any modification to the learning algorithm may affect the subset quality. Also, these methods are computationally expensive.

On the other hand, filter methods use intrinsic aspects of data to select relevant features. They are independent of learning algorithm used such as mutual information (MI) technique. It is a feature selection technique which uses MI score to assess which features convey more information [49]. The MI score is a measure of dependency between the output label (A) and input feature (B) and is given by:

$$I(A;B) = \iint_{AB} p(A,B) \log \frac{p(A,B)}{p(A)p(B)} dA dB$$

(7.5)

Here, $p(A)$ and $p(B)$ represents the marginal density functions, $p(A, B)$ denotes the joint probability density functions, A represent feature distribution and B represent the class distribution. If the input feature and target variable are independent of each other, MI score would become equal to 0. Higher value of MI score indicates that this feature is more discriminatory [41, 50, 51].

Another technique named Minimum Redundancy and Maximum Relevance (MRMR) is devised for microarray data [52]. It selects a subset of features that have the strongest correlation with a target class and the least association with each other. It ranks features using the minimal-redundancy-maximal-relevance criterion. To calculate relevance, the F-statistic or MI can be used, while redundancy can be estimated using the Pearson correlation coefficient or MI. Subhani et al. [53] selected the most relevant features using MRMR for stress classification.

7.5 Machine Learning Techniques

Machine Learning is a rapidly emerging field and have numerous applications in the medical domain. Clinical EEG analysis can be automated using machine learning techniques. Researchers have used different classifiers such as Logistic Regression (LR), Linear Discriminant Analysis (LDA), SVM, Random Forest (RF), Gradient Boosting (GB), k-Nearest Neighbors (KNN), etc.

The logistic regression [29] is a statistical analysis method used to model dichotomous variables given a set of independent variables. However, it can also be extended to a multiclass problem. It predicts the likelihood of an event occurring by fitting data to a logit function. It is a simple, efficient, and easy to implement classifier. But for high-dimensional data, it leads to overfitting.

LDA [54] is another widely used machine learning classifier. Assuming data is normally distributed and linearly separable classes, LDA draws a hyperplane and project the data onto it in such a way that the interclass variance is minimized and the intraclass distance is maximized. It is generally used for two class problems, but it can also be extended to problems with multiple classes. For multiple classes, it creates multiple linear discrimination functions representing several hyperplanes in the feature space. In [54], LDA is used for classification of EEG imagery tasks. Another study in [55] used LDA for deceit identification. LDA is not only a robust classifier, but it is also used for data visualization, dimensionality reduction and feature extraction. But it does not always provide good performance for non-linear classification.

Like LDA, SVM [56] is a linear classifier which uses discriminant hyperplanes to separate data items belonging to different classes. The hyperplane is optimized maximizes the distance between the hyperplane and the closest training data points known as support vectors. For non-linear data, it maps the feature space into a higher dimension using kernel function. This higher dimensional data is then classified using a linear decision boundary. Some of the most commonly used kernel functions include linear, radial basis function (RBF), polynomial and sigmoid. SVM classifier has been widely employed for diagnosis of various neurological disorders, cognitive processes [34] and BCI application [57]. It has a high generalization and thus prevents the model from over-fitting.

The KNN [34] is a supervised algorithm that assigns a class label to a new data sample based on the class of k-nearest training samples. It uses a distance metric such as Manhattan, Euclidean, Minkowski, hamming distance etc. to compute the similarity between an unseen point and its k neighbors. Studies [34, 57] used KNN for interpretation of EEG signals. It is robust to noise and simple to implement. But it has high computational cost. KNN saves training data, and all computation occurs at the time of classification. That is why it requires more memory compared to other classifiers.

Ensemble methods have also been used to boost the classification accuracy. Some of the most commonly used ensemble-based algorithms include RF, GB etc.

7.6 Deep Learning Techniques

Due to the ability to learn appropriate feature representations from raw data, deep learning has recently shown significant potential in interpreting EEG signals. It is a subfield of machine learning which provides an automated end-to-end learning from preprocessing to the classification of data samples while also achieving competitive performance on the objective task. The use of these networks in neuroimaging is on the rise, with recent studies using them to investigate cognitive tasks, diagnose disorders and human emotions detection.

Artificial Neural Network (ANN) refers to an architecture for processing information composed of a set of and is composed of interconnected nodes that mimic the biological neurons in a human brain. They are used for EEG based detection of autism [30], epileptic seizures [58], emotions [59], depression [37], Sleep Apnea [44] and BCI applications [60].

Convolutional neural networks (CNNs) are feed-forward neural networks capable of learning internal representations of data. Unlike machine learning classifiers, they are able to learn automatically without requiring any domain knowledge and features. The input data is passed through multiple convolutional and pooling layers. The convolutional layers consist of kernels or filters. These kernels convolve with the input data and generate output feature maps. For accurate classification, the hyperparameters of CNN should be tuned appropriately. Each convolution layer has an activation function that decides which neuron should be activated or not. Acharya et al. [61] presented a deep CNN architecture consisting of thirteen layers which classify EEG signals into normal, pre-ictal, and seizure classes. Nissimagoudar et al. [62] used a deep (CNN) to learn features. These features were then used to detect whether the car driver is alert while driving or in a drowsy state. Another research study [63] presented a CNN architecture which learns features from raw EEG signals to classify depressive and normal subjects. Oh et al. [64] also used CNN for the Parkinson's disease detection. Similarly, research study in [65] proposed a 23-layered CNN architecture for the classification of abnormal and normal EEG signals. Automatic feature extraction capabilities of deep learning networks are now used along with Machine learning classifiers for improved classification.

Another deep learning architecture is Recurrent Neural networks (RNN). They have the ability to capture information from the past inputs. In RNN, the neurons within the layer also share connections with each other. They can capture higher dimensional dependencies from time-series or sequential data, such as EEG signals. Traditional RNNs are quick in learning the short-term dependencies; however, due to vanishing and expanding gradient, they struggle to learn long-term dynamics. Long Short-term memory (LSTM) network is a form of RNN that can learn both long and short-term dependencies to solve vanishing and exploding gradient problems. It consists of three parts or gates namely forget, input and output gates. The forget gate decides whether the information coming from the previous layer is relevant or not. If not, then forget this information. The input gate learns the information from the input and the third part which is the output gate passes this information to the next cell. Zhang et al. [66] used LSTM for classifying hand movements. Recently, a hybrid architecture using both CNN and LSTM is designed which has shown significant improvement in terms of performance and classification accuracies.

7.7 Case Studies

7.7.1 Epilepsy Detection

Epilepsy is a neurological disorder which generate irregular and recurrent seizures. A seizure is an abnormal electrical activity that occurs suddenly in your brain. If not diagnosed, these seizures can even lead to death. Timely detection of these seizures is necessary in order to start medication and treatment. EEG is a widely used modality for screening epileptic patients. Manual examination of these highly complex and non-stationary signal is a quite laborious and time-consuming process. Therefore, [2] proposed a hybrid model of CNN and machine learning for automated detection of epileptic seizures.

7.7.1.1 Dataset

A publicly available dataset of CHB-MIT is used. This dataset consists of long duration EEG signals of 23 pediatric patients. These signals are recorded using 23 channels with a sampling rate of 256 Hz. The recorded signals were then split into 5 s segments consisting of 1280 sampling points. Here each segment makes an instance. Out of total 23 channels, they have considered only 22 channels because the data in 22nd and 23rd channel is almost similar. As, there are total 22 channels therefore, each segment consists of 1280 × 22 sampling points.

7.7.1.2 Methodology

As discussed previously, the EEG signals often get contaminated with noise and artifacts. Therefore, for signal denoising and filtration, they used Butterworth filter of order 2. The frequency content of a signal is confined between 0.5 and 50 Hz. In the relevant literature, we have observed that the deep learning architectures are most widely used for automatic learning of intrinsic aspects of data. In this study, CNN is used to classify the epileptic and non-epileptic patients. Before passing them to CNN, these filtered EEG signals were normalized between 0 and 1 using z-score normalization. Figure 7.4 shows the architecture CNN used in this study. Unlike machine learning classifiers, CNN can automatically learn from the data. CNN consists of two parts namely feature extraction and classification part. They consist of a stack of convolution and pooling layers which performs feature extraction. These convolution layers consist of kernels or filters which are convolved with the 1D data of EEG signals and generate feature maps. Different number of kernels are tried and their effect on the accuracy is observed. The number of kernels on which maximum accuracy is obtained are fixed.

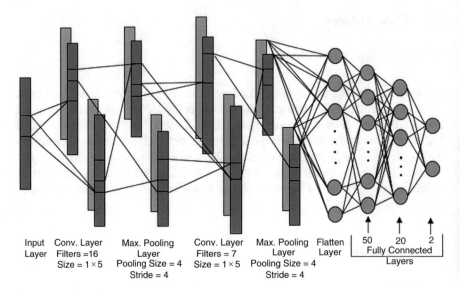

Input   Conv. Layer   Max. Pooling   Conv. Layer   Max. Pooling   Flatten   50   20   2
Layer   Filters =16   Layer   Filters = 7   Layer   Layer   Fully Connected
         Size = 1 × 5   Pooling Size = 4 Size = 1 × 5 Pooling Size = 4   Layers
                         Stride = 4   Stride = 4

Fig. 7.4 CNN Architecture for Epileptic Seizures Detection

Table 7.2 Summary of Classification Results for Epileptic Seizures Detection

Dataset	ANN	LR	RF	SVM	GB	KNN
CHB-MIT	91.6	88.5	90.5	92	92	94.9

These feature maps are then passed onto another layer known as the maximum pooling layer. The pooling layer selects the high-level features from these feature maps and reduces the dimensionality, number of parameters and amount of computation needed to process these features. The input data after passing through successive convolution and pooling layers reaches the flatten layer. The second part of a CNN is a classification part which consists of dense layers. These layers take 1D data as an input. But the feature maps are 2-dimensional. Therefore, the flatten layer is added to transform these 2D feature maps into a 1D feature vector. This feature map is then passed through three dense layers consisting of 50, 20 and 2 neurons, respectively. Note that the number of neurons in the last layer indicate the number of classes. A ten-fold cross-validation is used for training CNN model. The CNN based classification achieved 91.6% accuracy. Machine learning classifiers are very powerful, but they require features. Therefore, they extracted features from the flatten layer and sent them to different machine learning classifiers for classification. The results obtained are given in Table 7.2. When the features learnt by CNN are passed to KNN, the accuracy increased to 94.9%.

7.7.2 Schizophrenia Detection

Schizophrenia is a chronic mental illness which effect the daily activities of patients. The symptoms of this disease include hallucinations, delusions and other socio-psychological issues. Normally, it is diagnosed by conducting interviews and observing the symptoms. But this examination requires continuous monitoring of patients. Researchers have used different modalities to detect schizophrenic patients. Most of the researchers have used EEG modality due to its non-invasive nature along with a high temporal resolution. The study in [2] proposes a new model by fusing CNN and machine learning classifiers with the combination of only three channels.

7.7.2.1 Dataset

For analysis, researchers have used publicly available dataset collected from the Institute of Psychiatry and Neurology in Warsaw, Poland. The dataset consists of 15 minutes long EEG recordings from 28 patients including 14 SZ and 14 normal subjects. These signals are recorded using 19 channels with a sampling frequency of 250 Hz which are then divided into 20 sec segments. Each segment behaves as an instance consisting of 5000 sampling points. As there are total 19 channels, therefore each instance comprises of 5000×19 sampling points. All these instances are passed to a Butterworth filter for artifact removal. Then four datasets are created to study the effect of all channels, individual channels, different brain regions and selected channels on Schizophrenia detection.

7.7.2.2 Methodology

First of all, data is passed through a Butterworth filter and then applied normalization. Then they trained data of all nineteen channels on individual CNN networks. The number of kernels, kernel size, activation function, optimizer etc. are adjusted by varying them and observing their effect on the classification accuracy. There was total nineteen channels used which are Fp1, Fp2, F7, F3, Fz, F4, F8, T3, C3, Cz, C4, T4, T5, P3, Pz, P4, T6, O1, O2.

When the data of all these channels is grouped and trained on CNN, the model classified the instances with 97% accuracy. But, in this dataset, each instance consists of 5000×19 sampling points which is equal to 95,000. Training this high-dimensional data would take time to process. Therefore, CNN based channel selection is employed. Data of all the channels is individually trained on a CNN architecture. They observed that channels T4, Cz, T3 and C4 obtained highest accuracy as compared to the others which indicate that these channels contain more relevant information. From the combination of these channels, four different datasets have been created based on their classification accuracies. Table 7.3 shows the dataset created based on the combination of channels selected.

These datasets are then trained one by one on a CNN architecture. The hyperparameters are chosen by observing their effect on the classification accuracy. Different number of kernels of different sizes are tried. Similarly, the learning rate is increased from 0.01 to 0.0001. After trying different combinations of optimizers and learning rates, they found out that the Adam optimizer used with a learning rate of 0.001 is suitable. So, these parameters were fixed. Figure 7.5 shows the CNN architecture which is trained on selected channel dataset using ten-fold cross-validation.

Like previous case study, the features learnt by CNN are extracted from the flatten layer and passed to different machine learning classifiers. The results obtained are given in Table 7.4.

According to the results mentioned in the above table, when feature extractor of CNN is combined with logistic regression it achieved 98% accuracy. The sampling points or features are also reduced from 5000×19 to 5000×3.

7.8 Discussion

Accurate interpretation of EEG signals is a tedious process and might take years of training. This chapter discusses different machine learning techniques to automate clinical EEG signal analysis for different problems. There are two types of techniques presented in the literature: feature-based and end-to-end learning. Feature based learning requires manual extraction of features beforehand which are then passed to machine learning algorithms. Different combinations of signal processing, feature extraction and selection methods are used to extract more relevant features depending upon the problem. Table 7.5 shows a brief detail of the algorithms used for different problems. In all aforementioned studies based on feature-based learning, a non-linear analysis or an algorithm such as CWT, DWT, FFT, STFT etc. is required to extract features. The algorithm chosen might lose some critical information due to which it may work well on one dataset but fail on another dataset. Selection of the algorithm is quite difficult.

Deep learning or end to end feature learning is a subfield of machine learning which can significantly improve the categorization of EEG signals. Studies in [61–65] employed deep CNN to process EEG signals. The hidden layers have the ability

Table 7.3 Datasets based on Combination of Selected Channels [2]

Dataset name	Channels combination
A	T4, Cz
B	T4, C4, Cz
C	T4, T3, Cz
D	T4, T3, C4, Cz

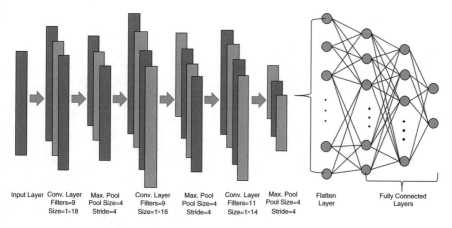

Input Layer | Conv. Layer Filters=9 Size=1×18 | Max. Pool Pool Size=4 Stride=4 | Conv. Layer Filters=9 Size=1×16 | Max. Pool Pool Size=4 Stride=4 | Conv. Layer Filters=11 Size=1×14 | Max. Pool Pool Size=4 Stride=4 | Flatten Layer | Fully Connected Layers

Fig. 7.5 CNN Architecture for Schizophrenia Detection [2]

Table 7.4 Classification Accuracy on "Selected_Channels" Dataset [2]

Datasets	CNN	LR	RF	SVM	GB
A	96.23	96.30	93.85	94.27	94.90
B	97.70	97.77	95.32	96.44	96.30
C	97.84	98.05	96.93	96.30	96.79
D	97	97	95	96	96

to capture the minute details from raw data without requiring feature extraction or selection algorithms. Due to high representational power, more hidden layers are required to learn details from raw EEG signals. Adding more hidden layers might improve the accuracy or might not depending upon the complexity of a problem and data size. Deeper architectures are more prone to overfitting. You can use any network depending upon your problem and the resources available. LSTM is another commonly used network to process time-series data. They have the advantage of being able to analyze lengthy input sequences without expanding the network size. But they require more parameters as compared to CNN.

Hassan et al. [2] employed a hybrid of CNN and ML algorithms in the thesis and presented two case studies epilepsy detection and schizophrenia detection which we have discussed here. This hybrid architecture uses the feature extraction capability of CNN and pass the learnt features to ML algorithms for classification. The model achieved the accuracy comparable to the other state-of-art accuracies for binary class problem without requiring any feature extraction and selection algorithm.

Table 7.5 Summary of research on EEG signals Classification

References	Problem	Preprocessing	Feature extraction and selection	Classification algorithm
[13]	Epileptic seizures detection	High-pass Butterworth filter	Tunable-Q wavelet transform (TQWT) framework Extracted statistical, entropy-based and fractal features	Ensemble-learning algorithms
[14]	Alcoholism detection	–	Wavelet transform PCA	Naive Bayes (NB), SVM, decision tree (DT), RF and GB
[19]	Epileptic seizure detection	Normalization	Extracted statistical features using DWT PCA, ICA and LDA	SVM
[23]	Automated artifacts identification	–	Wavelet multiresolution analysis ICA	SVM
[30]	Autism diagnosis	ICA and adaptive filtering	DWT + statistical features extraction	ANN
[44]	Sleep apnea classification	Infinite impulse response Butterworth band pass filter Hilbert Huang transform	Signal decomposition into five frequency bands Computed statistical features for every frequency band	SVM
[48]	Emotion recognition	–	RFE + PCA	Light gradient boosting machine
[50]	Arrythmia classification	Adaptive rate sampling Bandpass FIR filter	DWT + statistical features extraction MI-based feature selection	RF, SVM
[53]	Stress classification	Notch filter	Applied FFT and computed absolute power and relative power as features Feature selection using MRMR based on MI score	SVM
[54]	Motor imagery (MI) based BCI application	–	Computed PSD using FFT	LDA
[55]	Deceit identification	Bandpass filter	WPT + statistical features	LDA

(continued)

Table 7.5 (continued)

References	Problem	Preprocessing	Feature extraction and selection	Classification algorithm
[57]	Classification of mental tasks	Bandpass filter + Laplacian filter + normalization	Computed power spectral density from periodogram Channel selection	SVM
[61]	Epilepsy detection	Normalization	–	13-layered CNN
[62]	Driver state (alert/drowsy) detection	–	–	CNN
[63]	Depression diagnosis	–		13-layered CNN
[64]	Parkinson's disease detection	–	–	13-layered CNN
[65]	Epilepsy detection	Normalization		23-layered CNN
[66]	Classification of hand movements	Notch filter to remove 50 Hz power line interference + bandpass filter which allows a frequency range of 0.5–70 Hz + min-max normalization	Time-domain and frequency features	Attention-based LSTM network
Case studies	Epilepsy detection		CNN	KNN
	Schizophrenia detection		CNN Channel selection	LR

7.9 Conclusion

Biomedical signals provide a rich source of data to identify various diseases and identify events related to neurological state. EEG signals form an important part of a patient's medical data. This chapter gives an overview of machine learning methods used for EEG classification. To classify EEG data, a combination of different signal processing, feature extraction, and feature selection techniques are used. Numerous machine learning algorithms for the classification of EEG signals have been used in the literature.

The aim of biomedical signal processing is to remove the artifacts due to external and internal environments and transform raw data to a useful form. This transformation is basically feature extraction. Different studies have used different features depending upon the nature of the problem. Some studies extract time-domain features, for instance the mean and variance, whereas others observed that the hidden features become more apparent in frequency domain. In many cases, both time-domain and frequency domain features were considered useful. Overall, there are two major approaches to processing EEG signals in the literature – the first one involves using a combination of signal processing techniques, feature extraction methods, and feature selection algorithms to arrive at a set of derived features which can be used for classification and prediction. This is more efficient but may need domain knowledge for best effectiveness as the set of features may vary according to the problem and the data. The second approach leaves the cumbersome part of feature engineering to the deep learning classifier and uses a one-stop solution. The advantage is less human involvement but requires far more processing time and data to train the model.

Deep Learning architectures can automatically extract features but are complex in nature. For high-dimensional data, additional convolution layers are needed in case of raw EEG signals. More layers mean more parameters and more computations. However, with the addition of a few signal processing steps on the raw EEG data, the number of hidden layers can be significantly reduced. We have presented two case studies using hybrid of CNN and machine learning algorithm. A Butterworth bandpass filter is used for preprocessing of signals. The complex feature extraction part in conventional architectures have been replaced by the automated feature learning capability of CNN. Using this architecture, an accuracy of 94.9% and 98% is achieved for epilepsy and schizophrenia detection.

More research is needed to study the contribution of different channels in the interpretation of EEG signals. In this regard, there can be several further studies on EEG data and machine learning classifiers. For instance, multi-view learning can be a possible future direction where data from different channels are considered as views and a weighted multi-view classifier can automatically assess the contribution of each channel. Another aspect involves deeper study on the contribution of each channel or region of the brain.

7.10   Assignments

The following assignments are suggested for this chapter:

1. Download the Institute of Psychiatry and Neurology dataset. Select all 19 channels, i.e., Fp1, Fp2, F7, F3, Fz, F4, F8, T3, C3, Cz, C4, T4, T5, P3, Pz, P4, T6, O1, and O2. Run the CNN algorithm using parameters given in Sect. 7.7.1.2. Note the accuracy value and time taken using a ten-fold cross-validation strategy. Repeat the experiment with and without using Butterworth filter and Discrete Wavelet Transformation. Compare results and discuss the difference observed.
2. Repeat the experiment above but this time using only 4 channels, i.e., T4, T3, C4, Cz and the CNN architecture given in Fig. 7.5. What can be concluded about these channels?
3. CNN are popularly used deep learning techniques for processing ECG data. A CNN model can be separated into its two constituent parts- the convolution part, responsible for extracting relevant features, and the full connected layers used

for classification training. However, the feature extraction can also be done separately using sophisticated signal processing techniques and used as an input in different supervised machine learning classifiers. Download the CHB-MIT dataset comprising of 23 channels. Use the CNN architecture given in Fig. 7.4 along with ten-fold cross-validation for training the model. Separately, use DWT to generate 5 sub-bands as shown in Fig. 7.2 and extract the following statistical features – kurtosis, power spectrum, peak positive value, standard deviation, skewness, and peak negative value from the sub-bands and classify the data using SVM, ANN, and RF. Compare the results using CNN and feature selection + classification, using accuracy and time taken.

References

1. J.S. Kumar, P. Bhuvaneswari, Analysis of electroencephalography (EEG) signals and its categorization–a study. Procedia Eng. **38**, 2525–2536 (2012). https://doi.org/10.1016/j.proeng.2012.06.298
2. F. Hassan, *Applying Deep Learning Methods for EEG Classification - a Case Study of Epi Lepsy and Schizophrenia* (Master Thesis, Faculty of Computer Science and Engineering, Ghulam Ishaq Khan Institute of Engineering Sciences and Technology, 2022)
3. H. Akbulut, S. Güney, H.B. Çotuk, A.D. Duru, Classification of EEG signals using alpha and beta frequency power during voluntary hand movement, in *Scientific Meeting on Electrical-Electronics & Biomedical Engineering and Computer Science (EBBT)*, vol. 2019, (2019), pp. 1–4. https://doi.org/10.1109/EBBT.2019.8741944
4. N. Jatupaiboon, S. Pan-ngum, P. Israsena, Emotion classification using minimal EEG channels and frequency bands, in *The 2013 10th International Joint Conference on Computer Science and Software Engineering (JCSSE)*, (2013), pp. 21–24. https://doi.org/10.1109/JCSSE.2013.6567313
5. W. Peng, EEG preprocessing and Denoising, in *EEG Signal Processing and Feature Extraction*, ed. by L. Hu, Z. Zhang, (Springer, Singapore, 2019), pp. 71–87. https://doi.org/10.1007/978-981-13-9113-2_5
6. A. Suleiman, A.-B. Suleiman, A.-H. Fatehi, T. A. Fathi, "Features Extraction Techniques of EEG Signal for BCI Applications," 2013
7. P. Tangkraingkij, C. Lursinsap, S. Sanguansintukul, T. Desudchit, Personal identification by EEG using ICA and neural network. **6018**, 419–430 (2010). https://doi.org/10.1007/978-3-642-12179-1_35
8. M.N. Tibdewal, M. Mahadevappa, A.K. Ray, M. Malokar, H.R. Dey, Power line and ocular artifact denoising from EEG using notch filter and wavelet transform, in *2016 3rd International Conference on Computing for Sustainable Global Development (INDIACom)*, (2016), pp. 1654–1659
9. E. Maiorana, J. Solé-Casals, P. Campisi, EEG signal preprocessing for biometric recognition. Mach. Vis. Appl. **27**, 1–10 (2016). https://doi.org/10.1007/s00138-016-0804-4
10. A. Zabidi, W. Mansor, Y.K. Lee, C.W.N.F.C.W. Fadzal, Short-time fourier transform analysis of EEG signal generated during imagined writing, in *2012 International Conference on System Engineering and Technology (ICSET)*, (2012), pp. 1–4. https://doi.org/10.1109/ICSEngT.2012.6339284
11. M.A. Sohel, M. Naaz, M.A. Raheem, M.A. Munaaf, Design of discrete time notch filter for biomedical applications, in *Devices for Integrated Circuit (DevIC)*, vol. 2017, (*2017*), pp. 487–490. https://doi.org/10.1109/DEVIC.2017.8073997

12. N.W. Bin, S.A. Awang, C.Y. Fook, L.C. Chin, O.Z. Ying, A study of informative EEG channel and brain region for typing activity. *J. Phy. Confer. Series* **1372**(1), 012008 (2019). https://doi. org/10.1088/1742-6596/1372/1/012008

13. N. Ghassemi, A. Shoeibi, M. Rouhani, H. Hosseini-Nejad, Epileptic seizures detection in EEG signals using TQWT and ensemble learning, in *2019 9th International Conference on Computer and Knowledge Engineering (ICCKE)*, (2019), pp. 403–408. https://doi. org/10.1109/ICCKE48569.2019.8964826

14. N. Ahmadi, Y. Pei, M. Pechenizkiy, Detection of alcoholism based on EEG signals and functional brain network features extraction, in *IEEE 30th International Symposium on Computer-Based Medical Systems (CBMS)*, vol. 2017, (2017), pp. 179–184. https://doi.org/10.1109/ CBMS.2017.46

15. Z. Xue, J. Li, S. Li, B. Wan, Using ICA to remove eye blink and power line artifacts in EEG, in *First International Conference on Innovative Computing, Information and Control - Volume I (ICICIC'06)*, vol. 3, (2006), pp. 107–110. https://doi.org/10.1109/ICICIC.2006.543

16. G. Madhale Jadav, J. Lerga, I. Štajduhar, Adaptive filtering and analysis of EEG signals in the time-frequency domain based on the local entropy. *EURASIP J. Advanc. Signal Process.* **2020**(1), 7 (2020). https://doi.org/10.1186/s13634-020-00667-6

17. T.-P. Jung, C. Humphries, T.-W. Lee, S. Makeig, M. McKeown, V. Iragui, T.J. Sejnowski, Removing electroencephalographic artifacts by blind source separation. Psychophysiology **37**(2), 163–178 (2000)

18. Y. Xie, S. Oniga, A review of processing methods and classification algorithm for EEG signal. Carpathian J. Electron. Computer Eng. **13**(1), 23–29 (2020). https://doi.org/10.2478/ cjece-2020-0004

19. A. Subasi, M. Ismail Gursoy, EEG signal classification using PCA, ICA, LDA and support vector machines. Expert Syst. Appl. **37**(12), 8659–8666 (2010). https://doi.org/10.1016/j. eswa.2010.06.065

20. I. Winkler, S. Haufe, M. Tangermann, Automatic Classification of Artifactual ICA-Components for Artifact Removal in EEG Signals. *Behavioral Brain Funct.* **7**(1), 30 (2011). https://doi. org/10.1186/1744-9081-7-30

21. N. Mammone, F. La Foresta, F.C. Morabito, Automatic artifact rejection from multichannel scalp EEG by wavelet ICA. IEEE Sensors J. **12**(3), 533–542 (2012). https://doi.org/10.1109/ JSEN.2011.2115236

22. T. Radüntz, J. Scouten, O. Hochmuth, B. Meffert, EEG artifact elimination by extraction of ICA-component features using image processing algorithms. J. Neurosci. Methods **243**, 84–93 (2015). https://doi.org/10.1016/j.jneumeth.2015.01.030

23. C.Y. Sai, N. Mokhtar, H. Arof, P. Cumming, M. Iwahashi, Automated classification and removal of EEG artifacts with SVM and wavelet-ICA. IEEE J. Biomed. Health Inform. **22**(3), 664–670 (2018). https://doi.org/10.1109/JBHI.2017.2723420

24. A. Cimmino, A. Ciaramella, G. Dezio, P.J. Salma, Non-linear PCA neural network for EEG noise reduction in brain-computer Interface, in *Progresses in Artificial Intelligence and Neural Systems*, ed. by A. Esposito, M. Faundez-Zanuy, F. C. Morabito, E. Pasero, (Springer, Singapore, 2021), pp. 405–413. https://doi.org/10.1007/978-981-15-5093-5_36

25. S. Casarotto, A.M. Bianchi, S. Cerutti, G.A. Chiarenza, Principal component analysis for reduction of ocular artefacts in event-related potentials of normal and dyslexic children. Clin. Neurophysiol. **115**(3), 609–619 (2004). https://doi.org/10.1016/j.clinph.2003.10.018

26. K.I. Molla, T. Tanaka, T.M. Rutkowski, A. Cichocki, Separation of EOG artifacts from EEG signals using bivariate EMD, in *2010 IEEE International Conference on Acoustics, Speech and Signal Processing*, (2010), pp. 562–565. https://doi.org/10.1109/ICASSP.2010.5495594

27. M. Shahbakhti, V. Khalili, G. Kamaee, Removal of blink from EEG by Empirical Mode Decomposition (EMD), in *The 5th 2012 Biomedical Engineering International Conference*, (2012), pp. 1–5. https://doi.org/10.1109/BMEiCon.2012.6465451

28. R. Patel, S. Sengottuvel, M.P. Janawadkar, K. Gireesan, T.S. Radhakrishnan, N. Mariyappa, Ocular artifact suppression from EEG using ensemble empirical mode decomposition

with principal component analysis. Computers Elect. Eng. **54**, 78–86 (2016). https://doi.org/10.1016/j.compeleceng.2015.08.019

29. A. Subasi, E. Erçelebi, Classification of EEG signals using neural network and logistic regression. Comput. Methods Prog. Biomed. **78**(2), 87–99 (2005). https://doi.org/10.1016/j.cmpb.2004.10.009

30. R. Djemal, K. AlSharabi, S. Ibrahim, A. Alsuwailem, EEG-based computer aided diagnosis of autism Spectrum disorder using wavelet, entropy, and ANN. Biomed. Res. Int. **2017**, 1–9 (2017). https://doi.org/10.1155/2017/9816591

31. K. Bnou, S. Raghay, A. Hakim, A wavelet denoising approach based on unsupervised learning model. *EURASIP J. Advan. Signal Process.* **2020**(1), 1–26 (2020). https://doi.org/10.1186/s13634-020-00693-4

32. C.I. Salis, A.E. Malissovas, P.A. Bizopoulos, A.T. Tzallas, P.A. Angelidis, D.G. Tsalikakis, Denoising simulated EEG signals: A comparative study of EMD, wavelet transform and Kalman filter, in *13th IEEE International Conference on BioInformatics and BioEngineering*, (2013), pp. 1–4. https://doi.org/10.1109/BIBE.2013.6701613

33. Q. Zhao, B. Hu, Y. Shi, Y. Li, P. Moore, M. Sun, H. Peng, Automatic identification and removal of ocular artifacts in EEG—Improved adaptive predictor filtering for portable applications. IEEE Trans. Nanobioscience **13**(2), 109–117 (2014). https://doi.org/10.1109/TNB.2014.2316811

34. H.U. Amin, A.S. Malik, R.F. Ahmad, N. Badruddin, N. Kamel, M. Hussain, W. Chooi, Feature extraction and classification for EEG signals using wavelet transform and machine learning techniques. Australas. Phys. Eng. Sci. Med. **38**(1), 139–149 (2015). https://doi.org/10.1007/s13246-015-0333-x

35. M.K. Delimayanti, B. Purnama, N.G. Nguyen, M.R. Faisal, K.R. Mahmudah, F. Indriani, M. Kubo, K. Satou, Classification of brainwaves for sleep stages by high-dimensional FFT features from EEG signals. *Appl. Sci.* **10**(5), 5 (2020). https://doi.org/10.3390/app10051797

36. M. Rashid, N. Sulaiman, M. Mustafa, S. Khatun, B.S. Bari, The Classification of EEG signal using different machine learning techniques for BCI application, in *Robot Intelligence Technology and Applications*, (2019), pp. 207–221. https://doi.org/10.1007/978-981-13-7780-8_17

37. Y. Mohan, S.S. Chee, D.K.P. Xin, L.P. Foong, Artificial neural network for classification of depressive and normal in EEG, in *2016 IEEE EMBS Conference on Biomedical Engineering and Sciences (IECBES)*, (2016), pp. 286–290. https://doi.org/10.1109/IECBES.2016.7843459

38. R. Ramos-Aguilar, J.A. Olvera-López, I. Olmos-Pineda, S. Sánchez-Urrieta, Feature extraction from EEG spectrograms for epileptic seizure detection. Pattern Recogn. Lett. **133**, 202–209 (2020). https://doi.org/10.1016/j.patrec.2020.03.006

39. R. Upadhyay, P.K. Padhy, P.K. Kankar, Alcoholism diagnosis from EEG signals using continuous wavelet transform, in *2014 Annual IEEE India Conference (INDICON)*, (2014), pp. 1–5. https://doi.org/10.1109/INDICON.2014.7030476

40. W. Zhao, W. Zhao, W. Wang, X. Jiang, X. Zhang, X. Peng, B. Zhang, G. Zhang, A novel deep neural network for robust detection of seizures using EEG signals. Comput. Math. Methods Med. **2020**, 1–9 (2020). https://doi.org/10.1155/2020/9689821

41. S.M. Qaisar, S.F. Hussain, Effective epileptic seizure detection by using level-crossing EEG sampling sub-bands statistical features selection and machine learning for mobile healthcare. Comput. Methods Prog. Biomed. **203**, 106034 (2021). https://doi.org/10.1016/j.cmpb.2021.106034

42. H. Choubey, A. Pandey, A combination of statistical parameters for the detection of epilepsy and EEG classification using ANN and KNN classifier. SIViP **15**(3), 475–483 (2021). https://doi.org/10.1007/s11760-020-01767-4

43. S. Mian Qaisar, S. Fawad Hussain, Arrhythmia diagnosis by using level-crossing ECG sampling and sub-bands features extraction for mobile healthcare. *Sensors* **20**(8), 8 (2020). https://doi.org/10.3390/s20082252

44. V. Vimala, K. Ramar, M. Ettappan, An intelligent sleep apnea classification system based on EEG signals. *J. Med. Sys.* **43**(2), 36 (2019). https://doi.org/10.1007/s10916-018-1146-8
45. M.Y. Gokhale, D.K. Khanduja, Time domain signal analysis using wavelet packet decomposition approach. *Inter. J. Communicat. Network Syst. Sci.* **3**(3), 3 (2010). https://doi.org/10.4236/ijcns.2010.33041
46. W. Ting, Y. Guo-zheng, Y. Bang-hua, S. Hong, EEG feature extraction based on wavelet packet decomposition for brain computer interface. Measurement **41**(6), 618–625 (2008). https://doi.org/10.1016/j.measurement.2007.07.007
47. A.R. Hidalgo-Muñoz, M.M. López, I.M. Santos, A.T. Pereira, M. Vázquez-Marrufo, A. Galvao-Carmona, A.M. Tomé, Application of SVM-RFE on EEG signals for detecting the most relevant scalp regions linked to affective valence processing. Expert Syst. Appl. **40**(6), 2102–2108 (2013). https://doi.org/10.1016/j.eswa.2012.10.013
48. N. Roy, S. Aktar, M. Ahamad, M.A. Moni, A machine learning model to recognise human emotions using electroencephalogram, in *2021 5th International Conference on Electrical Information and Communication Technology (EICT)*, (2021), pp. 1–6. https://doi.org/10.1109/EICT54103.2021.9733675
49. S. Fawad Hussain, S. Mian Qaisar, Epileptic seizure classification using level-crossing EEG sampling and ensemble of sub-problems classifier. Expert Syst. Appl. **191**, 116356 (2022). https://doi.org/10.1016/j.eswa.2021.116356
50. S. Mian Qaisar, S.F. Hussain, *An Effective Arrhythmia Classification Via ECG Signal Subsampling and Mutual Information Based Subbands Statistical Features Selection* (J. Ambient. Intell. Human Comput., May, 2021), pp. 1–15. https://doi.org/10.1007/s12652-021-03275-w
51. S.F. Hussain, H.Z.-U.-D. Babar, A. Khalil, R.M. Jillani, M. Hanif, K. Khurshid, A fast non-redundant feature selection technique for text data. IEEE Access **8**, 181763–181781 (2020). https://doi.org/10.1109/ACCESS.2020.3028469
52. S.F. Hussain, F. Shahzadi, B. Munir, *Constrained Class-Wise Feature Selection (CCFS)*, vol 13 (Internat. J. Mac. Learn. Cybernet., Jun., 2022), pp. 3211–3224. https://doi.org/10.1007/s13042-022-01589-5
53. A.R. Subhani, W. Mumtaz, N. Kamil, N.M. Saad, N. Nandagopal, A.S. Malik, MRMR based feature selection for the classification of stress using EEG, in *2017 Eleventh International Conference on Sensing Technology (ICST)*, (2017), pp. 1–4. https://doi.org/10.1109/ICSensT.2017.8304499
54. M.R. Hasan, M.I. Ibrahimy, S.M.A. Motakabber, S. Shahid, Classification of multichannel EEG signal by linear discriminant analysis, in *Progress in Systems Engineering*, (Cham, 2015), pp. 279–282. https://doi.org/10.1007/978-3-319-08422-0_42
55. S. Dodia, D.R. Edla, A. Bablani, D. Ramesh, V. Kuppili, An efficient EEG based deceit identification test using wavelet packet transform and linear discriminant analysis. J. Neurosci. Methods **314**, 31–40 (2019). https://doi.org/10.1016/j.jneumeth.2019.01.007
56. S.F. Hussain, A novel robust kernel for classifying high-dimensional data using support vector machines. Expert Syst. Appl. **131**, 116–131 (2019). https://doi.org/10.1016/j.eswa.2019.04.037
57. E. Hortal, E. Iáñez, A. Úbeda, D. Planelles, Á. Costa, J.M. Azorín, Selection of the best mental tasks for a SVM-based BCI system, in *2014 IEEE International Conference on Systems, Man, and Cybernetics (SMC)*, (2014), pp. 1483–1488. https://doi.org/10.1109/SMC.2014.6974125
58. N. Kumar, K. Alam, A.H. Siddiqi, Wavelet transform for classification of EEG signal using SVM and ANN. Biomedical Pharmacol. J. **10**(4), 2061–2069 (2017)
59. A.Q.-X. Ang, Y.Q. Yeong, W. Wee, Emotion classification from EEG signals using time-frequency-DWT features and ANN. *J. Comput. Communicat.* **5**(3), 3 (2017). https://doi.org/10.4236/jcc.2017.53009
60. K. Amarasinghe, D. Wijayasekara, M. Manic, EEG based brain activity monitoring using Artificial Neural Networks, in *2014 7th International Conference on Human System Interactions (HSI)*, (2014), pp. 61–66. https://doi.org/10.1109/HSI.2014.6860449

61. U.R. Acharya, S.L. Oh, Y. Hagiwara, J.H. Tan, H. Adeli, Deep convolutional neural network for the automated detection and diagnosis of seizure using EEG signals. Comput. Biol. Med. **100**, 270–278 (2018). https://doi.org/10.1016/j.compbiomed.2017.09.017
62. P.C. Nissimagoudar, A.V. Nandi, H.M. Gireesha, Deep convolution neural network-based feature learning model for EEG based driver alert/drowsy state detection, in *Proceedings of the 11th International Conference on Soft Computing and Pattern Recognition (SoCPaR 2019)*, (Cham, 2021), pp. 287–296. https://doi.org/10.1007/978-3-030-49345-5_30
63. U.R. Acharya, S.L. Oh, Y. Hagiwara, J.H. Tan, H. Adeli, D.P. Subha, Automated EEG-based screening of depression using deep convolutional neural network. Comput. Methods Prog. Biomed. **161**, 103–113 (2018). https://doi.org/10.1016/j.cmpb.2018.04.012
64. S.L. Oh, Y. Hagiwara, U. Raghavendra, R. Yuvaraj, N. Arunkumar, M. Murugappan, U.R. Acharya, A deep learning approach for parkinson's disease diagnosis from EEG signals. Neural Comput. & Applic. **32**(15), 10927–10933 (2020). https://doi.org/10.1007/s00521-018-3689-5
65. Ö. Yıldırım, U.B. Baloglu, U.R. Acharya, A deep convolutional neural network model for automated identification of abnormal EEG signals. Neural Comput. & Applic. **32**(20), 15857–15868 (2020). https://doi.org/10.1007/s00521-018-3889-z
66. G. Zhang, V. Davoodnia, A. Sepas-Moghaddam, Y. Zhang, A. Etemad, Classification of hand movements from EEG using a deep attention-based LSTM network. IEEE Sensors J. **20**(6), 3113–3122 (2020). https://doi.org/10.1109/JSEN.2019.2956998

Chapter 8
Biomedical Signal Processing and Artificial Intelligence in EOG Signals

Alberto López and Francisco Ferrero

Abstract Electrooculography is a technique that detects and analyses eye movement based on electrical potentials recorded using electrodes placed around the eyes. The electrical signal recorded is named electrooculogram (EOG) and can be used as an alternative input for medical and human-computer interface systems. To implement an eye movement-based system, at least four main stages will be required: signal denoising, feature extraction, signal classification and decision-making. The first one after the EOG signal acquisition is signal denoising, which suppresses noise that could not be removed by the analogue filters. In this task, the slope of the signal edges, as well as the amplitudes of the signal to distinguish between different eye movements, must be preserved. After denoising, the second task is to extract the features of the EOG signal based mainly on the detection of saccades, fixations, and blinks. The next stage is the automatic identification of eye movements. This task, called signal classification, is essential for generating accurate commands, especially in real-time applications. This classification is carried out mainly using a combination of algorithms in artificial intelligence (AI). These types of algorithms are the most suitable for adaptive systems that require real-time decision-making supported by AI techniques. In some applications, EOG modelling, and compression are also applied as an additional signal processing stage.

A. López · F. Ferrero (✉)
Department of Electrical, Electronic, Communications and Systems Engineering, University of Oviedo, Gijón, Spain
e-mail: ferrero@uniovi.es

© The Author(s), under exclusive license to Springer Nature Switzerland AG 2023   185
S. Mian Qaisar et al. (eds.), *Advances in Non-Invasive Biomedical Signal Sensing and Processing with Machine Learning*, https://doi.org/10.1007/978-3-031-23239-8_8

.

8.1   Introduction

8.1.1   EOG Fundamentals

The electrooculogram (EOG) is the electrical signal produced by the potential difference between the cornea (the positive pole) and the retina (the negative pole). This potential difference is measured by placing surface electrodes near the eyes, and the process of measuring the EOG is called electrooculography.

The eye movements can be either saccades, smooth pursuits, vergence or vestibule-ocular, which can further be reflex or voluntary. Saccades are eye voluntary movements used in clinical studies to analyse eye movements. Smooth pursuits are also voluntary but are slower tracking eye movements that keep a moving stimulus on the fovea. Vergence and vestibulo-ocular movements have involuntary origins [1], so they are usually removed in EOG applications.

EOG-based human–computer interfaces (HCIs) offer disabled people a new means of communication and control as eye movements can easily be interpreted in EOG signals. In recent years, different types of HCI systems have been developed such as controlling the computer cursor, virtual keyboards, electric wheelchairs, games, hospital alarm systems, television control systems, home automation applications and smartphones [2–8]. Diabetic retinopathy or refractive disorders such as hypermetropia and myopia can be diagnosed early based on the EOG results [9]. EOG also provides reliable information to identify sleep stages and detect anomalies [10, 11].

Figure 8.1 shows a block diagram of the main stages to develop an EOG system. For the development of widely used EOG-based applications in the real world, it is necessary to provide accurate hardware and efficient software to implement the tasks shown in Fig. 8.1, which will be introduced in this chapter.

8.1.2   EOG Signal Measurement

Saccadic eye movements are the most interesting as they are voluntary and easily identifiable on the EOG. The most basic movements are up, down, right, and left. To distinguish between these eye movement classes, two pairs of bipolar electrodes and a reference electrode are positioned around the eyes as shown in Fig. 8.1.

The amplitude of the EOG signals has a mean range of 50–3500 µV and the frequency is between zero and about 50 Hz. Another issue to consider is that muscle noise spreads along with the signal bandwidth almost constantly, which makes it very difficult to completely remove it. The amplitude of the signal obtained using two electrodes to record the differential potential of the eye is directly proportional to the angle of rotation of the eyes within the range ± 30°. Sensitivity is on the order of 15 µV/° [12].

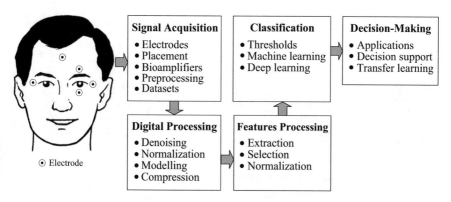

Fig. 8.1 Block diagram of the main stages that can make up a system based on EOG signals

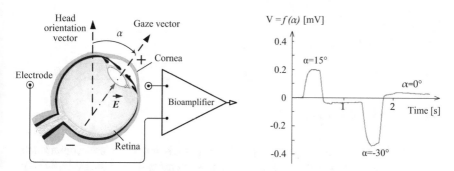

Fig. 8.2 Eye modelled as a dipole and an electrooculogram where two typical saccades with different amplitude depending on the gaze angle

Voluntary and involuntary blinks produce spikes in EOG signals that must be detected because they can be mistaken for saccades. Figure 8.2 shows EOG fundamentals by modelling the eye as a dipole and an electrooculogram where two typical saccades with different amplitudes depending on the gaze angle are represented.

Before any further analysis, a preprocessing step will be necessary to reduce mainly the base-line drift, the powerline interference and the electromyographic potential. For this task, analogue filters are usually used. Table 8.1 shows the most relevant commercial bio amplifiers used in EOG for experimental measurements.

On the other hand, several datasets are publicly available that offer signals which are already pre-processed and ready to be used. Some of the most widely used datasets in the literature are shown in Table 8.2, mostly related to sleep recordings.

Table 8.1 Most relevant commercial bio amplifiers used for EOG measurement along with their main characteristics

Name	Sampling rate	Num. of channels	Filtering	References
ADT26 PowerLab	100 Hz	10	0.1 to 2 kHz	[13]
Bluegain	1 kHz	2	0.1 to 30 Hz	[14]
ActiveTwo AD-box	64 Hz	8	Selectable	[15]
g.USBAmp	256 Hz	16	0.1 to 100 Hz	[16]
OtoScreen	200 Hz	2	0.02 to 70 Hz	[17]

Table 8.2 Summary of the most relevant EOG signal databases

Dataset name	Description	Num. of subjects	References
Physionet	Sleep	1893	[18]
Sleep-EDF-SC	Sleep	20	[18]
Sleep-EDF-ST	Sleep	22	[18]
Wisconsin	Sleep	1500	[19]
MASS	Sleep	200	[20]
Surrey-cEEGGrid	Sleep	12	[21]
SDRC	Sleep	22	[22]
UMALTA-EOG	Repetitive tasks	6	[23]

8.2 EOG Signal Denoising

After hardware acquisition and preprocessing, EOG signals are still contaminated by several noise sources that can mask eye movements and simulate eyeball events. Additional denoising must be done to remove unwanted spectral compo-nents to improve analogue filtering and remove other kinds of human biopotentials. Denoising must preserve the signal amplitudes and the slope of the EOG signals to detect blinks and saccades. In some cases, it is an additional feature while in others, it is considered an artefact that should be eliminated. In these latter cases, the blink artefact region is easily removed because blinking rarely occurs during saccades, instead, they usually occur immediately before and after the saccades. Another issue that needs to be considered in EOG noise removal is crosstalk or the interdependence between acquisition channels. Many changes in eye movements recorded by one channel generally appear in other EOG channels. The main strategy is to ignore those signals with a low amplitude.

Several methods are proposed in the literature to attenuate or eliminate the effects of artefacts on EOG signals. Digital filters are typically employed to reduce muscle artefacts and remove power line noise and linear trends. Adaptive filters, such as Kalman and Wiener filters are used to remove the effects of overlap frequencies over the EOG spectrum from electrocardiographic and electromyographic artefacts. In addition to linear filtering, the median filter is very robust in removing high-frequency noise, and preserving amplitude and the slope, without introducing any shift in the signal [11].

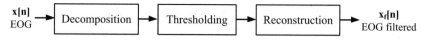

Fig. 8.3 General outline of the WT-based filtering procedure

Regression methods can learn signal behaviour by modelling colour noise that distorts the EOG signal and subtracting it. Due to the relationship between nearby samples, these methods include the nearby noise samples for the prediction of the given sample. The noise distribution characteristics are not considered in the regression models.

The wavelet transform (WT) is a powerful mathematical tool for noise removal. The WT consists of chopping a signal into scaled and displaced versions of a wavelet that is called "mother wavelet". From the point of view of signal processing, wavelets act as bandpass filters. The WT is a stable representation of transient phenomena, and therefore, conserves energy. In this way, the WT provides much more information about the signal than the Fourier transform because it allows to highlight its peculiarities by acting as a mathematical microscope.

Figure 8.3 shows the general scheme of the WT-based filtering procedure. The decomposition module is responsible for obtaining the wavelet coefficients of the EOG signal at the output of the conditioning stage. The thresholding stage consists of selecting an appropriate threshold for the wavelet coefficients so that those of lower values are eliminated because they correspond to noise and interference. Finally, the EOG signal is reconstructed through the coefficients not discarded in the previous stage. To do this, the reverse process of the wavelet transformation carried out in the first module is followed.

For a complete decomposition and reconstruction of the signal, it is necessary that the filters of the wavelet structures have a finite number of coefficients (finite impulse response filters) and that they are regular. In addition, it is also important to ensure that the filters have phase linearity, as this prevents the use of non-trivial orthogonal filters but allows the use of biorthogonal filters. It is very common to choose the Biorthogonal and Daubechies families for EOG signal processing [3, 24].

8.3 Compression

In some EOG applications, such as sleep studies, it is necessary to compress the signals because they can extend up to several gigabytes. Storage and transmission for remote health monitoring of this amount of data comes at a high cost. In these cases, compression techniques are needed for the transmission of the signal through the communication networks. An alternative is the Turning point compression algorithm reported in [25]. This algorithm reduces the effective sampling rate by half and saves the turning points that represent the peaks and valleys of the EOG signal. The main purpose of compressing data is to reduce the size while retaining the characteristic and useful features. Figure 8.4 shows the original, filtered, and compressed EOG signal using this technique.

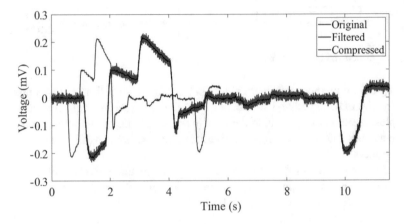

Fig. 8.4 Original, filtered, and compressed EOG signal using Turning point algorithm

8.4 EOG Feature Processing

EOG feature processing consists of selecting how many and which signal features are the most relevant for the application. An important issue is that the chosen features must be independent of each other to prevent collecting redundant data. By evaluating the EOG signals, it is possible to conclude that fixations have a stable slope whereas saccades and blinks increase quickly. The same happens for smooth eye movements and other features such as average speed, range, variance, and signal energy. Fixations are the slowest eye movements and saccades are the fastest [26]. The processing of informative, discriminatory, and independent features is a key step in preparing an appropriate collection of values for a classifier.

8.4.1 Feature Extraction

Feature extraction is the process of extracting features from the processed signals to obtain significant discrimination on several independent features. The goal is to find a space that makes the extracted features more independent and where they can be discriminated against. Feature extraction techniques can fall in the time domain, frequency domain, time-frequency domain, and nonlinear domain [27].

8.4.1.1 Time-Domain Features

Time-domain features represent the morphological characteristics of a signal. They are simply interpretable and suitable for real-time applications. The most popular time-based parameters are compiled in Table 8.3.

Table 8.3 Summary of the main time-domain EOG features, where x refers to the input signal, n is the nth sample of the signal, and N is the total number of samples

Feature name	Formula
Mean	$\mu = \dfrac{1}{N}\sum_{n=1}^{N} x_n$
Variance	$var = \dfrac{1}{N-1}\sum_{n=1}^{N}(x_n - \mu)^2$
Standard deviation	$std = (var)^{1/2}$
Skewness	$skew = \dfrac{E\left\lvert (x-\mu)^3\right\rvert}{\left(E\left\lvert (x-\mu)^2\right\rvert\right)^{3/2}}$
Kurtosis	$kurt = \dfrac{E(x-\mu)^4}{\left(E(x-\mu)^2\right)^4}$
Median	$M = \begin{cases} \dfrac{x_{\frac{N}{2}} + x_{\frac{N+1}{2}}}{2} & \text{for even } N \\ x_{\frac{N+1}{2}} & \text{for odd } N \end{cases}$
Threshold percentile	$Th - per = \dfrac{Th \times N}{100}$
Hjorth activity	$H_a = var(x)$
Hjorth mobility	$H_m = \sqrt{\dfrac{var\left(x\dfrac{dx}{dt}\right)}{var(x)}}$
Hjorth complexity	$H_c = \dfrac{var\left(x\dfrac{dx}{dt}\right)}{var(x)}$
Zero crossing rate	$ZCR = count\{n\lvert\,(x_n x_{n-1}) < 0\}$

- **Statistical features** are mean, variance, standard deviation, skewness, kurtosis, median and the 25th, and 75th percentile of the signal.
- **Hjorth features** are activity, mobility, and complexity parameters to measure the variance of a time series, the proportion of standard deviation of the power spectrum and change in the signal frequency, respectively.
- **Zero crossing rate features** refer to the number of times that a signal crosses the baseline. This parameter is very sensitive to additive noises.

Other time-domain EOG features for eye movements are amplitude, latency, deviation, velocity, slope, peak polarity, and duration.

8.4.1.2 Frequency Domain Features

The main features in the frequency domain are energy, power ratio, spectral frequency, duration ratio and power spectral density (PSD). The most popular methods to estimate the PSD are Autoregressive (AR), Moving average and Autoregressive moving average. In [28] AR was considered to extract features from the EOG signal. These methods are named the parametric method because the spectrum is estimated by the signal model. These approaches are suitable for signals with both low SNR and length. In the non-parametric methods, such as Periodogram and Welch, the PSD values are calculated directly from the signal samples in each signal window. In [29] a non-parametric statistical analysis is performed using Welch method. The features obtained by the Welch technique discriminate better due to the lower sensitivity of nonparametric methods to residual noise and motion artefacts compared to parametric and cumulant-based methods. The non-parametric methods based on the Fast Fourier transform are easy to implement. Another method used to extract the frequency domain features is the higher-order spectra, which represent the frequency content of a higher-order signal static.

8.4.1.3 Time-Frequency Features

EOG signals are non-stationary, and to transfer a signal from the time domain to the frequency domain, three main techniques are available:

- **Signal decomposition:** The aim of signal decomposition is to decompose the signals into a series of basic functions, and the most common methods are Short-Time Fourier and WT [3]. The first one is simple and well-known, however, for EOG signals, the second one is the most widely used. Continuous wavelet transforms have more separable features and the coefficients are more redundant than the discrete wavelet transforms within the same period.
- **Energy distribution:** Several methods are proposed for energy distribution: Choi–Williams distribution and Wigner-Ville distribution are the traditional nonlinear time-frequency methods widely used to analyse non-stationary signals. Hilbert–Huang transform is a more recent method to obtain momentary regularity of nonlinear and non-stationary signals such as EOGs [4].
- **Modelling:** The Gaussian mixture model (GMM) is used in some works to estimate the continuous probability density of the signal. The model parameters are estimated using the Expectation-Maximization algorithm such that the probability of observation is maximised. Figure 8.5 depicts the GMM model [8, 26, 30].

8.4.1.4 Non-Linear Features

Non-linear methods employed for EOG signal feature extraction fall into two main groups:

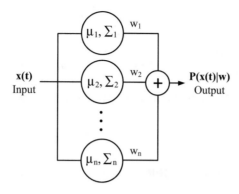

Fig. 8.5 GMM structure where three parameters must be estimated separately for each Gaussian function: mean vector (μ), covariance matrix (Σ) and weight (w). The weighted sum on these probabilities builds the output based on the input observations, $x(t) = \{x_1, ..., x_n\}$ where x_n is the nth observation or feature vector

- **Entropy and complexity-based methods.** Complexity methods are used to estimate the nonlinear dynamic parameters of EOG, electroencephalographic (EEG) and electromyographic (EMG) signals. Among complexity methods, entropy-based algorithms are robust estimators for evaluating the regularity of signals. Shannon's entropy method is the most famous one. However, in some cases, the data for the decision-making processes cannot be measured accurately and other methods have been proposed, such as Renyi's, Sample, Tsallis, Permutation, Multi scale and Approximate entropy [31].
- **Fractal-based methods.** They propose measuring the fractal dimension of the EOG irregular shape and determining the amount of self-similarity on the signal. The Correlation Dimension, Lyapunov exponent and Hurst exponent are examples of fractal-based methods. First, they map a signal into the phase space and then measure the self-similarity of its trajectory shape [32].

Both techniques are suitable for measuring the amount of roughness in the signal, in turn increasing the entropy of the signal with the irregularity. These techniques are only effective at detecting stage transitions, not for the signal bandwidth.

8.4.2   Feature Selection

After the feature extraction, feature selection techniques are applied to find a discriminative subset of features to reduce the number of features needed to feed and train subsequent classification models, for avoiding over-fitting and reducing the computational time [33].

Minimum redundancy maximum relevance is an algorithm for feature selection according to the criteria of minimum redundancy (least correlation between themselves) and maximum relevance (most correlation with the class). Redundancy can be computed by using Pearson's R for continuous features or mutual information for discrete ones. Relevance can be calculated using F-distribution under the null hypothesis for continuous features or mutual information for discrete ones [34].

Another selection method is named the Clear based feature selection (CBFS). CBFS computes the distance between the objective sample and the centroid of each class. Then, the algorithm compares the class of the closest centroid with the class of the target sample. [35] reports an efficient classification of EOG signals using this algorithm.

8.4.3   Feature Normalization

Feature normalization can be applied to reduce the effects of the individual variability and is performed over values for each feature separately. This process can prevent extremely high or low values from influencing any conclusions. [36] reports the procedure for feature normalization in an automatic sleep staging method. Another example of normalization is shown in [37] in which the original EOG signal, managed by a dynamic threshold (includes a positive and a negative threshold), would be transformed into a series of rectangular pulses that have −1 or 1 in their amplitude.

8.5   Classification

The automatic identification of eye movements (classification) is essential to generate accurate commands, especially in real-time applications. Classification techniques based on static or dynamic thresholds are also not easily generalisable, so methods based on artificial intelligence (AI) are needed. Many conventional machine learning algorithms and recently deep learning due to the increased computational power are truly becoming virtual assistants for clinicians to classify EOG features and improve medical diagnosis. The most widely used classifiers are herewith briefly commented.

The main parameters associated with classification performance are accuracy, precision, sensitivity, specificity, recall, F1 and F2 score, true positive rate, false-positive rate and Genni's or Mathew's correlation coefficient. Confusion matrices are also commonly used to compare the performance of different classification methods and avoid misleading when data is unbalanced.

8.5.1   Machine Learning Techniques

Conventional machine learning techniques include a wide variety of algorithms. All of them have shown great performance in EOG features' classification compared to threshold-based classification techniques proposed in some preliminary EOG-based systems. The main machine learning techniques used in EOG features' classification are briefly described below.

K-Nearest Neighbor (K-NN) is an algorithm that finds the nearest observations to the one it is trying to predict and classifies the observation of interest according to the majority of the surrounding data. The only parameter to set is the number of neighbouring points to consider in the vicinity to classify the different classes that are already known in advance.

Support vector machines are other conventional hierarchical supervised classifiers. They involve the adoption of a nonlinear kernel function to transform the input data into an optimal hyperplane for separating the features.

Decision trees are non-parametric supervised learning techniques that require little preprocessing and have a good runtime performance to handle tasks in real-time. The goal is to create a model that predicts the value of an objective variable according to various input variables [38].

Random Forest (RF) is one of the best algorithms for classifying large data with accuracy. RF is an ensemble of predictor trees such that each tree depends on the values of a random vector. This random vector is tested independently and presents the same distribution for each tree. Each tree is grown through bootstrap training. Figure 8.6 shows the general structure of RF. The classification is made from the vote of each tree in the ensemble and by selecting the most popular class among them [26]. [39] reports an automatic scoring of sleep stages classification using EOG signals.

Linear Discriminant Analysis (LDA) is a method of supervised classification in which two or more groups of variables are known a priori and new observations are classified into one of them according to their characteristics. The result is created on the nearest centre classifier applied to the LDA outputs. After training, the nearest centres calculate the distance between any point and each class. In [40], an LDA classifier was applied to EOG classification with good training and testing accuracy that could be used for disabled people.

Logistic Regression (LG) optimises a set of weights assigned to each input feature to provide the best classification performance using a training dataset. LG was used in the design of an omnidirectional robot controlled by eye movements because of its efficiency and the low computing resources needed [7].

GMM as a classifier learns the input features of each class and assigns a specific label to them. When a sample fits into the scheme of Fig. 8.5, the label that produces

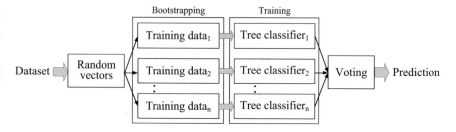

Fig. 8.6 Random Forest structure

the highest probability is assigned. The GMM provides a framework to model unknown distributional shapes. The key issue is to estimate how many components to include in the model.

A Hidden Markov Model (HMM) is a statical model in which the parameters are unknown. The training is done using maximum likelihood. HMM assesses the transition and emission probabilities from the observation sequence to the state sequence. This classifier can tolerate time warping of the input data. [8, 41] report a wheelchair navigation system based on an HMM for people with restricted mobility. Figure 8.7 shows an example of the transition of states of HMM.

Clustering is an unsupervised grouping classifier where the samples lack labels. The goal is to create groups with similar samples using criteria such as information, statistical measures, and distance metrics. Each eye movement has specific features; therefore, first grouping the signals into the two categories, centre gazes and non-centre gazes might be a useful step in some classification schemes. Figure 8.8 shows the application of this concept to the hierarchical clustering procedure for classifying eye movements.

Based on how the clusters are related to each other and the objects in the dataset, the first division of clustering algorithms can be established. In hard clustering, each object belongs to a single cluster, so the clusters would become a partition of the dataset. In soft (or fuzzy) clustering, the objects belong to the clusters according to a degree of trust or belonging (e.g., Fuzzy C-Means). Clustering can be classified by looking at how the object is related: flat clustering, hierarchical clustering, graph-based clustering, and density-base clustering. Examples of these clusters can be found in [26, 42].

Even EOG signals from the same eye movement can differ in amplitude and time and thus, produce errors in recognition. The Dynamic time wrapping algorithm can

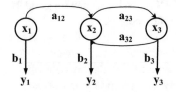

Fig. 8.7 Example of HMM architecture, where 'x' refers to hidden states, 'y' refers to observable outputs, 'a' are transition probabilities, and 'b' are the output probabilities

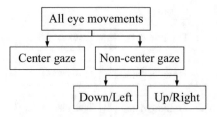

Fig. 8.8 Hierarchical clustering procedure to classify eye movements

solve this problem by breaking the problem recursively into subproblems, storing the results and later using those results when needed. For large datasets, this algorithm employs a lot of time for training the model [8, 43].

Artificial neural network (ANN) has numerous applications for pattern classification in the medical field to easily interpret the EOG signals and diagnose the problem more accurately. An ANN comprises several highly interconnected processing elements called neurons, which are organized into layers. These layers have a geometry and functionality linked to the human brain. ANNs include three layers: input, hidden and output as depicted in Fig. 8.9 [44].

8.5.2 Deep Learning Techniques

Deep learning (DL) replicates the functioning of the human brain regarding sending information from one neuron to another and handling a great amount of data. DL produces more insight knowledge than machine learning techniques as it can learn multiple levels of representation from raw data using unsupervised learning and model more complex relationships. The nucleus of DL is the ANN with multiple nonlinear hidden layers. DL offers robust computing power and enormous datasets, as they generally use a greater number of recordings to develop and evaluate their methodologies than the traditional machine learning classification methods.

A convolutional neural network (CNN) is an ANN class composed of a convolution layer to filter the extraction of features, a pooling layer to reduce the size of the analysed data, a fully connected layer, and a loss function to calculate the errors between the current and the desired network output. Back propagation is applied to update weights for convolutional layers and pooling filters cascade. Figure 8.10 shows an example of a deep neural network for eye movement classification.

CNN requires fewer parameters than the conventional neural network, therefore CNN can be applied for solving regression problems. For example, in [45] CNN was used to eliminate eye blinking artefacts, and in [46], the authors used CNN for drowsiness detection based on EOG signals.

The recurrent neural network (RNN) is basically an ANN developed under the premise that humans always consider the past when making decisions. RNN

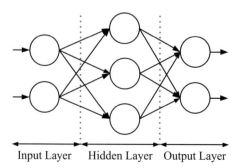

Input Layer   Hidden Layer   Output Layer

Fig. 8.9 Basic architecture of multilayer feed-forward ANN where the circles represent an artificial neuron

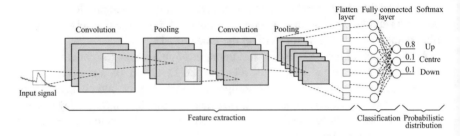

Fig. 8.10 Deep neural network for detection/classification of EOG features

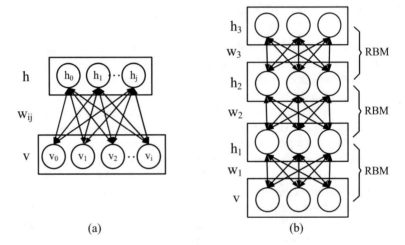

Fig. 8.11 Examples of (**a**) RBM and (**b**) DBN. v visible layer, w weights, h hidden layer

automatically stores past information through a loop within its architecture. Based on this fact, in [47], an RNN was considered for real-time eye blink suppression in EEG recordings.

The time distributed convolutional neural network (TDConvNet) is a DL model comprising two main stages: a one-dimensional CNN epoch encoder, to extract the time-invariant features from raw EOG signals, and another one-dimensional CNN stage, to infer labels from the sequence of epochs. TDConvNet was applied to classify the sleep stages of polysomnography signals [48].

Unsupervised pre-training algorithms initialise the parameters such that the optimisation process ends up with a higher speed of training. In [49, 50], two pre-training methods were presented for EOG signals: restricted Boltzmann machine (RBM) and deep belief networks (DBN). Figure 8.11a shows an example of the RBM system. The relation between the input and output layers allows the network to be trained much faster. RBM can be extended if the output layer of one RBM is the input layer for another RBM, as shown in Fig. 8.11b.

Long short-term memory (LSTM) deep networks are developed to obtain long-term dependencies in the data. LSTM algorithm as a classifier uses three kinds of gates to configure the data entering a network: input, forget and output. The more important formations can be saved between data segments using two forward and backward LSTMs. This architecture of two LSTMs, named Bidirectional long short-term memory (Bi-LSTM), presents each forward and backward training sequence in two separate LSTM layers, connected to the equal output layer.

Since the large length of the data can cause a leakage gradient problem, Gated Recurrent Unit (GRU) networks can be used to learn the representation of the EOG signal. This recurrent neural layer not only allows the improvement of the memory capacity but also eases the training since they retain the information within the unit while a sequence flows in the gating unit [51].

8.6 Decision-Making

The major difficulty in classification and subsequent decision-making is the variability of the data. Hence the importance of having large datasets that allow the creation of generalisable models and the learning process. The classification methods must be adapted to each user based on the previous actions and the results derived from them. Eye movements and blinks (voluntary and involuntary) are considered commands in the EOG-based systems and are used as input in different medical diagnostic systems and operation interfaces, such as serious games, home automation or communication and mobility solutions.

Some of the EOG-based communication solutions also include text-to-speech modules. These multilingual speech synthesisers are one of the recent forms of AI. They convert the stream of digital text selected by eye movements and blinks into natural-sounding speech. EOG can also be found in the design of industry-oriented robotic arms. In these systems, decision-making based on the results of previous commands improves real-time usability to provide the user with a reasonable degree of control.

8.6.1 Intelligent Decision Support Systems

Intelligent decision support systems (IDSS) use AI tools to improve the decision-making related to complex problems that involve a large amount of data in real-time. ANNs, Fuzzy logic, Expert systems, Case-based reasoning (CBR), and Intelligent agents (IA) can be considered IDSS. This section is a brief introduction to some of these techniques related to bio-signals for medical applications.

Fuzzy logic is a very promising technology within the medical decision-making application. Its main challenge is obtaining the required fuzzy data, even more when one must produce such data from patients. Usually, Fuzzy logic is used for the classification of the EOG and EEG signals, but they need calibration parameters obtained previously during the user training. [52] is an example of a Fuzzy logic-based controller for wheelchair motion control using the EOG technique.

An Expert system tries to solve human problems by embedding human knowledge in the computer. A typical application of expert systems is to filter ocular artefacts hidden in EEG signals without affecting clinically important EEG information [53]. Another application is reported in [54] for multichannel sleep data analysis.

ANNs have the advantage of executing the trained network quickly, which is a key issue for signal processing applications. However, the ANN algorithm is iterative and suffers from convergence problems. ANN has many practical applications, for example, ANN can be used for the diagnosis of a subnormal eye through the analysis of EOG signals [44].

To solve a new problem, CBR compares that problem with earlier solved problems and adjusts their well-known solutions instead of starting from scratch [55]. A CBR problem requires recovering relevant cases from the memory of cases, choosing the best cases, developing a solution, assessing the solution, and storing in the memory the newly solved case. A CBR system was used to classify ocular artefacts in EEG signals [56].

Alexa and Siri are examples of IA. They gather data from the internet without the help of the user. In the field of biomedical application, IA is used to diagnose, treat, and manage problems associated with dementia and Alzheimer's [57]. In these cases, the agents may be any methodologies with decision-making abilities such as patient analysts, signal processing, neural network models and Bayesian systems. The information of each agent can be shared with other agents.

In the last ten years, Multi-Agent System (MAS) has gained interest due to the advances in AI, wireless sensor networks and sensors. In MAS, a larger problem can be divided into smaller subproblems. A task can be delegated among different agents, and each agent produces the output according to its task. Then, all outputs are joined and converted into the final answer to the complete problem. The interaction between agents increases the speed of problem resolution. MAS is a research topic in complex medical applications [58].

8.6.2   Learning Approaches

Learning approaches try to overcome the problems related to training data of the classification models in many EOG studies. Another important challenge is to improve the automatic classification.

Two of these learning approaches are Transfer learning (TL) and Deep transfer learning. These are powerful methods that reuse previously trained models as the starting point. This approach avoids the needed large training dataset and saves time, while, at the same time, does not reduce the accuracy of the assessment. Figure 8.12 outlines the TL from the source to the target domains [59]. The base

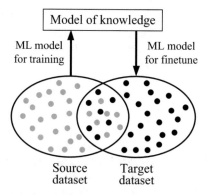

Fig. 8.12 Transfer learning from the source to the target domains

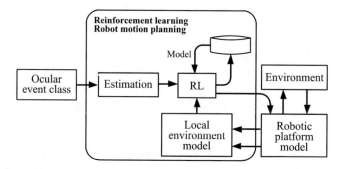

Fig. 8.13 Q-learning reinforcement learning algorithm applied to robot motion planning based on eye movements

model is trained using the data from the source domain and then fitted to the data from the target domain to complete the transfer of knowledge and make EOG-based systems more reliable and accurate. Through transfer learning, the classification performance improves significantly in all learning cases for temporal models trained only on the target domains.

Due to the limited ability of the EOG signals to adapt to the characteristics of each user, a Reinforcement Learning (RL) algorithm is included, which allows adapting the interface to the user. The RL algorithm allows the adaptation of the user's commands to the responses in the interfaces controlled by EOG. This algorithm is usually implemented in computer serious games as a moderator of the intensity of user commands given experience [60].

A model-free Q-learning method was proposed in [61] for the planning of robot motion through the user EOG signals, including obstacles surrounding the robotic platform. Figure 8.13 depicts the navigation approach in a simplified way.

Learning vector quantization (LVQ) is a supervised classification algorithm frequently used to recognise eye movements in EOG-based systems. LVQ is an artificial neural network that lets us choose how many training instances to latch onto and learns exactly what those instances should look like. EOG features can be considered as training data to build a network for recognition. Despite not being particularly powerful compared to other methods, it is simple and intuitive for the recognition of eye movements [62].

8.7 Discussion

Considering the articles published in the last decade, we can say that for EOG signal denoising, wavelet transform is the most useful technique for data preprocessing because this mathematical tool is better focused on transient and high-frequency phenomena. For EOG feature selection, the CBFS allows reducing redundant features and increases the precision and accuracy of the neural network-based classifier. EOG compression improves the signal transmission with fewer data from the original signal. As a result, the size of memory is reduced, which is an important feature for large polysomnogram signals.

EOG signal classification can be done automatically using any conventional classification algorithm. K-NN is the typical classification algorithm based on supervised ML that offers better performance and simplicity. K-NN employs the complete dataset to train "every point", which is why the required memory is higher than other classifiers. Therefore, K-NN is recommended for small datasets with fewer features.

CNN is a very efficient classification method in EOG signal processing, especially for EOG-based HCIs. CNN yields models of significantly higher correlation coefficients than the traditional K-NN classification algorithm for large datasets. The RL layer is used to help the user by selecting proper actions, and at the same time, learning from previous behaviours. For example, to prevent collisions in a robotic platform or improve wheelchair navigation. Deep transfer learning can be used for a relatively small amount of data for sleep stage classification and models.

The development of sophisticated AI-based models together with the availability of larger datasets will allow better interpretation of EOG. This will result in the design of more efficient systems that also present an improvement in the decision-making stage.

8.8 Conclusions

This chapter introduced and discussed signal processing in electrooculographic signals, which is a challenging problem due to the wide variability in the morphology and features of electrooculograms within the population. The key aspect is to find the technique that presents the best overall performance in each of the basic signal processing stages that are divided: denoising, feature extraction, classification, and decision-making. Some applications require the processing of large electrooculograms lasting several hours to monitor the health status of patients. Such scenarios also bring the need for powerful artificial intelligence-based techniques for classification and modelling, as well as compression of the signal for efficient decision and storage.

References

1. E. Kowler, Eye movements: The past 25 years. Vis. Res. **51**(13), 1457–1483 (2011). https://doi.org/10.1016/j.visres.2010.12.014
2. A. López, F.J. Ferrero, D. Yangüela, C. Álvarez, O. Postolache, Development of a computer writing system based on EOG. Sensors **17**, 1505 (2017). https://doi.org/10.3390/s17071505
3. A. López, M. Fernández, H. Rodríguez, F.J. Ferrero, O. Postolache, Development of an EOG-based system to control a computer serious game. Measurement **127**, 481–488 (2018). https://doi.org/10.1016/j.measurement.2018.06.017
4. G. Teng, Y. He, H. Zhao, D. Liu, J. Xiao, S. Rankumar, Design and development of human computer interface using electrooculogram with deep learning. Artif. Intell. Med. **102**, 101765 (2021). https://doi.org/10.1016/j.artmed.2019.101765
5. Q. Huang, S. He, Q. Wang, Z. Gu, N. Peng, K. Li, Y. Zhang, M. Shao, Y. Li, An EOG-based human–machine interface for wheelchair control. IEEE Trans. Biomed. Eng. **65**(9), 2023–2032 (2017). https://doi.org/10.1109/tbme.2017.2732479
6. R. Zhang, S. He, X. Yang, X. Wang, K. Li, Q. Huang, Z. Yu, X. Zhang, D. Tang, Y. Li, An EOG-based human-machine interface to control a smart home environment for patients with severe spinal cord. IEEE Trans. Biomed. Eng. **66**(1), 89–100 (2018). https://doi.org/10.1109/tbmc.2018.2834555
7. F.D. Pérez-Reynoso, L. Rodríguez-Guerrero, J.C. Salgado-Ramírez, R. Ortega-Palacios, Human–machine interface: multiclass classification by machine learning on 1D EOG Signals for the Control of an Omnidirectional Robot. Sensors **21**(17), 5882 (2021). https://doi.org/10.3390/s21175882
8. F. Fang, T. Shinozaki, Electrooculography-based continuous eye-writing recognition system for efficient assistive communication systems. PLOS One **13**(2), e0192684 (2018). https://doi.org/10.1371/journal.pone.0192684
9. D. Kumar, K. Priyadharsini, Analysis of CNN model based classification of diabetic retinopathy diagnosis, in *Proceedings of International Conference on Secure Cyber Computing and Communication (ICSCCC)*, (2021)
10. A. López, F.J. Ferrero, O. Postolache, An affordable method for evaluation of ataxic disorders based on electrooculographic signals. Sensors **19**, 3756 (2019). https://doi.org/10.3390/s19173756
11. R.A. Becerra-García, R.V. García-Bermúdez, G. Joya-Caparrós, A. Fernández-Higuera, C. Velázquez-Rodríguez, M. Velázquez-Mariño, F.R. Cuevas-Beltrán, F. García-Lagos, R. Rodríguez-Labrada, Data mining process for identification of non-spontaneous saccadic movements in clinical electrooculography. Neurocomputing **250**, 28–36 (2017). https://doi.org/10.1016/j.neucom.2016.10.077
12. R.J. Leigh, D.S. Zee, *The neurology of eye movements. Encyclopedia of biomedical engineering*, 5th edn. (Oxford, New York USA, 2015)
13. PowerLab 26 Series. ADInstruments. [Online]. Available: https://www.adinstruments.com/products/powerlab/35-and-26-series
14. BlueGain Cambridge Research Systems. BlueGain EOG Biosignal Amplifier. [Online]. Available: http://www.crsltd.com/tools-for-vision-science/eye-tracking/bluegain-eog-biosignal-amplifier/

15. ActiveTwo AD-box. Biosemi. [Online]. Available: https://www.biosemi.com/ad-box_activetwo.htm
16. g.USBAMP Research. G.Tec. [Online]. Available: https://www.gtec.at/product/gusbamp-research/
17. C. Velázquez-Rodríguez, R.V. García-Bermudez, F. Rojas-Ruiz, R. Becerra-García, Automatic glissade determination through a mathematical model in electrooculographic records, in *Proceedings of Lecture Notes in Computer Science*, (2017)
18. A.L. Goldberger, L.A. Amaral, L. Glass, J.M. Hausdorff, P.C. Ivanov, R.G. Mark, J.E. Mietus, G.B. Moody, C.K. Peng, H.E. Stanley, Physiobank. Physiotool. Physionet Circulat. **101**(23), e215–e220 (2000). https://doi.org/10.1161/01.cir.101.23.e215
19. G.Q. Zhang, L. Cui, R. Mueller, S. Tao, M. Kim, M. Rueschman, S. Mariani, D. Mobley, S. Redline, The national sleep research resource: towards a sleep data communications. J. Am. Med. Inform. Assoc. **25**(10), 1351–1358 (2008). https://doi.org/10.1093/jamia/ocy064
20. C. O'Reilly, N. Gosselin, J. Carrier, T. Nielsen, Montreal archive of sleep studies: An open-access resource for instrument benchmarking & exploratory research. J. Sleep Res. **1**(24), 628–635 (2014). https://doi.org/10.1111/jsr.12169
21. A. Sterr, J.K. Ebajemito, K.B. Mikkelsen, M.A. Bonmati-Carrion, N. Santhi, C. Della Monica, L. Grainger, G. Atzori, V. Revell, S. Debener, D.J. Dijk, M. De Vos, Sleep EEG derived from behind-the-ear electrodes (ceegrid) compared to standard polysomnography: A proof of concept study. Front. Hum. Neurosci. **12**(452), 1–9 (2018). https://doi.org/10.3389/fnhum.2018.00452
22. M. Rezaei, H. Mohammadi, H. Khazaie, EEG/EOG/EMG data from a cross sectional study on psychophysiological insomnia and normal sleep subjects. Mendeley Data **V4** (2017). https://doi.org/10.17632/3hx58k232n.4
23. N. Barbara, T.A. Camilleri, K.P. Camilleri, A comparison of EOG baseline drift mitigation techniques. Biomed. Sign. Proces. Cont. **57**(540), 101738 (2020). https://doi.org/10.1016/j.bspc.2019.101738
24. A. Banerjee, A. Konar, D.A. Timbarewala, R. Janarthanan, Detecting eye movement direction from stimulated electro-oculogram by Intelligent Algorithms, in *Proceedings of International Conference on Computing Communication & Networking Technologies (ICCCNT)*, (2012)
25. A. López, F.J. Ferrero, J.R. Villar, EOG signal compression using turning point algorithm, in *Proceedings of IEEE International Instrumentation and Measurement Technology Conference (I2MTC)*, (2021)
26. R. Boostani, F. Karimzadeh, M. Nami, A comparative review on sleep stage classification methods in patients and healthy individuals. Comput. Methods Prog. Biomed. **140**, 77–91 (2017). https://doi.org/10.1016/j.cmpb.2016.12.004
27. K. Mehta, A Review on different methods of EOG signal analysis. Internat. J. Innovat. Res. Sci. Eng. Technol. **5**(2), 1862–1865 (2016). https://doi.org/10.15680/IJIRSET.2016.0502128
28. A. Banerjee, S. Dattab, M. Palb, A. Konarb, Tibarewalaa, DN Janarthananc R Classifying electrooculogram to detect directional eye movements, in *Proceedings of International Conference on Computational Intelligence: Modeling Techniques and Applications (CIMTA)*, (2013)
29. S. D'Souza, N. Sriraam, Statistical based analysis of electrooculogram (EOG) signals: A Pilot Study. Internat. J. Biomed. Clin. Eng. **2**(1), 12–25 (2013). https://doi.org/10.4018/ijbce.2013010102
30. A. López, F.J. Ferrero, S.M. Qaisar, O. Postolache, Gaussian mixture model of saccadic eye movements, in *Proceedings of Medical Measurements and Applications (MeMeA)*, (2022)
31. H. Wang, H. Wu, T. Li, Y. He, P. Chen, A. Bezerianos, Driving fatigue classification based on fusion entropy analysis combining EOG and EEG. IEEE Access **7**, 61975–61986 (2019). https://doi.org/10.1109/ACCESS.2019.2915533
32. G.R.M. Babu, S. Gopinath, E. Arunkumar, An intelligent EOG system using fractal features and neural networks. Test Eng. Manag. **83**, 9920–9925 (2020)
33. S. Mala, K. Latha, Feature selection in categorizing activities by eye movements using electrooculograph signals, in *Proceedings of Science Engineering and Management Research (ICSEMR)*, (2014)

34. C. Ding, H. Peng, Minimum redundancy feature selection from microarray gene expression data. J. Bioinforma. Comput. Biol. **3**(2), 185–205 (2005). https://doi.org/10.1142/S0219720005001004
35. S. Mala, K. Latha, Efficient Classification of EOG using CBFS feature selection algorithm, in *Proceedings of International Conference on Emerging Research in Computing Information, Communication and Applications (ERCICA)*, (2013)
36. C.-E. Kuo, G.-T. Chen, Automatic Sleep staging based on a hybrid stacked LSTM Neural Network Verification Using Large-Scale Dataset. IEEE Access **8**, 111837–111849 (2020). https://doi.org/10.1109/ACCESS.2020.3002548
37. Z. Lv, X.-P. Wu, M. Li, D.-X. Zhang, Development of a human computer interface system using EOG. Health **1**(1), 39–46 (2009). https://doi.org/10.4236/health.2009.11008
38. P. Babita Syal, P. Kumari, Comparative analysis of KNN, SVM, DT for EOG based human computer interface, in *Proceedings of International Conference on Current Trends in Computer, Electrical, Electronics and Communication (CTCEEC)*, (2017)
39. M.M. Rahman, M.I.H. Bhuiyan, A.R. Hassanb, Sleep stage classification using single-channel EOG. Comput. Biol. Med. **102**, 211–220 (2018). https://doi.org/10.17605/OSF.IO/SCGJX
40. F. Anis, M. Mustafa, N. Sulaiman, M. Rashid, B. Sama, M. Islam, M. Hasan, N. Ali, The classification of Electrooculogram (EOG) through the application of Linear discriminant analysis (LDA) of selected time-domain signals, in *Proceedings of Innovative Manufacturing, Mechatronics & Materials Forum (IM3F)*, (2020)
41. F. Aziz, H. Arof, N. Mokhtar, M. Mubin, HMM based automated wheelchair navigation using EOG traces in EEG. J. Neural Eng. **11**(5), 1–11 (2014). https://doi.org/10.1088/1741-2560/11/5/056018
42. N. Flad, T. Fomina, H. Buelthoff, L. Chuang, Unsupervised clustering of EOG as a viable substitute for optical eye tracking, in *Proceedings of Eye Tracking and Visualization (ETVIS)*, (2015)
43. Z. Lv, X.P. Wu, M. Li, D. Zhang, A novel eye movement detection algorithm for EOG driven human computer interface. Pattern Recogn. Lett. **31**(9), 1041–1047 (2010). https://doi.org/10.1016/j.patrec.2009.12.017
44. L. Jia, N. Alias, Comparison of ANN and SVM for classification of eye movements in EOG signals. J. Phys. **971**, 1–11 (2018). https://doi.org/10.1088/1742-6596/971/1/012012
45. M. Jurczak, M. Kolodziej, A. Majkowski, Implementation of a convolutional neural network for eye blink artifacts removal from the electroencephalography signal. Front. Neurosci. **16**, 782367 (2022). https://doi.org/10.3389/fnins.2022.782367
46. X. Zhu, W.L. Zheng, B.L. Lu, X. Chen, S. Chen, C. Wang, EOG-based drowsiness detection using convolutional neural networks, in *Proceedings of International Joint Conference on Neural Networks (IJCNN)*, (2014)
47. A. Erfanian, B. Mahmoudi, Real-time ocular artifact suppression using recurrent neural network for electro-encephalogram based brain-computer interface. Med. Biol. Eng. Comput. **43**, 296–305 (2005). https://doi.org/10.1007/BF02345969
48. M. Dutt, M. Goodwin, C.W. Omlin, Automatic sleep stage identification with time distributed convolutional neural network, in *Proceedings of International Joint Conference on Neural Networks (IJCNN)*, (2021)
49. B. Xia, Q. Li, J. Jia, J. Wang, U. Chaudhary, A. Ramos-Murguialday, N. Birbaumer, Electrooculogram based sleep stage classification using deep belief network, in *Proceedings of International Joint Conference on Neural Networks (IJCNN)*, (2017)
50. P. Kawde, G.K. Verma, Deep belief network based affect recognition from physiological, in *Proceedings of Uttar Pradesh Section International Conference on Electrical, Computer and Electronics (UPCON)*, (2017)
51. I. Niroshana, X. Zhu, Y. Chen, W. Chen, Sleep stage classification based on EEG, EOG, and CNN-GRU deep learning model, in *Proceedings of IEEE International Conference on Awareness Science and Technology (iCAST)*, (2019)
52. N.M.M. Noor, S. Ahmad, Implementation of Fuzzy logic controller for wheelchair motion control based on EOG data. Appl. Mech. Mater. **661**, 183–189 (2014). https://doi.org/10.4028/www.scientific.net/amm.661.183

53. M.T. Hellyara, E.C. Ifeachora, D.J. Mappsa, E.M. Allen, N.R. Hudson, Expert system approach to electroencephalogram signal processing. Knowl.-Based Syst. **8**(4), 164–175 (1995). https://doi.org/10.1016/0950-7051(95)96213-B
54. T.G. Chang, J.R. Smith, J.C. Principe, An expert system for multichannel sleep EEG/EOG signal analysis. ISA Trans. **28**(1), 45–51 (1989). https://doi.org/10.1016/0019-0578(89)90056-6
55. I. Watson, F. Marir, *Case-based reasoning: A review* (Cambridge University, 2009)
56. S. Barua, S. Begum, M.U. Ahmed, P. Funk, Classification of ocular artifacts in EEG signals using hierarchical clustering and case-based reasoning, in *Proceedings of International Conference on Case-Based Reasoning (ICCBR)*, (2014)
57. H.B. Abdessalem, A. Byrns, C. Frasson, Optimizing Alzheimer's disease therapy using a neural intelligent agent-based platform. International Journal of Biosensors & Bioelectronics. Inter. J. Biosens. Bioelectron. **11**(2), 70–96 (2021). https://doi.org/10.4236/ijis.2021.112006
58. T.P. Filgueiras, P.B. Filho, Intelligent agents in biomedical engineering: a systematic review. Inter. J. Biosens. Bioelectron. **6**(5), 123–128 (2020). https://doi.org/10.15406/ijbsbe.2020.06.00200
59. H. Phan, O.Y. Chén, P.K. Zongqing, I. McLoughlin, A. Mertins, M. De Vos, Towards more accurate automatic sleep staging via deep transfer learing. IEEE Trans. Biomed. Eng. **68**(6), 1787–1798 (2021). https://doi.org/10.1109/TBME.2020.3020381
60. J. Perdiz, L. Garrote, G. Pires, U.J. Nunes, A Reinforcement learning assisted eye-driven computer game employing a decision tree-based approach and CNN classification. IEEE Access **9**, 46011–46021 (2021). https://doi.org/10.1109/ACCESS.2021.3068055
61. L. Garrote, J. Perdiz, G. Pires, U. Nunes, Reinforcement learning motion planning for an EOG-centered robot assisted navigation in a virtual environment, in *Proceedings of IEEE International Conference on Robot and Human Interactive Communication (RO-MAN)*, (2019)
62. P. Zhang, M. Ito, S.-I. Ito, M. Fukumi, Implementation of EOG mouse using Learning vector quantization and EOG-feature based methods, in *Proceedings of Conference on Systems, Process & Control (ICSPC)*, (2013)

Chapter 9
Peak Spectrogram and Convolutional Neural Network-Based Segmentation and Classification for Phonocardiogram Signals

Anam Abid and Zo-Afshan

Abstract Heart diseases are one of the contributing reasons for the human loss in the world. The Phonocardiogram (PCG) provides information for the exact and timely detection of Cardiovascular Diseases (CVDs). Digital stethoscopes record the heart sound and store it as a PCG signal for the identification of abnormal sounds. This chapter discusses heart sound segmentation and classification algorithms to diagnose the abnormal symptoms of the heart. Firstly, the breakdown of heart signal into "S1", "systole", "S2", and "diastole" states is performed using multi-level threshold values for peak detection. Phonocardiograms are the non-stationary signals for which the identification of the exact location of the peaks is difficult. Using the multi-level threshold method for peak detection and with the peak spectrogram generation, the identification of the peak locations is improved to 91.2%. Subsequently, features of the generated peak spectrograms are extracted from these four states to perform the naming of PCG as "normal" or "abnormal" using a traditional "Support Vector Machine" (SVM) and "Convolutional Neural Network". The developed algorithms are tested on the PhysioNet2016 heart sound challenge dataset. The results show the suitability of the developed methods for the identification of "normal" and "abnormal" PCG for CVDs identification and scored an accuracy of 93.3%.

A. Abid (✉)
Department of Mechatronics Engineering, University of Engineering and Technology, Peshawar, Pakistan
e-mail: anam.abid@uetpeshawar.edu.pk

Zo-Afshan
Department of Electrical and Computer Engineering, Air University, Islamabad, Pakistan
e-mail: zoafshan@mail.au.edu.pk

9.1   Introduction

Medical Signal Processing, an emerging field, has come into the limelight and shown a vital role in the identification of solutions for various diseases. Along with the recent advancement, it is now realized that various medical issues require intelligent systems and assistance. Particularly, "Deep Learning" algorithms i.e., "Convolutional Neural Networks" (CNN), "Long-Short Term Memory", and "Recursive Neural Networks", have had a great impact on biomedical fields. These systems are supposed to work like a human, think like a human, possess the decision-making ability, and also explain how to take action. The quintessence of designing an intelligent system of this kind is Deep Learning Convolutional Neural Network: convolution that extracts dominant features and neural networks that are designed to recognize patterns and adapt the environmental changes to cope with real-time scenarios.

An intelligent system has made nearly impossible tasks into reality. It is frequently advantageous to use multi-disciplinary computing techniques and methodologies in cooperation rather than exclusively. One such synergistic construction of an intelligent system is the prelude of this chapter. In particular, the integration of two complementary approaches: Signal Processing and Machine Learning, results in an innovative approach for the analysis and early detection of cardiovascular disease through phonocardiogram (PCG) signals.

Agreeing to the "World Health Organization" (WHO), CVDs are one of the most important reasons for death in the world. From the statistics reported by WHO, 17.9 million people lost their lives in 2017 alone due to CVDs [1]. Considering the severity of the situation, there is a dire need for an automated system that can be used for the evaluation of heart conditions and timely detection of any abnormality.

9.1.1   Auscultation

The heart system comprises of "heart", "blood vessels", and "blood", whereas the heart is its most important organ. Therefore, the functioning and monitoring of the heart become crucial to avoid a heart attack, angina, or stroke. A heart abnormality originates due to the constriction or complete blockage of the blood vessels and may result in serious complications. Auscultation is a medical screening process in which a medical expert/physician listens to the sounds/murmurs of the body organs by using a stethoscope. During heart sound auscultation, heartbeats present very useful information for the recognition of abnormalities. However, only a handful of skilled medical experts can correctly identify heart abnormality by listening to the heart sounds. Biomedical signal processing and artificial intelligence techniques have been facilitating doctors and cardiologists in heart abnormality diagnosis over the last few decades.

9.1.2 Phonocardiogram Signal

Stethoscopes are considered essential screening instruments for the diagnosis of heart and lung pathologies. With the development of digital stethoscopes, the process of auscultation of heart sounds becomes easier and more convenient. Digital stethoscopes record the heart sound and store them for the identification of heart abnormalities. A Phonocardiogram (PCG) signal (refer to Fig. 9.1) consists of various events like "S1" sound, "S2" sound, and "murmurs" [2, 3]. "S1" and "S2" correspond to the primary PCG components (i.e., systolic and diastolic activities of the heart respectively) which are important for heart sound segmentation. In particular, each heart sound segment contains different characteristics. In segmented data analysis, the information from each heart sound segment is retrieved for an in-depth analysis and heart disease detection [4]. Consequently, in unsegmented data analysis methods, the entire PCG signal is given as input. A discussion on segmented and unsegmented PCG data analysis is given in the following section.

The heart pumping process represents a synergetic combination of mechanical and electrical activities which form a certain set of activities over the entire cycle. The blood is circulated with efficient coordination of atria and ventricles with each other. The cardiac cycle includes two phases: Systole (the contraction phase) and Diastole (the relaxation phase). During systole, contraction of atria or ventricles occurs and the blood is pushed to the arteries whereas during diastole, relaxation of heart muscles occurs and the blood is supplied to the heart. The systole period represents the contraction of the right and left ventricles and discharge of blood into the aorta and pulmonary artery which is allowed through the opening of the aortic and pulmonic valves while the atrioventricular valves remain closed during the systole period to prevent the blood flow into the ventricles. Diastole represents the relaxation of left and right ventricles. The blood runs through the mitral and tricuspid valves. Left and right atria contract at the end of the diastole period pushing an extra

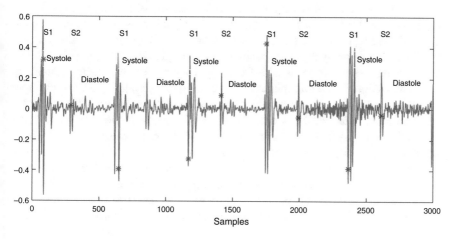

Fig. 9.1 Visualization of a phonocardiogram signal

amount of blood into the ventricles. The generated electrical signal during the heart pumping process force the blood flow between heart chambers and throughout the body. The heart produces sounds as a result of the heart beating and blood flow through it during the cardiac cycle. Also, the vibrations are produced with the closure of heart valves creating turbulence, which is audible and can be listened to through a stethoscope during cardiac auscultation by the examiner. The heart sounds are distinct and unique which gives valuable acoustic information about the heart condition. Normally in adults, there are two heart sounds, i.e., "Lub" and "Dub", generated due to the closing of the semilunar and atrioventricular valve.

There are two normal primary heart sounds, i.e., "S1" and "S2", associated with heart valves closing. S1 is also called first heart sounds or "Lub". S1 is generated by the closing of tricuspid and bicuspid valves during the start of the systole period. The vibrations are produced as a result of turbulence during ventricles contraction in systole and they could be easily heard with a stethoscope placed at the heart vertex. It has two parts: M1 which is caused by mitral valve closing and T1 which is caused by tricuspid valve closure. M1 occurs before T1 with an approximate 25–45 cycles per second whereas it elapses for an interval of around 0.14–0.15 s [4].

S2 is also known as second heart sound or "Dub". S2 is produced by semilunar valve closure during the end of the systole or early diastole period. S2 is best heard with the stethoscope placed in the aortic area. It has two components: A2 caused by the aortic valve closure and P2 caused by the closure of the pulmonary valve. Generally, S2 sound is louder and high-pitched as compared to S1 sound with a frequency falling in the range of 40–70 Hz. In addition, its duration is relatively longer which elapses for an interval of around 0.11–0.12 s [4].

9.1.3   PCG Signal Acquisition

PCG signals are correlated with the mechanical activity of the heart and provide a means of visualization for better analysis. PCG signals provide the most valuable qualitative and quantitative heart-related attributes. PCG signal acquisition process is categorized as one-channel acquisition and multiple-channel acquisition. In the one-channel case, the PCG signal is fragmented using the actual signal without any prior knowledge. In the multiple-channel scenario [5], certain signals for example an electrocardiogram, photoplethysmogram, and carotid pulse are simultaneously obtained along with PCG. As a result, the performance of the multiple-channel acquisition setup is more effective than its one-channel counterpart. Nonetheless, simultaneous acquisition of multiple signals (modalities) becomes expensive and unmanageable, especially when conditions are ambulatory. Hence, field experts prefer one-mode segmentation methods over multiple-channel counterparts [6–8].

The rest of the chapter is organized as follows. Section 9.2 discusses the recent work carried out for PCG segmentation and classification. Section 9.3 discusses the quality assessment and pre-processing of the PCG signal and Sect. 9.4 presents a threshold-based peak detection method. Section 9.5 details the proposed segmentation techniques i.e., identification of "S1" and "S2" states by (i) calculating statistical features, and (ii) converting 1D PCG signals into their 2D spectrogram respectively. Section 9.6 discusses the final labeling of PCG signal into "S1", "systole", "S2", and "diastole" states, followed by PCG classification. In Sect. 9.7 experiment and results are presented based on the developed methods. Sections 9.8 and 9.9 present a comparison study, discussions, and conclusions of the chapter respectively.

9.2 Related Work

Automated analysis of a PCG signal can be classified into various steps. The typical approach involves (i) pre-processing, (ii) segmentation, and (iii) classification. In pre-processing PCG signal is filtered and extra noise spikes are removed to make the signal more appropriate for starting the analysis process. Most of the heartbeat segmentation methods follow a similar preprocessing approach, starting with noise reduction by applying filters and the normalization of the signal using the absolute maximum. This is followed by the application of envelope detection methods, such as the Hilbert Transform, Homomorphic Envelope, Wavelet Transform, Shannon Energy, and Power Spectral Density [9]. In the unsegmented PCG signal processing approach, deep features are obtained from the unsegmented PCG chunks, and deep learning algorithms are employed for classification.

9.2.1 Segmentation

In earlier works, the rule of thumbs and facts-based distinction was used to differentiate between "S1" and "S2", (i.e., interval lengths). Other techniques [10, 11] involve PCG energy calculation. Gomes [11] designed a system that changes the phonocardiogram signal into individual segmentation fragments. In [10], the Shannon envelope of the signal is extracted from the overlapping fragments of the entire signal. Threshold-based peak detection is performed in each window/fragment. Heart sound signals are mainly known as non-stationary signals. Hence, by applying energy-based calculation methods only, better results cannot be obtained. Considering this issue, researchers combined these methods with some transforms, for instance, Short Time Fourier Transform [12], Wavelet Transform [13, 14]. In [14], a wavelet-transform-based segmentation algorithm was employed to extract temporal, time, and frequency domain attributes of PCG. In [15], the authors used an advanced mode of decomposition method for PCG segmentation using various modes of the decomposed PCGs and variational mode decomposition. Other than these techniques, neural networks have also been applied for heart sound segmentation [16]. Specifically, a neural network algorithm was proposed for PCG segmentation using a Hidden Markov Model. Features extracted for the PCG classification were the time and frequency domains representing the underlying characteristics of the phonocardiogram signal. The inter-patient differences challenge was addressed in [17] where the main focus is to compare the heart sounds within and across the patient's PCG dataset using "Dynamic Time Warping" (DTW). The combination of DTW and "Mel Frequency Cepstral Coefficients" (MFCC) features was given to an SVM classifier. As compared to MFCC, DTW-based features computed in an unbiased dataset condition performed well. In [18] heart sound recordings are classified by first performing the heart sound segmentation, followed by 1D waveforms transformation into 2D time-frequency heat maps using MFCC, and finally, classification was performed using CNN.

9.2.2 Extracted Features and Classifiers

After the segmentation of PCG signals as "S1" and "S2", these segments are passed to the feature (distinctive attribute of an item) extraction stage, followed by the classification stage. For PCG classification features are extracted to analyze the changes in the signal over time and frequency contents within the signal. In the segmentation-based heart sound analysis approach, different features are calculated at two different stages. At first, the features are extracted to find the S1 and S2, and in the second stage (i.e., classification) features are extracted to classify the signal as normal and abnormal. Some common features are mean, median, kurtosis, energies, entropy, spectral edges, etc.

Some classification methods are based on clustering like K-Means [19]; others use statistical analysis like Hidden Markov Model [20], K-Nearest Neighbor [21], etc. Machine learning (ML) models are applied to PCG databases with several feature extraction approaches [22–24]. In [9], Springer used a modified form of the Hidden Markov Model (the Hidden Semi Markov Model) for the classification of PCGs. Similarly in [25], Kaur used fuzzy K-NN, Bayesian, and Gaussian mixer Model-based KNN for the classification. In [26], two stages were employed, the first stage performed segmentation using SVM, and "Artificial Neural Networks" (ANN) were used for the final classification of PCGs. Most of the recent studies employed classification techniques like "multi-layer perceptron" (MLP) [27], SVM [28], CNN [18], etc. The above-mentioned methods use different preprocessing techniques to segment PCG signals and extract suitable features from the PCG segments using techniques such as Short Time Fourier Transform [12], Wavelet Transform [13, 14], DTW [17], MFCC [29], etc. These ML methods are subjective and time-consuming due to the handcrafted feature selection process. In addition, deep features using deep neural networks [30, 31], spectrograms of heart sounds [32, 33], and a continuous wavelet transform-based scalogram [34] were also used for PCG analysis.

The existing research work conducted on CVD identification using ML and deep learning on different medical databases has contributed to the detection of heart sound abnormalities and most of them achieved significant results. The proposed study is focused on spectrogram-based segmentation of PCG using CNN.

9.2.3   Unsegmented PCG Classification

The second approach for the PCG classification does not involve segmentation. Researchers have opted for this approach to directly classify the PCG signals into normal and abnormal classes skipping the intermediate segmentation stage. In [35] authors performed the classification of heart sound without segmentation using 5 categories of features that include "Linear Predictive Coefficient", Entropy-based features, MFCC, wavelet transform, power spectral density. From the set of 40 features, 18 features were chosen using one of the search algorithms (called wrapper-based) for the feature selection. In this method, a sequential forward selection search was used. A total of 20, 2-layer feed-forward ANNs were used for the classification (25 neuron nodes per hidden layer). In the output layer, 4 neurons were used for two classification tasks at the same time, two for normal vs. abnormal and two for good vs. bad. In [36] authors classify the heart sound recording as normal or abnormal by extracting the morphological features of the PCG signals. Several features are extracted from both temporal and spectral domains, and the classification is performed using an SVM. In another approach [37], wavelet entropy at a wavelet scale of 1.7 and with a threshold of 7.8 was employed. The heart signal was recorded for 5 seconds, and then wavelet coefficients were calculated. Afterward, wavelet energy and entropy were calculated and it was passed to the criterion function which used a threshold for signal classification. Another CNN-based PCG classification approach [38] employed Power Spectral Density (PSD) features with a window of 150 ms. These spectrograms were fed to the network for the classification task. SVM, logistic regression, and random forest were also applied for PCG classification and their results were compared. Another method using temporal dynamics of the signal using Markov features along with other statistical and frequency domain features was presented in [39]. These features were trained over the ensemble of artificial neural networks and gradient boosting trees.

9.3   Quality Assessment and Pre-processing of PCG Signals

In a real-world environment, during auscultation, the recorded PCG signal is often contaminated with noise. It is always necessary to check the suitability of the PCG signal before carrying out any kind of processing. For this purpose, firstly quality assessment of the PCG signal is carried out [16] in which the suitability of the signal is tested based on evaluation criteria. If the PCG signal fails the criteria, it is declared as "unsure" and no further processing is carried out for that PCG signal. The details of quality assessment and pre-processing stages are discussed in this section.

9.3.1   Evaluation Criteria

The classification task requires the determination of a heart sound recording as normal, abnormal, or unsure (due to the high content of noise). For this purpose, three measures of quality assessment are taken [16]. If any of the criteria does not meet, the signal is not called suitable. These criteria are; (i) root mean square of successive differences, (ii) number of counted normal peaks in the specified size window, and (iii) number of zero crossings in the whole PCG signal. PCG signal is tested over these criteria, and the suitable signal is passed on to the next step. On the other hand, if any criterion fails, the PCG signal will be declared as "unsure" and no further processing will be carried out for that PCG signal.

9.3.2   Filtering and Spike Removal

Heart sound recording and analysis are generally employed as an effective and low-cost alternative for heart abnormality screening. Nonetheless, there are a few challenges involved in this process. Firstly, the accurate localization of primary heart sounds (i.e., "S1" and "S2") is very important for the detection of any heart abnormality as it provides the basis for the upcoming classification stage. Another challenge is the vulnerability of heart sounds from different noise sources. In particular, external noises present in the nearby setting of the signal acquisition arrangement (e.g., human speech, noise generated by appliances and devices), measurement noise due to the involvement of sensors, and other components data acquisition system. In contrast, internal noises (coming from the patient body), for instance, sounds originating from lungs and other body parts, speech, etc. may also deteriorate the desired PCG signal. Consequently, it is the foremost task to remove the undesired noises from the acquired signal using appropriate noise filtering methods.

Filters play an essential role in the field of signal processing. A filter is a special type of process which is used to remove the unwanted part of the signal, suppress the effect of unwanted or unnecessary signal, or restore the original signal from corruption. Normal PCG signals have low frequencies, ranging from 40 Hz to 200 Hz. Murmurs and extra heart sounds have frequency ranges up to 400 Hz. In literature the usage of Butterworth and Chebyshev filters [17, 28, 40] and their variants are found quite often. These linear filters are used for the separation of noise from the signal using different cutoff frequencies provided that the signal does not overlap in the frequency domain. In this study, the PCG signal is resampled to 1 kHz and the resampled signal is filtered with a Butterworth low-pass filter with a cut-off frequency of 400 Hz and order 4. After that output of the first filter is passed to a Butterworth high-pass filter with a cut-off of 25 Hz.

Noisy spikes are then removed from the filtered signal to make the PCG signal clean from extra spikes other than the actual peaks of the heartbeat. Some common spike removal methods are Nonlinear Median filters, Schmidt spike removal function [20], etc. After that envelope of the PCG using the Hilbert transform is extracted and it is normalized using the mean and standard deviation values of the extracted PCG envelope. Researchers also suggest calculating the Shannon Energy [10] for PCG envelope calculation.

9.4 Single and Multi-Level Threshold-Based Peak Detection Methods

During PCG signal segmentation, a signal is segmented into its fundamental heart sounds, i.e., "S1" and "S2". Therefore, the localization is threefold; the identification of all peaks present in the normalized PCG, extraction of true peaks, and removal of false peaks. Firstly, the local maxima function is employed to identify the location of all peaks, called candidate peaks, from the normalized envelope of the PCG signal. The second step is the determination of true peaks which becomes difficult due to the sub-par quality of the PCG acquisition process. Generally, clinical settings or ambulatory conditions affect the recorded signal quality due to the presence of external and observational noise. In such situations, a specific single-threshold is not a suitable measure for extracting true peaks for the reason that signals usually have a "Signal to Noise ratio" (SNR) of a different range. Due to the degraded performance of single-threshold techniques, employment of one perfect, global threshold value for the determination of true peaks i.e., "S1" and "S2", is not possible. Another associated challenge of a one-specific threshold is the determination of the threshold level. For instance, by selecting a low threshold value, peaks in systole/diastole intervals are also selected along with true peaks. In contrast, by selecting a high threshold value sometimes the misdetection of "S1" peaks from the PCG signal increases considerably, however, the peaks in systole and diastole intervals are not detected anymore. This is because the signal with a high SNR performs well with a low threshold value and a signal with low SNR requires a high threshold value. In literature, a multi-threshold algorithm [28] is suggested to find out the candidate peaks for S1 and S2 from the pool of all detected peaks. The summary of the multi-threshold algorithm is shown in Fig. 9.2.

The proposed method employs multiple threshold levels for true peak selection namely, "moderate-level (MLT)", "high-level (HLT)", and "low-level (LLT)". These levels are applied in sequence and the criterion for the selection of a threshold is a count of candidate peaks, 'count', occurring in a pre-defined window size (0.2 s in our case). To begin with, the 'count' is computed with MLT (0.1 in our case). When 'count' is above the specified upper limit (sp1), HLT is incorporated. Similarly, when 'count' is below the specified lower limit (sp2), LLT is employed. Afterwards, true peaks fulfilling the requirements i.e., equal to or above the updated threshold are selected using the freshly updated threshold. Over each candidate peak, a window of 1 ms with overlapping of 0.5 ms is placed to segment that particular portion of the signal.

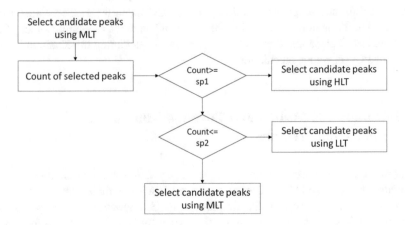

Fig. 9.2 Multi-Level threshold algorithm

9.5   Segmentation Methods of PCG Signals

In the proposed methodology, two approaches are employed for the classification of "S1" and "S2":

- Segmentation based on statistical features and Support Vector Machine (SVM)
- Segmentation based on Peak Spectrogram and Convolutional Neural Networks (CNN)

Both approaches are discussed in detail in this section.

9.5.1   Segmentation Based on Statistical Features and Support Vector Machine

In this approach, a total of 11 features obtained from both time and frequency domains are extracted from the windowed PCG segments (wS) and complete heart sound (HS). A list of these features is mentioned in Table 9.1. These features provide statistical values for the classification of "S1" and "S2". Different classifiers are trained using these 11 features namely K-Nearest-Neighbor (KNN), ANN, and SVM. Accuracy results obtained from all mentioned classifiers are given in Sect. 9.8.

Table 9.1 Proposed features for heart sound peak classification

1. SD of 'wS'/SD of heart 'HS'
2. μ of 'wS'/μ of 'HS'
3. S of 1st-level approximation coefficient of 'HS'
4. S of 1st-level detail coefficients of 'HS'
5. S of 2nd-level approximation coefficient of 'HS'
6. Spectral edge frequency of 'HS'
7. Spectral S for dyadic bands of 'HS'
8. Fractional dimensions of 'HS'
9. Hjorth parameters of 'HS'
10. Skewness of 'HS'
11. Kurtosis of 'HS'

Note: SD, Standard deviation; μ, Mean; S, Entropy

9.5.2   Segmentation Based on Spectrograms and Convolutional Neural Network

Convolutional Neural Network (CNN) works better on 2D data. On the other hand, the signal acquired during auscultation is 1D. To make it useful for CNN, in this approach, Short Time Fourier Transform of PCG segment determined after which 1D signal is converted into a 2D peak spectrogram. The time-domain representation of "S1" and "S2" and their respective spectrograms are shown in Fig. 9.3.

These peak spectrograms are fed to a CNN which classifies them into "S1" and "S2". The architecture used for the CNN model is shown in Fig. 9.4. At the end of this step, all candidate peaks are assigned with their respective labels, like "S1" or "S2". This information is used in the next phase of the proposed methodology to get fully labeled cardiac cycles in the PCG signal.

9.6   Post-processing and Classification of PCG Signals

9.6.1   Post-processing and PCG Labeling

In this step, the marked positions of "S1" and "S2" along with the duration distribution provided by Schmidt et.al [20]. are utilized to label the systole and diastole regions in the PCG signal. A fully labeled PCG signal with states "S1", systole, "S2", and diastole is obtained after the post-processing. The example of a labeled PCG signal obtained after segmentation is presented in Sect. 9.7.

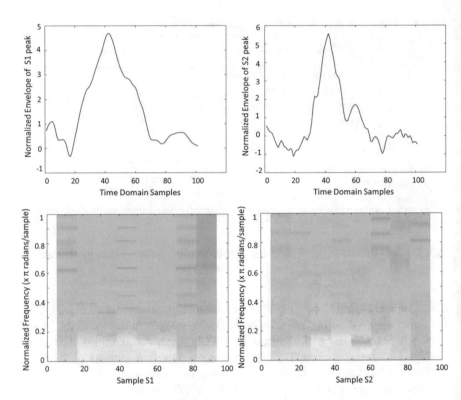

Fig. 9.3 Peak Spectrogram generation using short-time-Fourier-transform

9.6.2 PCG Classification

In this step, features are extracted utilizing post-processed state labels for PCG signals that are used to train the classifier. A total of 50 features are extracted (20 time-domain, 30 frequency-domain). A list of these features is given in Table 9.2. These features are used to train SVM. As mentioned earlier, for segmentation, two approaches were proposed. Both of them follow the same classification step separately and their accuracies are reported in Sect. 9.7.

9.7 Experimentation on the PhysioNet2016 Challenge Dataset

This section discusses the experiments and the obtained results of the proposed method implementation. A detailed description of the results obtained in each step is given below.

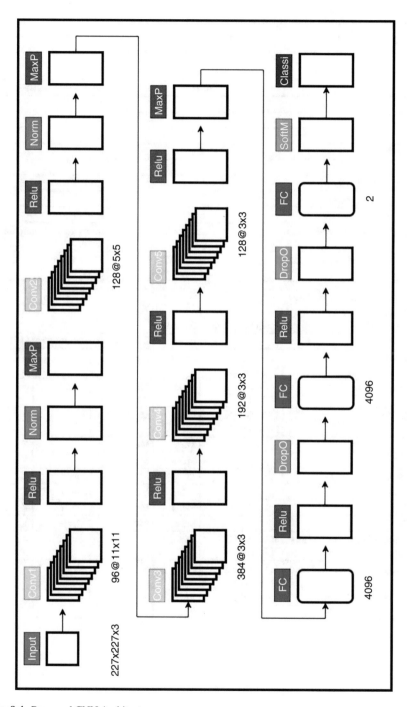

Fig. 9.4 Proposed CNN Architecture

Table 9.2 Proposed features for SVM Classifier Training

Time-Domain Features

Interval/ Interval Ratio	Features	
	Mean	Standard Deviation
R-R	X	X
S1	X	X
S2	X	X
Systole	X	X
Diastole	X	X
Systole, R–R ratio	X	X
Diastole, R–R ratio	X	X
Systole, diastole ratio	X	X
Systole period, S1 period ratio	Mean absolute amplitude ratios	Mean absolute amplitude ratios
Diastole period, S2 period ratio	Mean absolute amplitude ratios	Mean absolute amplitude ratios

Frequency-Domain Features

Segments/ Segments Ratio	Frequency Band	Features			
		Power	Band Power	Amplitude	Q-factor
Cardiac Cycle	150–350 Hz 200–400 Hz	Mean	Mean	–	–
Systole	150–350 Hz 200–400 Hz	Mean	Mean	–	–
Diastole	150–350 Hz 200–400 Hz	Mean	Mean	–	–
S1		Mean	Mean	–	X
S2		Mean	Mean	–	X
Systole		Mean	Mean	Mean	X
Diastole		Mean	Mean	Mean	X
S1		Mean	Mean	Mean	X
S2		Mean	Mean	Mean	X
Cardiac Cycle, systole ratio	100–300 Hz 200–400 Hz	Average	–	–	–
Cardiac Cycle, diastole ratio	100–300 Hz 200–400 Hz	Average	–	–	–
Diastole, systole ratio	100–300 Hz 200–400 Hz	Average	–	–	–

9.7.1 Dataset

The proposed methodology is implemented on the PhysioNet2016 challenge dataset [41]. In this dataset, a total of 3226 data samples of PCG recording both from healthy and pathological patients were collected. 1610 instances of the total data samples are used for training and 1616 samples are used for testing. The physioNet dataset consists of multiple sub-datasets including A, B, C, D, E, and F. The audio recordings present in each sub-dataset are 409, 488, 29, 53, 2137, and 110 respectively. A 50-50% split training-testing strategy is incorporated in this study. The actual number of recordings used for training are 204, 244, 14, 26, 1067, and 55 and for testing 205, 244, 15, 27, 1070, and 55 respectively. For segmentation, "S1" and "S2" labels for each PCG signal sample are obtained using the Springer Algorithm [9] which are compared with the segmentation results of the developed method.

9.7.2 Results of Pre-processing

After obtaining the suitable (classifiable) signals the preprocessing techniques are performed. First, the signal is passed through the low pass and high pass filters. Furthermore, the removal of spikes is carried out using a Schmidt spike removal function. Followed by the extraction of the envelope using the Hilbert transform. Finally, the resultant signal is normalized using simple mean and standard deviation formula. The results of different preprocessing operations are illustrated in Fig. 9.5. Figure 9.5a shows a smaller chunk of the original (classifiable) signal. Figure 9.5b shows the signal obtained after filtering and spike removal operations. It is clear that after preprocessing the signal became smooth and spikes were removed. Furthermore,

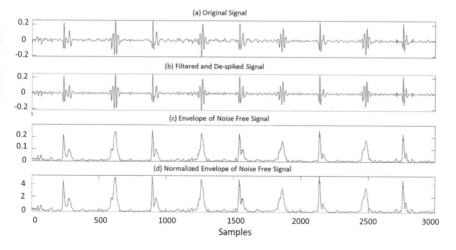

Fig. 9.5 Pre-processing results

Fig. 9.5c shows the obtained envelope of the preprocessed signal which contains useful information regarding the "S1" and "S2" activities. Finally, a normalized envelope of the processed signal is obtained as shown in Fig. 9.5d.

9.7.3   Results of Segmentation

In this stage, true peaks are extracted from the preprocessed signal. Firstly all peaks are identified using peak finders which are called the candidate peaks for the "S1" and "S2". Afterward, a multi-level threshold is employed for the identification of the true peaks. Consequently, true peaks are selected from the pool of peaks which are sent to the feature extractor to classify them as "S1" and "S2" based on their features. The results of the peak finder stage illustrating the candidate peaks are given in Fig. 9.6a. Subsequently, the candidate obtained using the starting threshold is given in Fig. 9.6b. Afterward, true peaks are detected and false peaks are eliminated using the developed multi-level threshold, as shown in Fig. 9.6c.

Classification of peaks is performed using a spectrogram of obtained true peaks. The windowing procedure is applied to obtain the true peak, and its spectrogram is obtained using Short Time Fourier Transform. These spectrograms are fed as input to the convolutional neural network which learns features in 100 iterations and trains its model. Final testing of the model is performed on unseen samples of spectrogram which classify them as "S1" and "S2". The spectrogram and CNN combination gives an overall segmentation accuracy of 91.20% as compared to SVM and ANN classifiers. Figure 9.7 illustrates the peak identification results where the true peaks are labeled based on the peak spectrograms.

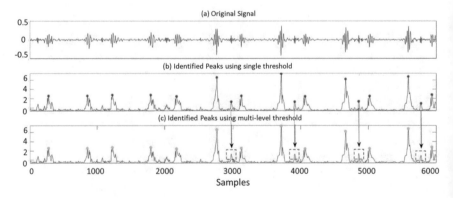

Fig. 9.6 True peak detection results based on multi-level threshold

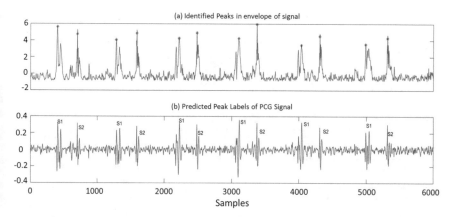

Fig. 9.7 Predicted labels using peak spectrogram and convolution neural network

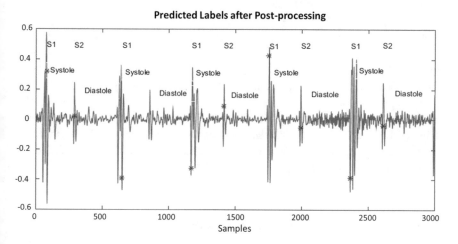

Fig. 9.8 Predicted label after post-processing

9.7.4 Results of Post-processing

After the assignment of "S1" and "S2" peaks by the classifier, a post-processing step is required. This completes one cycle as "S1", "systole", "S2", and "diastole" as shown in Fig. 9.8.

9.7.5 Results of PCG Segmentation

The state sequences (i.e., "S1", systole, "S2", diastole) obtained after post-processing are forwarded to the final stage in which features are extracted based on the intervals between the states, their ratios, mean, standard deviation, amplitudes,

Table 9.3 Segmentation results on the PhysioNet 2016 challenge dataset

Classifier	Accuracy (%)	Sensitivity (%)	Specificity (%)
CNN (Proposed)	91.20	94.05	88.53
SVM	87.57	92.08	83.08
ANN	82.01	87.33	76.93

Table 9.4 Comparison Analysis on the PhysioNet 2016 challenge dataset

Approach	Technique	Score/Accuracy
Proposed Methodology I	SVM without spectrogram	86.89
Proposed Methodology II	SVM with spectrogram	93.33
Classifying Heart Sound Recording Using Deep Convolutional Neural Network [18]	CNN	88%
Morphological Determination of Pathological PCG Signal by Time and Frequency Domain Analysis [36]	SVM	81%
PCG Classification using Neural Network Approach [16]	ANN	79%

and other power-energy features. The classifier employed for this purpose is the SVM which performs the binary classification. In another set of experiments, PCG signal segmentation was performed using the developed spectrogram and CNN-based segmentation approach. Afterward, PCG signal classification is performed using an SVM classifier and the classification result are shown in Table 9.3 which shows that with the incorporation of spectrogram and CNN combination the PCG classification accuracy improves.

9.8   Comparison Analysis and Discussions

In this section, a comparison study is presented between the proposed approach and the state-of-the-art counterparts on the same datasets i.e., PhysioNet 2016, as discussed in Sect. 9.7. Comparison results with other classifiers (i.e., Artificial Neural Networks, Convolutional Neural networks, and Support Vector Machine) are also shown in Table 9.4. In [16] PCG signal is classified using Hidden Markov Model (HMM) for extracting features and ANN focusing only on the statistical features which results in an accuracy of 79%. Support Vector Machine with Time and Frequency domain features is employed in [38] for analysis of PCG signals and it obtained an accuracy of 81%. In [18] the emphasis is on the state-of-the-art CNN, and this approach leads to an accuracy of 88%. In this chapter, two different classification approaches were presented. In the Proposed Methodology I, PCG signals were analyzed under the category of segmented approach using a multi-level threshold, extracting the time and frequency domain features along with the Support

Vector Machine for final classification with the accuracy of 86.89%. In the Proposed Methodology II, the same strategy was followed except that segmentation was carried out using a CNN along with the SVM as a final classifier, resulting in the highest accuracy of 93.33%.

9.9 Conclusions

Phonocardiograms are the non-stationary signals which make the task of identifying the exact location of the peaks difficult. Using the multi-threshold method for peak detection and with the peak spectrogram, the identification of the peak locations was improved. Also, PCG signal classification into normal and abnormal was improved to 93.33% with our developed method. The segmentation and classification results reported for our developed approach using peak spectrogram and state-of-the-art convolutional neural network have an accuracy of 91% and 93.33% respectively.

Classification of PCGs can be bettered by calculating advanced features which extract the information of signal in more depth or by using deep learning models. In this paper, separate methods are used for PCG segmentation and classification. Nonetheless, there can be a possibility to use a unified framework for segmenting and classifying PCG both. In addition, instead of binary classification non-binary classification can be performed to find out the exact CVD in future endeavors.

References

1. H. Mehrtash, R. Laing, V.J. Wirtz, Comparative analysis of essential medicines for cardiovascular diseases in countries of the WHO Eastern Mediterranean region. East. Mediterr. Health. J. **24**(5), 427–434 (2018)
2. M.W. Arnaudin, J.J. Mintzes, Students' alternative conceptions of the human circulatory system: A cross-age study. Sci. Educ. **69**(5), 721–733 (1985)
3. A.J. Weinhaus, K.P. Roberts, Anatomy of the human heart, in *Handbook of Cardiac Anatomy, Physiology, and Devices*, 2nd edn., (2005), pp. 59–85
4. Q. Mubarak, M.U. Akram, A. Shaukat, A. Ramazan, Quality Assessment and Classification of Heart Sounds Using PCG Signals. no. February, (2018), pp. 1–11
5. N.K. Al-Qazzaz, I.F. Abdulazez, S.A. Ridha, Simulation recording of an ECG, PCG, and PPG for feature extractions. J. Al-Khwarizmi Eng. J. **10**(4), 81–91 (2014)
6. S.I. Malik, M.U. Akram, I. Siddiqi, Localization and classification of heartbeats using robust adaptive algorithm. Biomed. Signal Process. Control **49**, 57–77 (2019)
7. S. Ari, K. Hembram, G. Saha, Detection of cardiac abnormality from PCG signal using LMS based least square SVM classifier. Expert Syst. Appl. **37**(12), 8019–8026 (2010)
8. C.D. Papadaniil, L.J. Hadjileontiadis, Efficient heart sound segmentation and extraction using ensemble empirical mode decomposition and kurtosis features. IEEE J. Biomed. Heal. Informatics **18**(4), 1138–1152 (2014)
9. D.B. Springer, L. Tarassenko, G.D. Clifford, Logistic regression-HSMM-based heart sound segmentation. I.E.E.E. Trans. Biomed. Eng. **63**(4), 822–832 (2016)

10. F. Chakir, A. Jilbab, C. Nacir, A. Hammouch, A. Hajjam, Detection and identification algorithm of the S1 and S2 heart sounds, in *International Conference on Electrical and Information Technologies (ICEIT)*, (2016), pp. 418–420

11. E.F. Gomes, P.J. Bentley, M. Coimbra, E. Pereira, Y. Deng, Classifying heart sounds: Approaches to the PASCAL challenge, in *Heal. 2013 – Proceedings of the International Conference Heal. Informatics*, (2013), pp. 337–340

12. K.N. Khan, F.A. Khan, A. Abid, T. Olmez, Z. Dokur, Deep learning based classification of unsegmented phonocardiogram spectrograms leveraging transfer learning. Physiol. Meas. **42**, 095003 (2021)

13. Z. Dokur, T. Ölmez, Feature determination for heart sounds based on divergence analysis, in *19th Digital Signal Processing*, (2009), pp. 521–531

14. B. Bozkurt, I. Germanakis, Y. Stylianou, A study of time-frequency features for CNN-based automatic heart sound classification for pathology detection. Comput. Biol. Med. **100**, 132–143 (2018)

15. K.A. Babu, B. Ramkumar, M.S. Manikandan, S1 and S2 heart sound segmentation using variational mode decomposition, in *IEEE Region 10 Conference (TENCON)*, (2017), pp. 1629–1634

16. I. Grzegorczyk, M. Soliński, M. Łepek, A. Perka, J. Rosiński, J. Rymko, K. Stępień, J. Gierałtowski, PCG Classification Using a Neural Network Approach, in *Conference on Computing in Cardiology*, (2016), pp. 1–4

17. J. Gonz, C.P. Phoo, J. Wiens, Heart Sound classification based on temporal alignment techniques, in *Computing in Cardiology Conference (CinC)*, (2016), pp. 1–4

18. J. Rubin, R. Abreu, A. Ganguli, S. Nelaturi, I. Matei, K. Sricharan, Classifying heart sound recordings using deep convolutional neural networks and mel-frequency cepstral coefficients, in *Computing in Cardiology Conference (CinC)*, (2016), pp. 1–4

19. Z. Xiong, T. Liu, G. Tse, M. Gong, P.A. Gladding, B.H. Smaill, M.K. Stiles, A.M. Gillis, J. Zhao, A machine learning aided systematic review and meta-analysis of the relative risk of atrial fibrillation in patients with diabetes mellitus. Front. Physiol. **9**, 835 (2018)

20. S.E. Schmidt, C. Holst-Hansen, C. Graff, E. Toft, J.J. Struijk, Segmentation of heart sound recordings by a duration-dependent hidden Markov model. Physiol. Meas. **31**(4), 513–529 (2010)

21. J. Park, K. Lee, K. Kang, Arrhythmia detection from heartbeat using k-nearest neighbor classifier, in *IEEE International Conference on Bioinformatics and Biomedicine*, (2013), pp. 15–22

22. F. Safara, S. Doraisamy, A. Azman, A. Jantan, A.R.A. Ramaiah, Multi-level basis selection of wavelet packet decomposition tree for heart sound classification. Comput. Biol. Med. **43**(10), 1407–1414 (2013)

23. J. Li, L. Ke, Q. Du, Classification of heart sounds based on the wavelet. Entropy **21**(5), 472 (2019)

24. S. Patidar, R.B. Pachori, Classification of cardiac sound signals using constrained tunable-Q wavelet transform. Expert Syst. Appl. **41**(16), 7161–7170 (2014)

25. J.M. Keller, M.R. Gray, J.A. Givens, A fuzzy k-{NN} neighbor algorithm. IEEE Trans. Syst. Man Cybern. **SMC-15**(4), 580–585 (1985)

26. S.K. Randhawa, M. Singh, Classification of heart sound signals using multi-modal features. Procedia Comput. Sci. **58**, 165–171 (2015)

27. H.M. Hadi, M.Y. Mashor, M.Z. Suboh, M.S. Mohamed, Classification of heart sound based on s-transform and neural network, in *10th International Conference on Information Science, Signal Processing and their Applications*, (2010), pp. 189–192

28. A.A. Zo-Afshan, F. Hussain, Localization of phonocardiogram signals using multi-level threshold and support vector machine, in *2019 IEEE 19th International Symposium on Signal Processing and Information Technology, ISSPIT 2019*, (2019), pp. 1–5

29. F.A. Khan, A. Abid, M.S. Khan, Automatic heart sound classification from segmented/unsegmented phonocardiogram signals using time and frequency features. Physiol. Meas. Pap. **41**, 055006 (2020)

30. F. Demir, A. Şengür, V. Bajaj, K. Polat, Towards the classification of heart sounds based on convolutional deep neural network. Health Inf. Sci. Syst. **7**(16) (2019)
31. H. Alaskar, N. Alzhrani, A. Hussain, F. Almarshed, The implementation of pretrained AlexNet on PCGClassification, in *International Conference on Intelligent Computing*, (2019), pp. 784–794
32. K. Wołk, A. Wołk, Early and remote detection of possible heartbeat problems with convolutional neural networks and multipart interactive training. IEEE Access **7**, 145921–145927 (2019)
33. R. Yamashita, M. Nishio, T.K. Do RKG, Convolutional neural networks: an overview and application in radiology. Insights Imaging **9**, 611–629 (2018)
34. S.A. Singh, S. Majumder, Classification of unsegmented heart sound recording using KNN classifier. J. Mech. Med. Biol **19**, 1950025 (2019)
35. C. Potes, S. Parvaneh, A. Rahman, B. Conroy, Ensemble of feature: Based and deep learning: Based classifiers for detection of abnormal heart sounds, in *2016 Computing in Cardiology Conference (CinC)*, vol. 43, (2017)
36. M.A. Goda, P. Hajas, Morphological determination of pathological PCG signals by time and frequency domain analysis. Comput. Cardiol. **2010**(43), 1133–1136 (2016)
37. P. Langley, A. Murray, Abnormal heart sounds detected from short duration unsegmented phonocardiograms by wavelet entropy. Comput. Cardiol. **2010**(43), 545–548 (2016)
38. G. Clifford, C. Liu, D. Springer, B. Moody, Q. Li, R. Abad, J. Millet, I. Silva, A. Johnson, R. Mark, Classification of normal/abnormal heart sound recordings: The PhysioNet/computing in cardiology challenge 2016, in *2016 Computing in Cardiology Conference (CinC)*, vol. 43, (2017), pp. 3–6
39. S. Vernekar, S. Nair, D. Vijaysenan, R. Ranjan, A novel approach for classification of normal/ abnormal phonocardiogram recordings using temporal signal analysis and machine learning. Comput. Cardiol. **2010**(43), 1141–1144 (2016)
40. A. Bouril, D. Aleinikava, M.S. Guillem, G.M. Mirsky, S. Llc, U.P. De València, Automated classification of Normal and abnormal heart sounds using support vector machines. Comput. Cardiol. **43**, 549–552 (2016)
41. G.D. Clifford, I. Silva, B. Moody, Q. Li, D. Kella, A. Shahin, T. Kooistra, D. Perry, R. Mark, The PhysioNet/computing in cardiology challenge 2015: Reducing false arrhythmia alarms in the ICU. Comput. Cardiol. **2010**(42), 273–276 (2015)

Chapter 10
Eczema Skin Lesions Segmentation Using Deep Neural Network (U-Net)

Humaira Nisar, Ysin Ren Tan, and Kim Ho Yeap

Abstract Atopic Eczema is a skin condition that causes dry, itchy, and inflamed skin. The treatment of eczema requires detection of the infected region and grading of eczema symptoms. Dermatologists assess eczema visually and use special forms to record their findings. This process is tiresome and uses a great deal of time. In addition, it introduces inter-observer and intra-observer variability in the results. Hence in this work a fully automated method is developed to segment eczema skin lesions. A five-stage U-Net is trained to perform segmentation on the eczema dataset that consists of 84 images of different severity levels. Four different color spaces i.e., the RGB color space, HSV color space, YCbCr color space and CIELAB color space are employed for the segmentation analysis. In addition, the effect of color space normalisation technique and Adaptive Light Compensation (ALC) for illumination compensation are also examined. For performance evaluation five metrics are used namely, accuracy, sensitivity, specificity, Positive Predictive Value (PPV) and Negative Predictive Value (NPV). The highest average segmentation accuracy of 87.44% is achieved by using 16 channels in the first stage of convolution layer with 512×512 image dimension after training for 500 epochs, using ALC as pre-processing, G color channel from RGB space and mathematical morphology-based post-processing methods.

10.1 Introduction

Eczema is commonly known as atopic dermatitis. It is among the well-known skin diseases that effects the quality of life of people in different age groups ranging from children to adults. The symptoms include various degrees of inflammation on

H. Nisar (✉) · Y. R. Tan · K. H. Yeap
Department of Electronic Engineering, Faculty of Engineering and Green Technology,
Universiti Tunku Abdul Rahman, Kampar, Malaysia
e-mail: humaira@utar.edu.my; ysinren97@1utar.my; yeapkh@utar.edu.my

S. Mian Qaisar et al. (eds.), *Advances in Non-Invasive Biomedical Signal Sensing and Processing with Machine Learning*, https://doi.org/10.1007/978-3-031-23239-8_10

the skin, reddish patches, rashes, and itchiness. The problem with eczema is that it is not totally curable, rather it requires continuous treatment and home care to heal the infected skin region and prevent further infection.

The treatment of eczema requires detection of the infected area. The grading of eczema is based on the size of the infected area and the severity index [1]. This process is time-consuming and requires an expert dermatologist to evaluate it. Visual assessment may suffer from inter-rater well as intra-rater variability depending on the experience level of dermatologists as well as their working condition and burn out. Hence it is recommended to automate the process using computer-based technology which may result in improving the grading quality and speed of assessment. The first step in eczema severity grading is the segmentation of the infected region. Skin lesion segmentation is one of the toughest jobs for a computer system. This is because image segmentation requires pixel-wise classification to determine the region of the infected skin lesion.

Recent advances in computer technology allows for the medical diagnosis to be carried out with the aid of machines hence assisting the medical health professionals in their tedious tasks of diagnosing and grading different diseases. Therefore, the focus of this chapter is on segmenting eczema skin lesions using deep learning models.

10.1.1   Eczema Area and Severity Index Measurement

One of the methods used by dermatologists to identify and grade the severity levels of eczema is by using Eczema Area and Severity Index (EASI) [1] standard. This is a grading standard to determine the severity index of eczema with the help of the area of the infected region and the severity of the infection [2]. In this method the human body is divided into four main regions: head and neck, trunk, upper limb and lower limbs, and the area score is calculated according to percentage coverage of the eczema skin lesions. The area score has seven levels; the area score 0 corresponds to <1% infected region, 1 is for 1–9% infected area, 2 is for 10–29%, 3 is for 30–49%, 4 is for 50–69%, 5 is for 70–89% and 6 is for 90–100%. The severity/intensity score is graded based on four parameters; redness, thickness, scratching and lichenification into 0 with none, 1 with mild, 2 with moderate and 3 with severe intensity [1].

The calculation of the area and severity scores is a time-consuming process and needs lots of expertise as well. In addition to EASI method there are also other methods of eczema assessment which are Atopic Dermatitis Severity Index (ADSI); body surface area (BSA); Six Area, Six Sign Atopic Dermatitis (SASSAD); SCORing Atopic Dermatitis (SCORAD); Physician Global Assessment (PGA); Patient Dermatology Life Quality Index (DLQI); Oriented Eczema Measure (POEM); and pruritus Numerical Rating Scale (NRS) [3].

10.1.2   Segmentation

The first step for the automated detection of the eczema lesion is to acquire an image of the lesion and then segment this lesion from the background skin. This process is known as image segmentation. Segmentation is a very important process in image processing. There are a lot of segmentation methods to handle images of different modalities and different level of details. The existing image segmentation methods can be classified into 7 groups, as summarized in Table 10.1 [4].

Threshold-based segmentation makes use of intensity variation between the background and region of interest (ROI) to separate the image into intended regions. Global thresholding method looks at the overall intensity across the image and assigns threshold value to separate background and the intended region. Edge-based segmentation algorithm isolates the intended segmentation region from the background by detecting the edge or discontinuity of the intended object through derivative (first or second derivative) of intensity value. It determines the boundary of the object by examining the rapid change of intensity value within an image.

Region-based segmentation techniques assign classes to each pixel by determining whether the pixel is in a neighbourhood of the region through calculating the connectivity of pixel with initial seeds. The initial seeds are random points chosen to form regions with the surrounding pixels. Clustering algorithm makes use of mean, variance, and distance between clusters to classify pixels in images. Pixels with intensity value closest to the distance, mean or variance of one cluster are assigned to the respective cluster. The number of clusters is set at the beginning of the segmentation process based on the intended output.

Watershed based segmentation operates by assigning 'basin' based on intensity topology of image and classify pixels based on the drainages which separate all the basins. The drainage represents the edge in images and the basin represents different regions in the images. Partial differential equation (PDE) based method reduces noise in an image and performs edge detection by using different orders of PDE. For

Table 10.1 Image segmentation methods

Segmentation Methods	Algorithms
Thresholding	Otsu Thresholding
	Local Adaptive Thresholding
Edge Detection	Sobel Operator
	Roberts Operator
Region-Based	Seeded Region Growing
Clustering	K-means Clustering
	Hierarchical Clustering
	Gaussian Mixture Model
Watershed	Marker-based Watershed
Partial Differential Equation	Lavenberg and Marquardt Minimization
Neural Network	Fully Convolutional Networks
	Recurrent Neural Networks

example, second order PDE is suitable for edge detection and fourth order PDE is suitable for noise reduction. Neural network-based methods perform segmentation by extracting the features in each region of the object and classify pixels based on a supervised learning technique. A training set consists of original images and ground truth images are used to train the weight of each node in the neural network and validation set is used to verify the accuracy of segmentation.

10.2 Deep Learning Approach in Segmentation

The main features to differentiate deep learning with other machine learning techniques or traditional methods is the multiple layers of neural network in the model. It utilises the powerful computing, analysing, and processing capabilities of deep layers of the network to overcome the limitation or blind spot of humans in performing these tasks.

10.2.1 Neural Network

The neural network is inspired from the biological structure of the human brain which processes information through an infinite number of neurons. The neurons work together to transmit information from one end to the other end at the junctions known as synapses. Neural network mimics the operation of a human neuron. Figure 10.1 shows the architecture of a neural network; the basic components of the neural networks are the numerous circles interconnected with each other, these are known as nodes or neurons. Each neuron is responsible for a certain feature or information. Weights are assigned to each neuron to represent the significance of the

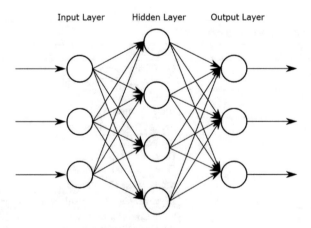

Fig. 10.1 Architecture of a neural network

features owned by the respective neuron. The input layer is normally represented by a vector, array or tensor that holds the input information whether in sequence or random.

When the input information propagates through the neural network, each neuron imparts some influence on the information according to the weights and features carried by them. The output layers are shaped according to the intended output pattern. It may be a predicted value, a probability of an event happening or a simple binary representation of yes and no.

The powerful aspect of neural network is derived from its capability to continuously monitor and update the weight of each neuron to obtain the optimal results through supervised learning. At the instance where the information propagates through the neural network and reaches the output node, a cost function is implemented to determine the difference between the predicted value and the actual value. After that, the difference or error is backpropagated to each neuron and the weight of each neuron is updated in such a way to achieve the optimal output accuracy.

10.2.2   Convolutional Neural Network (CNN)

Convolutional neural network (CNN) is a modification of the basic neural network structure with the intention to utilize it in image processing, especially for classification. The fundamental architecture of CNN is shown in Fig. 10.2. There are four main operations in the CNN model; convolution, pooling, flattening and fully connected layer. Convolutional layers in CNN are responsible for extracting features from an image by performing simple 2-D convolution either with zero padding or without it. The results of the convolution are numerous feature maps that hold different feature channel of the original image. Each convolution operation is followed

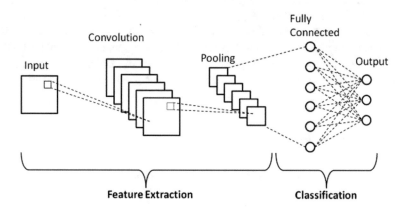

Fig. 10.2 Basic architecture of a CNN

by a rectification operation, which improves the non-linearity within each feature channels [5].

Pooling performs down scaling by reducing the size of the feature map and it sends only the important data to next layers in CNN. It thus reduces the pixel density of the image. Flattening layer is an intermediate layer that converts all the 2-D arrays from pooled feature maps into a single linear vector. The fully connected layer is the final layer that contains all the information required to determine the expected output, by applying normalization function such as SoftMax function. In a multi-class problem SoftMax specifies decimal probabilities to each class (the sum of all probabilities should be equal to 1.0).

10.2.3 Region-Based CNN (R-CNN)

The basic CNN structure has its limitations. Its applications are usually limited to image classification. When it comes to segmentation, the CNN architecture as shown in Fig. 10.2 is not very useful. This is because CNN is responsible for extracting features from images and classify them based on the similarities among the features from all images. While in segmentation, the image dataset normally shares similar general features. For example, the whole image dataset is about human skin. The focus of CNN is on the features in the images while segmentation requires to focus on differentiating features within images, or more accurately, features represented by each pixel or group of pixels.

Region-based CNN (R-CNN) is an alternative to deal with the shortcomings of the CNN model. Instead of focusing on inter-image features, R-CNN method is specifically designed to perform convolution on randomly selected regions of the image to create values for region-specific details [6]. This allows localization and detection to take place as R-CNN model focuses on features within the images. There is a simple example to illustrate R-CNN outcomes, imagine that the algorithm randomly selected three regions and one of them is the ROI. The R-CNN would provide a label for ROI, for example, a car, while the other two regions may be labelled as background. The architecture of R-CNN is shown in Fig. 10.3. R-CNN is more promising when it comes to image segmentation. Table 10.2 lists down the methods proposed by researchers to perform skin lesion segmentation based on R-CNN model. Their pros and cons are analyzed and summarized.

10.2.4 Fully Convolutional Network (FCN)

Another method for image segmentation using deep learning is Fully Convolutional Neural Network. FCN blends the encoder-decoder structure with CNN architecture to form a network that is suitable for segmentation. Encoder-decoder network is one of the branches in deep learning that takes the output size or output channel like the

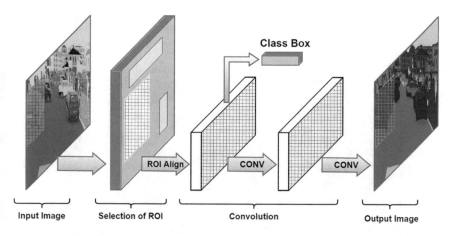

Fig. 10.3 Basic architecture of a R-CNN

Table 10.2 R-CNN based segmentation algorithms

Model	Dataset	Advantage	Disadvantage
R-CNN (Girshick et al., 2015) [7]	ILSVRC2013	Able to perform segmentation	Time consuming, Poor region selection algorithm Low accuracy,
Fast R-CNN (Girshirk, 2015) [6]	PASCAL VOC 2007	Efficient segmentation	Poor region selection algorithm, Low accuracy
Faster R-CNN (Ren et al., 2015) [8]	PASCAL VOC 2007	Time efficient	Poor region selection algorithm, -Low accuracy
Mask R-CNN (He et al., 2017) [9]	COCO 2015, COCO 2016	High accuracy segmentation	–
SSD (Liu et al., 2016) [10]	PASCAL VOC, COCO, ILSVRC	Grid-based region selection algorithm	Required extra network to perform segmentation

input channel. The autoencoder structure has strong application in compressing and encoding information and recovering it [11]. The architecture of the encoder-decoder algorithm is shown in Fig. 10.4.

When the encoder-decoder structure blends with the CNN architecture shown in Fig. 10.2, it forms a perfect architecture for segmentation. As shown in Fig. 10.5, FCN takes the input which is same as the size of the original image and performs convolution on features within the image without padding. At the final stage, reconstruction of image maximizes the possibility to obtain high accuracy in segmentation since the reconstructed image preserves most of the pixel information and allows evaluation of accuracy to be performed at the same size as of the original image [12]. Some common deep learning models implemented by researchers to

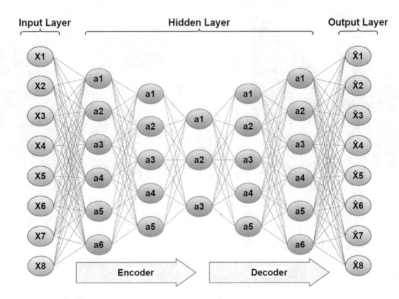

Fig. 10.4 Encoder-decoder architecture

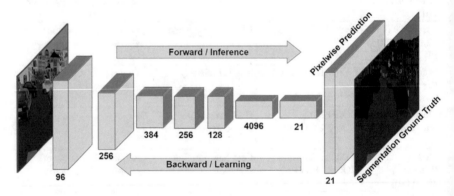

Fig. 10.5 FCN architecture

perform skin lesion segmentation are shown in Table 10.3. The pros and cons are listed by analyzing the performance of each model.

10.2.5 Summary of Lesion Segmentation Literature

There are many methods proposed in the literature for skin lesion segmentation using machine and deep learning. Many methods are proposed for Melanoma lesion segmentation using different neural network models [17–27]. Abraham and Khan (2018) proposed U-Net and Attention U-Net as the methods to carry out

Table 10.3 FCN based segmentation algorithms

Model	Dataset	Advantage	Disadvantage
FCN (Long et al., 2015) [12]	PASCAL VOC 2011	Able to perform segmentation	Large dataset required
SegNet (Badrinara. et al.,2017) [13]	PASCAL VOC12	Efficient segmentation	Not suitable for biomedical images
DeepLab (Chen et al., 2017) [14]	PASCAL VOC 2012	Time efficient suitable for large object segmentation	Not suitable for biomedical images
U-Net (Ronneberger et al., 2015) [15]	ISBI 2012 Challenge	Feasible for small dataset. Suitable for biomedical image segmentation	Up sampling phase limitation due to transpose convolution technique
R2U-Net (Alom et al.,2018) [16]	Skin cancer lesion, Lung cancer, retina blood vessel	Feasible for small dataset. Suitable for biomedical image segmentation	Complex network architecture

segmentation [17, 18]. A dice score of 0.838 for U-Net and 0.856 for Attention U-Net was achieved. Yuan (2017) [18] proposed Convolutional-deconvolutional Network to segment melanoma images and recorded mean Intersection over Union (IoU) of 78.40% while Bi et al. (2017) [20] using Multiscale Resnet to perform segmentation on melanoma dataset and achieves 79.40% IoU.

For eczema segmentation, traditional machine learning approaches have been used by previous researchers. Ch'ng et al. (2014) reported 84.60% accuracy by using K-means [28] and using a semi-automatic bi- level k-means with CSN-I Green channel and adaptive light compensation (ALC) as pre-processing method, a highest average segmentation accuracy of 86.07% is achieved [29]. Nisar et al. (2020) proposed a fully automatic method of eczema lesion segmentation using feature ranking and SVM with CSN-I RGB color space [30]. An accuracy of 84.43% was achieved with Green-channel. Nisar et al. (2020) proposed another eczema segmentation method using U-Net [31] on the same dataset with a slightly higher accuracy of 85.16% with Green channel of RGB color space.

Table 10.4 summarizes segmentation methods of skin diseases including melanoma (skin cancer) and eczema. Hence from Table 10.4 we can see that the average segmentation performance of melanoma lesion segmentation using deep learning model is 75–85%. FCN based network including U-Net, FCN and FCRN shows promising performance in lesions segmentation compared to other families of deep learning model. For eczema lesion segmentation, the traditional methods show the highest accuracy of 86.07% and a simple U-Net based method gives an accuracy of 85.16% [31]. Based on the performance of deep learning network in melanoma segmentation, it is recommended to try deep learning models for eczema lesion segmentation to design a fully automated segmentation process without the tedious task of feature extraction.

Table 10.4 Skin lesion segmentation algorithms

Author	Dataset	Segmentation Model	Accuracy
Abraham and Khan (2018) [17]	Melanoma	U-net	0.838 ± 0.026 (Dice)
Abraham and Khan (2018) [17]	Melanoma	Attention U-net	0.856 ± 0.007 (Dice)
Yuan (2017) [18]	Melanoma	CDNN	0.784
Li and Shen (2018) [19]	Melanoma	FCRN	0.753
Bi et al. (2017) [20]	Melanoma	MResNet-Seg (Multi-scale)	0.794
Goyal and Yap (2017) [21]	Melanoma	FCN	0.785 (Dice)
Vesal, Ravikumar, Maier (2018) [22]	Melanoma	Skinnet	0.7667
Wen (2017) [23]	Melanoma	FCN	0.82
Attia et al. (2017) [24]	Melanoma	CNN + RNN	0.93
Yuan, Chao, Lo, (2017) [25]	Melanoma, PH2	FCN	0.836
Izadi et al. (2018) [26]	DermoFit, (Melanoma)	GANs + UNet	0.812
Tang et al. (2019) [27]	ISBI 2016 (Melanoma)	Multistage UNet+Context Information Fusion Structure+Deep Supervision	0.853
Ch'ng et al. (2014) [28]	Eczema	K-means	0.846
Ch'ng et al. (2014) [29]	Eczema	2 Levels k-means	0.8607
Nisar et al. (2020) [30]	Eczema	SVM, NBC, KNN CSN-1 RGB, Green channel	0.844,0.833, 0.835
Nisar et al. (2020) [31]	Eczema	UNET RGB, Green channel	0.852

10.3 Methodology

This section explains the complete method to perform segmentation of eczema skin lesions. The flow of the process includes pre-processing, image augmentation, segmentation, post-processing, and performance evaluation. Figure 10.6a provides an overview of the work flow. After image acquisition, ground truth images are prepared for evaluation as shown in Fig. 10.6b. Image pre-processing and augmentation are carried out before applying the neural network to segment the skin lesions. Performance evaluation is carried out at the end of the segmentation process.

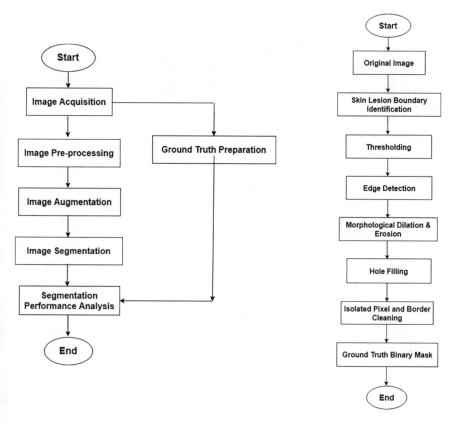

Fig. 10.6 (**a**) Overview of workflow (**b**) Ground truth binary mask preparation

10.3.1   Image Acquisition and Ground Truth Preparation

A total of 84 images in jpg format are a acquired using a Digital Single Lens Reflex (DSLR) camera. The images were obtained from the Raja Permaisuri Bainun Hospital, Ipoh and were provided voluntarily. The images in the dataset are composed of three severity levels, mild, moderate, and severe.

The ground truth for the skin lesions was manually drawn for performance assessment. This was done with the help of GNU Image Manipulation Program (GIMP) (The GIMP team, 2014). The ground truth was verified by the dermatologist. Figure 10.7 shows original images of different severity levels and a ground truth image. The lesion is surrounded by the black border that is manually drawn and verified by the dermatologist. It separates the normal skin region from the region of interest (ROI) i.e. the lesion. For performance evaluation, the ground truth images are further transformed into a binary image. The algorithm to transform the ground truth image into binary form is shown in the Fig. 10.6b.

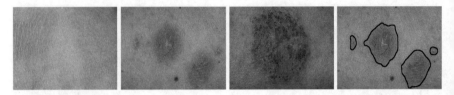

Fig. 10.7 Original Images. (**a**) Mild (**b**) Moderate (**c**) Severe and (**d**) ground truth image

10.3.2 *Image Pre-processing*

Deep learning approach requires different pre-processing pipeline as compared to the traditional approach. It involves two major steps, data structure preparation and pre-processing which includes light compensation and color model conversion.

10.3.2.1 Data Structure Preparation for Supervised Learning Methods

Supervised learning methods require dataset to be split into two or more parts, namely training set and validation set. Dataset is split into training and validation set by generating random seed and applying the random splitting function to the original dataset. The procedure to implement data structure preparation is outlined as follows:

- Read image from original dataset folder
- Generate random seed
- Apply dataset splitting function
- Create directory separating training and validation set following a hierarchical structure
- Save training and validation dataset into the corresponding directory

In this work, the splitting ratio for the training set and validation set is 7:3 instead of conventional ratio 8:2. This is due to the small dataset size.

Deep neural network model for segmentation often accepts a specific size of input images, therefore all the images including ground truth images are resized to 512 by 512.

10.3.2.2 Adaptive Light Compensation (ALC)

The image segmentation may be affected by non-uniform illumination. ALC proposed by Ch'ng et al. [28] is applied on eczema images to decrease the effect of non-uniform illumination. In ALC the value of the luminance component which isdenoted by Y is extracted from the input image and Y_{avg} is computed. To achieve good luminance, a high value of 200 and low value of 80 is obtained empirically from the images. Finally, a luminance factor is computed for image correction as given in Eq. (10.1).

$$Luminance\ Factor = \begin{cases} 80/Y_{avg}; & \text{if } Y_{avg} < 80 \\ 1\ ; & \text{if } 80 < Y_{avg} < 200 \\ 200/Y_{avg}; & \text{if } Y_{avg} > 200 \end{cases}$$

$$(10.1)$$

10.3.2.3   Color Model Conversion

Different color models have been used in this study which are RGB, HSV, YCbCr, CIElab [32]. In addition, color space normalization I technique is also applied on RGB color model [29].

10.3.3   Data Augmentation

Data augmentation is deep learning specific technique to handle the problem of a small dataset. For applications such as biomedical imaging, it is difficult to obtain large datasets as it requires lots of time as well as ethical issues are involved. Geometrical transformation is used for image augmentation. However, image augmentation is challenging for segmentation. This is due to the reason that segmentation dataset consists of both the original image and ground truth image, where segmentation dataset normally is limited due to the tedious ground truth preparation process. Data augmentation for segmentation is more tedious than conventional form as it requires transformation of both the original image and corresponding ground truth image simultaneously. The parameters assigned for augmentation are listed in Table 10.5.

Table 10.5 Image augmentation parameters

Parameters	Tuning Range
Horizontal flip	Yes
Vertical flip	Yes
Brightness range	0.5
Shear range	0.2
Rotation range	0.2
Zoom range	0.2

10.3.4 Image Segmentation

10.3.4.1 U-Net Architecture

The proposed method to handle segmentation task is U-Net proposed by Ronneberger et al. (2015) [15] from the University of Freiberg. U-Net is a deep neural network under the FCN family. Figure 10.8 shows the architecture of the U-Net.

As the name suggests, U-Net is a U-shape network composed of three main parts: down sampling path, up sampling path and bottleneck. Each of the stage in down sampling path consists of two 3×3 convolution layers, Rectified Linear Unit (ReLU) layers and one 2×2 max-pooling layer. The feature channels double while going through each convolution set until reaching the bottleneck.

The up sampling (path) is performed through transpose convolution where the feature channel is halved at each stage and concatenated with the similar layer of the cropped image at down sampling path. The up-sampling path is created to reconstruct the image so that the mask can be analyzed at the same size as the original image. After 33 output layers, an extra 1 by 1 convolution layer is added to generate the output segmentation map.

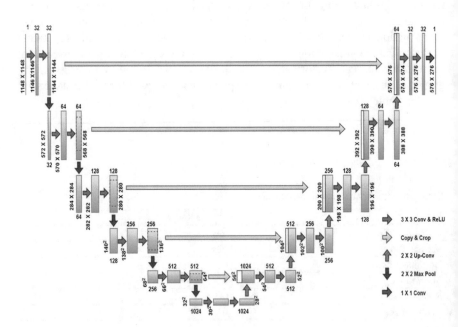

Fig. 10.8 U-Net architecture

10.3.4.2 U-Net Implementation

The procedure to implement U-Net can be divided into three steps; building the network, training network and validating the network. The first step of building U-Net involves constructing down sampling path using convolution, pooling, and rectifier function. Combination of these functions forms the first five layers of U-Net. After that reconstruction path is built by applying transpose convolution, pooling, and concatenation function. Five layers of reconstruction path forms the symmetrical structure of the U-shape network. Training network uses the training set of images and masks to train the network for several epochs. For each epoch, the network is validated either through accuracy, loss, or dice coefficient. Weights of the network are updated based on the validation coefficient. The network is trained and validated until the validation coefficient reaches a certain limit or no improvement is achieved for successive epochs. Validation network includes the process of applying the test set to the trained network to verify the performance of the network. Problems such as overfitting and underfitting or poor performance may occur in this stage, therefore validation process is important. Verification of network is simply checking the performance analysis parameters such as accuracy, sensitivity, and specificity of segmentation.

In this work 5 layers U-Net is used to perform segmentation. 3×3 convolution kernels followed by 2×2 max pooling kernels are used in each layer. The convolution layers' channels used are $(16, 32, 64, 128, 256)$. The parameters to keep track of the training process are accuracy and loss. The images are resized to 512×512 before applying to the model as the model only accepts symmetrical input images. The loss function used in this U-Net model is binary cross-entropy and the optimizer used is Adam optimizer. Eq. 10.2 shows the binary cross-entropy loss function. The results are obtained based on the training parameters of 50 epochs and 300 steps per epoch. The steps involved in implementing U-Net are shown in Fig. 10.9 and the parameters used are listed in Table 10.6.

$$H_p(q) = \frac{1}{N}\sum_{i=1}^{N} y_i \cdot \log\left(p\left(y_i\right)\right) + \left(1 - y_i\right) \cdot \log\left(1 - p\left(y_i\right)\right) \tag{10.2}$$

$$H_p(q) = \frac{1}{N}\sum_{i=1}^{N} y_i \cdot log\left(p(y_i)\right) + (1 - y_i) \cdot log\left(1 - p(y_i)\right) \tag{10.2}$$

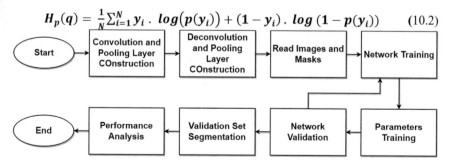

Fig. 10.9 Implementing U-Net

Table 10.6 Parameters used to build U-Net

Parameters	Value
Network Layers	5
Convolution Kernel Size	3×3
Max. pooling kernels	2×2
Number of convolution channels	(16,32,64,128,256)
Image Dimension	512×512
Steps per epoch	300
Training epoch	50
Loss Function	Binary cross-entropy
Optimizer	Adam

10.3.5 Image Post Processing

After image segmentation the next step is to remove unwanted noise like holes and broken links/edges. This is carried out using morphological image processing. Hole filling and morphological dilation is carried out using a disk shape structuring element to perform postprocessing.

10.3.6 Segmentation Performance Analysis

The segmentation results are evaluated using the following metrics as given in Eqs. 10.3, 10.4, 10.5, 10.6, and 10.7.

$$Accuracy = \frac{TP + TN}{TP + TN + FP + FN} \tag{10.3}$$

$$Sensitivity / Recall = \frac{TP}{TP + FN} \tag{10.4}$$

$$Specificity = \frac{TN}{FP + TN} \tag{10.5}$$

$$PPV = \frac{TP}{FP + TP} \tag{10.6}$$

$$NPV = \frac{TN}{TN + FN} \tag{10.7}$$

Validation accuracy determines the degree of correctness based on the pixels of foreground and background segmented when compared with the ground truth. In other words, it determines how much regions are classified correctly. Sensitivity denotes the detection rate of the region of interest (ROI), which is the eczema lesions in this work. In other words, out of the correct lesions depicted in ground truth image, how much is correctly segmented as lesion. Specificity provides information about the correct rejection rate of normal skin i.e., background in the image. In other words, how much normal skin region or background is correctly segmented as background. The PPV determines the precision of segmentation, which is the percentage of correct eczema region out of the regions segmented as lesions. While NPV determines the correct rejected region out of the regions rejected.

10.4   Results and Discussion

10.4.1   Image Pre-processing for Ground Truth Images

Image pre-processing phase turns the mask of the ground truth images into binary ground truth. This ground truth images serve as the golden images for performance evaluation after segmentation. Figure 10.10. shows a sample binary mask of ground truth. The black color indicates the eczema skin region while the white color label represents normal skin region.

10.4.2   Image Segmentation

The algorithm is tested using different color channels from different color models. In addition, for illumination correction ALC is applied. After image augmentation and illumination correction, image segmentation is performed using U-Net architecture and the results are evaluated based on individual color spaces, ALC method, as well as the effect of varying training epochs, steps per epochs and kernel number.

 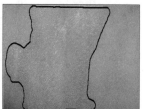 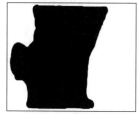

Fig. 10.10 Sample images from the dataset. (**a**) Original image. (**b**) Marked ground truth (**c**) Ground truth binary mask

10.4.2.1 Color Channels

Table 10.7 shows the average segmentation performance for RGB, HSI, YCbCr, CIELAB and CSN-I RGB channels monitored using accuracy. From the table, it is observed that the green channel achieves the highest average segmentation accuracy of 85.16% followed by GrayScale and Lightness channel, while the Value Channel recorded the highest average segmentation sensitivity and NPV, which are 90.92% and 91.28% respectively followed by Red and CSN-I Red Channels. In addition, Hue channel provides the highest average segmentation specificity followed by Blue and CSN-I blue. Lastly Blue channel also has highest PPV of 89.75% followed by Lightness and Green channels.

Table 10.8 shows the average segmentation performance for all channels monitored using loss. From the table 10.8, it is observed that the Grayscale achieves the highest average segmentation accuracy of 84.90% followed by Lightness and Y channels, while the C_b channel recorded the highest average segmentation sensitivity of 97.74% followed by A* and CSN-I Red channels. In addition, Hue channel provides the highest average segmentation specificity of 100% followed by Blue and CSN-I Blue channels. Highest average segmentation PPV is given by Blue channel of 87.9% followed by Green and Y channels and lastly highest NPV is given by CSN-I Red of 93.07% followed by Red and Value channels.

Summarizing Tables 10.7 and 10.8, and compiling results for different channels with the segmentation accuracy higher than 70%, it is seen that the Green Channel obtained highest accuracy of 85.16%, CSN-I Red channel provides the highest

Table 10.7 Average segmentation performance for different color channels monitored using accuracy

Color Channel	Validation Accuracy (%)	Sensitivity (%)	Specificity (%)	PPV (%)	NPV(%)
Grayscale	84.59	81.18	85.55	78.10	88.31
Red	76.05	90.72	65.40	64.81	92.62
Green	85.16*	75.51	89.39	84.10	86.39
Blue	82.13	59.93	93.69	89.75	81.39
Hue	63.29	3.84	99.72	–	62.74
Saturation	74.83	59.21	80.14	69.65	79.77
Value	74.97	90.94	63.65	63.50	91.28
Y	81.32	85.67	77.01	73.28	90.07
Cb	65.64	77.99	56.74	54.55	84.75
Cr	45.54	85.99	21.63	40.41	71.63
Lightness	84.31	81.60	84.41	78.72	88.80
A*	53.98	65.55	49.01	44.59	69.49
B*	53.38	70.95	43.78	43.60	70.54
CSN-I Red	80.41	87.50	74.73	70.78	91.01
CSN-I Green	74.95	67.10	80.15	71.76	80.68
CSN-I Blue	67.86	31.04	90.21	67.58	69.01

(*refers to highest accuracy, and highlight refers to top 3 values)

Table 10.8 Average segmentation performance for different channels monitored using loss

Color Channel	Validation Accuracy (%)	Sensitivity (%)	Specificity (%)	PPV (%)	NPV(%)
Grayscale	84.90*	80.87	86.19	79.40	88.54
Red	76.87	92.04	66.28	64.39	92.49
Green	84.78	74.29	90.30	84.11	85.12
Blue	79.12	47.00	96.67	87.90	76.45
Hue	62.01	0.36	100	0	61.94
Saturation	51.10	83.34	30.87	42.54	79.09
Value	78.04	89.06	69.12	69.30	90.64
Y	83.08	75.06	86.96	81.42	85.47
Cb	44.68	97.74	11.79	40.40	80.27
Cr	36.98	50.60	30.64	28.73	50.05
Lightness	84.18	79.12	86.40	79.86	86.69
A*	41.01	94.91	7.73	38.77	67.99
B*	61.28	62.93	60.95	50.10	71.55
CSN-I Red	76.59	92.13	62.05	64.89	93.07
CSN-I Green	75.71	59.17	85.27	79.94	78.61
CSN-I Blue	67.01	27.89	90.26	–	67.93

(*refers to highest accuracy, and highlight refers to top 3 values)

average segmentation sensitivity of 92.13%. While blue channel from RGB color space recorded the highest average segmentation specificity of 96.67% and PPV of 89.75% respectively. The CSN-I red channel achieves highest average segmentation NPV of 93.07%. Overall, the comparison between different color spaces summarizes that RGB color space is indeed the best to perform eczema skin lesions segmentation. While the green channel is the best channel among all the color channels as it gives the highest average segmentation accuracy.

Figure 10.11 shows the segmentation results for a simple image using all channels. By observation, the blue channel provides the best segmentation results as the boundary and the regions of the eczema lesion and normal skin are well defined. Grayscale and green channels provide satisfied output masks as the boundary of the infected region and normal skin region is outlined clearly although there are some holes in the eczema lesions. While the red channel exhibit poor segmentation performance in this simple image as it missed the main area of the infected region. For HSV channels only the value channel provides acceptable segmentation results, where the segmentation output provides a clear boundary and the eczema lesion. Hue and saturation channel are unable to perform segmentation on this dataset. Both channels classified most of the pixels as a normal skin region and could not localize the infected region on skin. For YC_bC_r model, only Y channel provides acceptable segmentation results, with a clear boundary and the regions of infected skin. The result is not perfect as there are still little regions wrongly labelled as infected although it is normal skin. C_b and C_r channel both are unable to perform segmentation on this dataset. For LAB channels, only the lightness channel provides acceptable segmentation results, with a clear boundary and the eczema skin

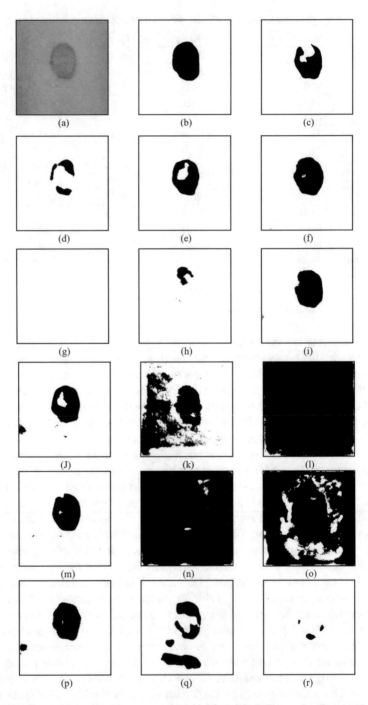

Fig. 10.11 Simple lesion and Segmented Images (**a**) Original Image. (**b**) Ground Truth. (**c**) Grayscale (**d**) Red Channel. (**e**) Green Channel. (**f**) Blue Channel (**g**) Hue Channel. (**h**) Saturation Channel. (**i**) Value Channel (**j**) Y Channel. (**k**) C_b Channel. (**l**) C_r Channel. (**m**) Lightness Channel. (**n**) A* Channel. (**o**) B* Channel (**p**) CSN-I Red channel. (**q**) CSN-I Green channel. (**r**) CSN-I Blue channel

lesion. A* and B* channels are unable to perform segmentation on this dataset. Both channels classified most of the pixels as the normal skin region and could not localize the infected region on the skin. For CSN-I RGB channels, CSN-I red and CSN-I green channel provides acceptable segmentation results, where the segmentation output of CSN-I red channel provides a clear boundary for eczema lesion. CSN-I green channel can identify a small region of eczema lesion and there are some mislabeled regions as well. CSN-I blue channel is unable to perform segmentation on this dataset. It classified most of the pixels as the normal skin and cannot localize the eczema lesion.

Figure 10.12 shows the results for all channels on a complex image. All RGB channels can segment the normal skin region and eczema skin legion at a satisfying level, but the green channel and grayscale image provide detailed segmentation of the boundary. Overall, green channel provides the highest accuracy as well as detailed segmentation on both simple and complex images. For HSV model, only the value channel provides acceptable segmentation with a clear boundary. Hue and saturation channels are unable to perform segmentation on this dataset. For YC_bC_r model, only Y channel provides acceptable segmentation results with a clear boundary of eczema lesion. However, a small region is wrongly labelled as eczema lesion although it is normal skin. C_b and C_r channels are unable to perform segmentation on this dataset. For LAB channels, only the lightness channel provides acceptable segmentation results with a clear boundary of eczema lesion. A* and B* channels are unable to perform segmentation on this dataset. For CSN-I RGB channels, CSN-I red and CSN-I green channels provide acceptable segmentation results, where CSN-I red channel gives a clear boundary and eczema skin lesion. CSN-I green channel only identifies the main eczema lesion but it cannot clearly define the boundary between normal skin and eczema lesion. CSN-I blue channel is unable to perform segmentation.

10.4.2.2   Adaptive Light Compensation Technique (ALC)

Tables 10.9 and 10.10 show the average segmentation performance for ALC RGB channel monitored using accuracy and loss respectively. It is observed that the accuracy improved after applying ALC technique to all the channels. The ALC green channel achieves highest average segmentation accuracy of 86.55%. ALC grayscale channel has the highest average segmentation sensitivity and NPV of 85.66% and 90.06% among all ALC RGB channels. The ALC blue channel provides the highest average segmentation specificity and PPV of 93.99% and 90.64% respectively. However, when CSN-I is applied along with ALC then the accuracy values decreased for all channels.

Table 10.10 shows the average segmentation performance for ALC RGB channel monitored using loss. The ALC green channel achieves highest average segmentation accuracy of 86.59%. ALC grayscale channel provides the highest average segmentation sensitivity of 88.30%. The ALC blue channels provide the highest

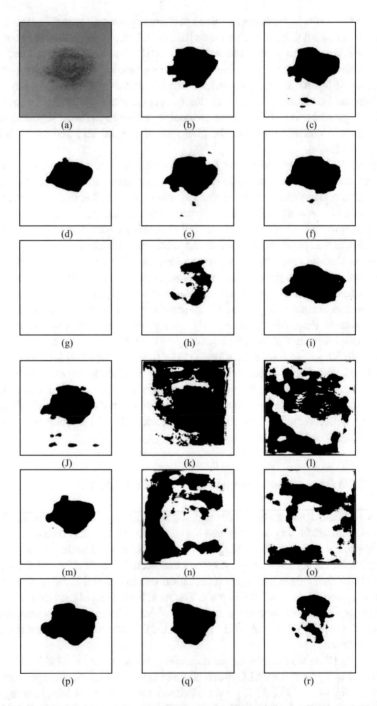

Fig. 10.12 Complex lesion and Segmented Images. (**a**) Original Image. (**b**) Ground Truth. (**c**) Grayscale. (**d**) Red Channel. (**e**) Green Channel. (**f**) Blue Channel (**g**) Hue Channel. (**h**) Saturation Channel. (**i**) Value Channel (**j**) Y Channel. (**k**) C_b Channel. (**l**) C_r Channel. (**m**) Lightness Channel. (**n**) A* Channel. (**o**) B* Channel (**p**) CSN-I Red channel. (**q**) CSN-I Green channel. (**r**) CSN-I Blue channel

Table 10.9 Average segmentation performance for different channels with ALC and monitored using accuracy

Color Channel	Validation Accuracy (%)	Sensitivity (%)	Specificity (%)	PPV (%)	NPV(%)
Grayscale	84.59	81.18	85.55	78.10	88.31
Red	76.05	90.72	65.40	64.81	92.62
Green	85.16	75.51	89.39	84.10	86.39
Blue	82.13	59.93	93.69	89.75	81.39
ALC Grayscale	84.38	85.66	81.65	76.10	90.06
ALC Red	78.01	49.87	91.41	85.36	77.70
ALC Green	86.55*	72.73	93.05	89.18	85.08
ALC Blue	83.47	62.28	93.99	90.64	82.30
ALC CSN1 Red	74.46	36.22	96.47	–	73.32
ALC CSN1 Green	79.55	56.90	90.08	83.60	80.84
ALC CSN1 Blue	65.50	20.45	93.09	59.97	65.27

(*refers to highest accuracy, and highlight refers to top 2 values)

Table 10.10 Average segmentation performance for different channels with ALC and monitored using loss

Color Channel	Validation Accuracy (%)	Sensitivity (%)	Specificity (%)	PPV (%)	NPV(%)
Grayscale	84.90	80.87	86.19	79.40	88.54
Red	76.87	92.04	66.28	64.39	92.49
Green	84.78	74.29	90.30	84.11	85.12
Blue	79.12	47.00	96.67	87.90	76.45
ALC Grayscale	82.85	88.30	77.34	72.78	91.55
ALC Red	75.78	41.44	93.02	0	75.40
ALC Green	86.59*	69.89	94.18	90.98	84.77
ALC Blue	80.74	51.67	95.99	97.08	78.98
ALC CSN1 Red	71.73	27.65	97.69	–	70.07
ALC CSN1 Green	80.67	59.48	91.07	84.80	81.35
ALC CSN1 Blue	70.83	24.94	96.82	87.66	68.08

(*refers to highest accuracy, and highlight refers to top 2 values)

average segmentation PPV of 97.08%. Whereas by combining ALC with CSN I, only Red channel achieved a highest specificity of 97.69%.

Figure 10.13 shows the segmentation accuracy for ALC RGB Channels Monitored for a simple image. By observation, the grayscale channel provides the best segmentation results as the boundary and the regions of eczema lesion and normal skin are well defined. Green channels provide satisfied output as the boundary of the eczema region and normal skin region is outlined clearly. While the red channel and blue channel exhibits poor segmentation performance in this simple image as it missed the main lobe of the infected region. For segmentation using

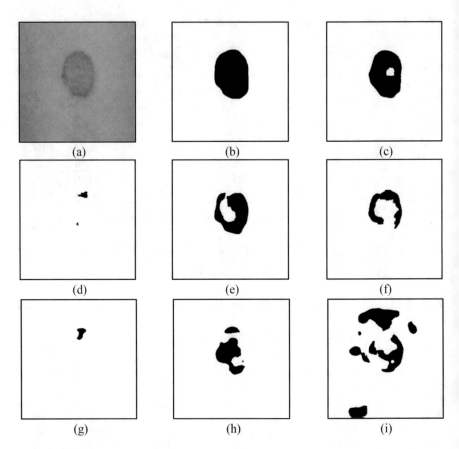

Fig. 10.13 Simple lesion and Segmented Images (**a**) Original image. (**b**) Ground truth. (**c**) ALC Grayscale. (**d**) ALC Red channel. (**e**) ALC Green channel. (**f**) ALC Blue channel (**g**) ALC CSN I Red channel. (**h**) ALC CSN I Green channel. (**i**) ALC CSN I Blue channel

ALC CSN-I RGB channels on a simple image, none of the three channels provide good segmentation results as the boundary and the regions of the eczema lesion and normal skin could not be defined by any of the channels.

Figure 10.14 shows the segmentation accuracy for ALC RGB Channels Monitored for a complex image. By observation, grayscale, green and blue channels provide good segmentation results as the boundary and the eczema skin and normal skin are well defined. Grayscale channel provides extra details on the boundary of normal skin and eczema lesion. While the red channel exhibits poorer segmentation performance in this complex image as it cannot identify and localize the eczema lesion. For ALC CSN-I RGB channels on a complex image, by observation, ALC CSN-I green channel provides the better segmentation output among three channels as it can localize the eczema skin lesion as well as the boundary of the normal skin and eczema lesion. ALC CSN-I red and ALC CSN-I blue channels do not provide good segmentation.

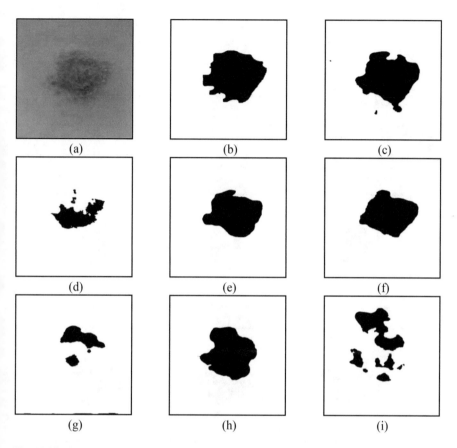

Fig. 10.14 Complex lesion and Segmented Images (**a**) Original image. (**b**) Ground truth. (**c**) ALC Grayscale. (**d**) ALC Red channel. (**e**) ALC Green channel. (**f**) ALC Blue channel (**g**) ALC CSN I Red channel. (**h**) ALC CSN I Green channel. (**i**) ALC CSN I Blue channel

10.4.3   Post-processing

After image segmentation the next step is to remove unwanted noise like holes, small gaps from it using morphological image processing. Hole filling and morphological dilation is carried out using a disk shape structuring element with radius 1 pixel is applied to the connected area with size larger than 500 pixels to perform postprocessing. This step helps to improve the overall segmentation quality as seen from Table 10.11 and Fig. 10.15.

Table 10.11 Average segmentation performance after post processing (PP)

Color Channel	Validation Accuracy (%)	Sensitivity (%)	Specificity (%)	PPV (%)	NPV(%)
Green (Before PP)	85.16	75.51	89.39	84.10	86.39
Green (After PP)	85.52	79.08	87.45	82.52	88.20
ALC Green (Before PP)	86.55	72.73	93.05	89.18	85.08
ALC Green (After PP)	87.44*	77.10	91.78	88.11	86.76

(*refers to highest accuracy, and highlight refers to top 2 values)

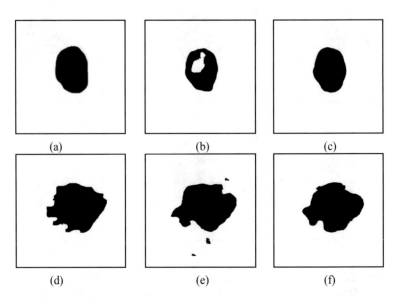

Fig. 10.15 Segmentation before and after post processing (**a**) Simple image ground truth. (**b**) Green channel (without post-processing). (**c**) Green channel (with post-processing). (**d**) Complex image ground truth. (**e**) Green channel (without post-processing). (**f**) Green channel (with post-processing)

10.4.4 Analysis of the Effect of Varying Kernel Number in Convolution Layer

Table 10.12 shows the average segmentation performance of U-Net with different kernel numbers of convolution layers. Results show that with 16 kernels at the first stage, the highest average segmentation accuracy of 85.99% is achieved. With 2 kernels at the first stage, the accuracy is the lowest, which is 47.92%. Figure 10.16 shows the segmentation results of a simple image when the number of kernels at each convolution layers are varied. By observation, 8 and 16 kernels at first stage provides good segmentation as the boundary of eczema lesion and normal skin regions are clearly defined in addition to good localization of eczema lesion.

Table 10.12 Average segmentation performance of U-Net with different Kernel numbers

Kernel No. at each stage	Validation Accuracy (%)	Sensitivity (%)	Specificity (%)	PPV (%)	NPV(%)
2,4,8,16,32	47.92	64.19	37.21	38.66	62.94
4,8,16,32,64	80.83	60.67	91.50	84.24	79.49
8,16,32,64,128	82.71	84.85	81.15	75.12	88.93
16,32,64,128,256	85.99*	79.29	89.09	83.96	87.96
32,64,128,256,512	85.36	73.99	91.15	87.10	86.34

(*refers to highest accuracy, and highlight refers to top value)

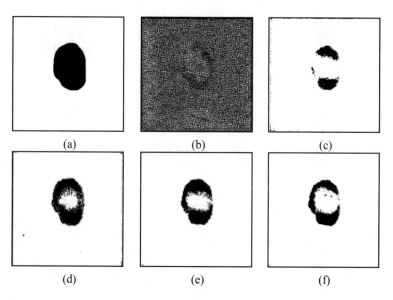

Fig. 10.16 Simple Lesion and segmented images with different kernel sets (**a**) Ground truth. (**b**) 2,4,8,16,32. (**c**) 4,8,16,32,64. (**d**) 8,16,32,64,128. (**e**) 16,32,64,128,256. (**f**) 32,64,128,256,512

Figure 10.17 shows the segmentation results on a complex image when the number of kernels at each convolution layers are varied. By observation, all kernel sets except the one with 2 kernels at first stage result in good segmentation as the boundary of the eczema skin lesion and normal skin regions are clearly defined in addition to good localization of the eczema lesion.

10.4.5 Analysis of the Effect of Varying Steps per Epoch

Table 10.13 shows the average segmentation performance of U-Net when varying steps per epoch in the training process. Results show that when 500 steps per epoch is used in training, the output has the highest average segmentation accuracy, which

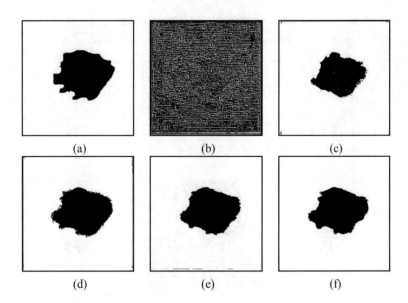

Fig. 10.17 Complex Lesion and segmented images with different kernel (**a**) Ground truth. (**b**) 2,4,8,16,32. (**c**) 4,8,16,32,64. (**d**) 8,16,32,64,128. (**e**) 16,32,64,128,256. (**f**) 32,64,128,256,512

Table 10.13 Average segmentation performance of U-Net with different steps per epoch

Steps per Epoch	Validation Accuracy (%)	Sensitivity (%)	Specificity (%)	PPV (%)	NPV(%)
1	48.78	46.10	49.77	36.34	60.39
10	69.18	55.72	75.65	57.54	73.35
50	80.59	64.04	88.99	78.88	81.39
100	83.80	76.93	85.63	78.70	87.46
300	85.99	79.29	89.09	83.96	87.96
500	86.41*	80.83	88.73	84.00	88.53
1000	86.17	72.04	93.09	89.54	86.03

(*refers to highest accuracy, and highlight refers to top value)

is 86.41%. when one step per epoch is used in training, the average segmentation accuracy is the lowest, which is 48.78%.

Figure 10.18 shows the segmentation result of simple image when steps per epochs at the training stage are varied. It is observed that when 300 onwards steps per epoch are used in training, it provides very good segmentation as the boundary of eczema lesion and normal skin regions are clearly defined in addition to good localization of eczema lesion and less noise. With one step per epoch the output binary mask is full of noise. Figure 10.19 shows the segmentation result of a complex image when steps per epochs at the training stage are varied. By observation, when 300 onwards steps per epoch are used in training, it provides best

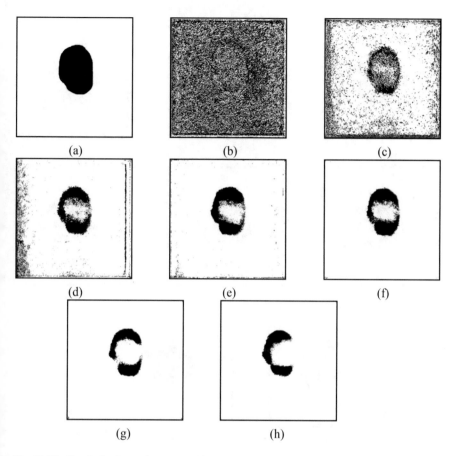

Fig. 10.18 Simple Lesion and segmented images with different step sizes per epoch (**a**) Ground truth. (**b**) 1 step. (**c**) 10 steps. (**d**) 50 steps. (**e**) 100 steps. (**f**) 300 steps. (**g**) 500 steps. (**h**) 1000 steps

segmentation result as the boundary of eczema skin lesion and normal skin region are clearly defined in addition to good localization of eczema lesion and less noise.

10.4.6 Analysis of the Effect of Varying Number of Epochs

Table 10.14 shows the average segmentation performance of U-Net when varying the number of training epochs. Results show that when training epochs are 500, the highest average segmentation accuracy, which is 87.44% is achieved. Figure 10.20 shows the segmentation results on a simple image when training epochs are varied. By observation, when 10 epochs are used in training, it provides the very good segmentation of the eczema skin lesion and the boundary between eczema lesion and normal skin regions are clearly defined. When 500 epochs are used in training, it

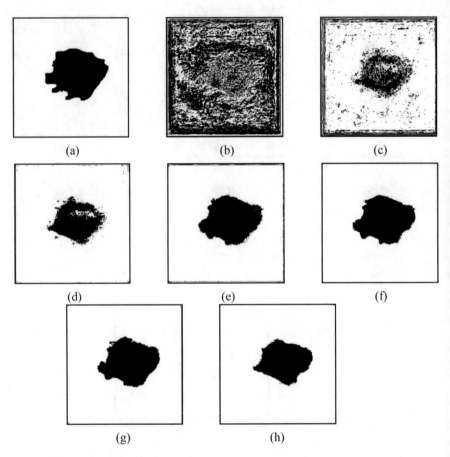

Fig. 10.19 Complex Lesion and segmented images with different step sizes per epoch (**a**) Ground truth. (**b**) 1 step. (**c**) 10 steps. (**d**) 50 steps. (**e**) 100 steps. (**f**) 300 steps. (**g**) 500 steps. (**h**) 1000 steps

Table 10.14 Average segmentation performance of U-Net with different number of epochs

No. of Epochs	Validation Accuracy (%)	Sensitivity (%)	Specificity (%)	PPV (%)	NPV(%)
1	85.99	79.29	89.09	83.96	87.96
5	86.90	74.72	93.61	89.54	86.15
10	87.00	76.38	92.25	87.77	86.22
25	85.60	77.50	87.78	81.82	87.15
50	86.59	69.89	94.18	90.98	84.77
500	87.44*	78.10	91.34	87.35	87.19

(*refers to highest accuracy, and highlight refers to top value)

also provides the very good segmentation on the boundary between the eczema skin lesion and normal skin in addition to sufficient coverage of eczema skin lesion. Notice that other training epochs including 1, 5, 25 and 50 provide moderate result

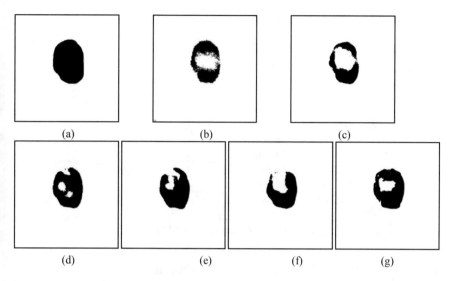

Fig. 10.20 Simple Lesion and segmented images with different number of epochs (**a**) Ground truth. (**b**) 1 epoch. (**c**) 5 epochs. (**d**) 10 epochs. (**e**) 25 epochs. (**f**) 50 epochs. (**g**) 500 epochs

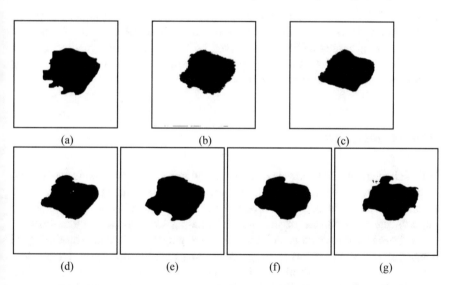

Fig. 10.21 Complex Lesion and segmented images with different number of epochs (**a**) Ground truth. (**b**) 1 epoch. (**c**) 5 epochs. (**d**) 10 epochs. (**e**) 25 epochs. (**f**) 50 epochs. (**g**) 500 epochs

as there is either discontinuity at the boundary between lesion and normal skin region or there is insufficient coverage of lesion. Figure 10.21 shows the segmentation result on complex image when training epochs are varied. By observation, all training epochs provide good segmentation result as there is no noise and discontinuity at the boundary between the eczema lesion and normal skin region.

Table 10.15 Average segmentation performance comparison of different algorithms

Algorithm	Color Channel	Classifier	Accuracy (%)	Sensitivity (%)	Specificity (%)
[30] Fully Automatic	CSN-I G	SVM	84.43	84.98	84.28
Semi Automatic	CSN-I G	2-level K-Means	88.28*	81.76	90.37
Fully Automatic	CSN-I G	Fuzzy C Means 5 clusters	87.36	78.6	91.37
	CSN-I G	K Means 5 clusters	87.51	79.23	90.07
Proposed Fully Automatic	RGB G	U-Net	87.44	77.10	91.78

(*refers to highest accuracy, and highlight refers to top 2 values)

10.4.7 Comparison of Machine Learning and Deep Learning Methods

Table 10.15 shows a comparison of the proposed method with other state of the art segmentation algorithms available in the literature. It is observed that the highest segmentation accuracy 88.28% is achieved by a semi automatic method and the second highest accuracy is achieved by the proposed method in this work with is 87.44% and this method is fully automatic.

10.5 Conclusions

In this chapter, detailed analysis of eczema skin lesion segmentation is carried out. A deep learning network based on U-Net architecture was built and implemented to segment eczema lesions. Several image processing techniques were incorporated to improve the performance of the model including Color Space Transformation, Color Space Normalisation, Adaptive Light Compensation and Morphological image processing. From the results, green channel achieves the highest average segmentation accuracy among all the color channels from different color spaces including RGB, HSV, CIELAB and YCbCr and CSN-I RGB. Adaptive Light Compensation (ALC) technique and post processing significantly improved the segmentation performance of deep learning U-Net model. Final a segmentation accuracy of 87.44% is achieved with a fully automatic segmentation method.

Here are some recommendations to further improve the overall segmentation performance.

- Building a more sophisticated deep learning segmentation model. From the literature review it is observed that to segment biomedical images with a small dataset Variants of U-Net may be suitable. The model chosen in this chapter is U-Net, but R2U-Net may also provide a better result.

- Another possible improvement is using powerful and specific artificial intelligence training hardware to handle the training process. In this work due to the limitation of GPU memory, the number of iterations, the number of convolution channels and the layers of the model were restricted, thus it directly affects the highest performance of deep learning model. A tensor core GPU or AI chips are recommended to significantly improve the performance.

References

1. J.M. Hanifin, M. Thurston, M. Omoto, R. Cherill, S.J. Tofte, M. Graeber, The eczema area and severity index (EASI): Assessment of reliability in atopic dermatitis. EASI Evaluator Group. Exp Dermatol. **10**(1), 11–18 (2001)
2. M.J. Ridd, D.M. Gaunt, R.H. Guy, N.M. Redmond, K. Garfield, S. Hollinghurst, N. Ball, L. Shaw, S. Purdy, C. Metcalfe, Comparison of eczema severity measures. Br. J. Dermatol. **179**(2), e99–e99 (2018)
3. M.J. Gooderham, R. Bissonnette, P. Grewal, P. Lansang, K.A. Papp, C.H. Hong, Approach to the assessment and management of adult patients with atopic dermatitis: A consensus document. Section II: Tools for assessing the severity of atopic dermatitis. J. Cutan. Med. Surg **22**(1_suppl), 10S–16S (2018)
4. D. Kaur, Y. Kaur, Various image segmentation techniques: A review. Int. J. Comput. Sci. Mob. Comput. **3**(5), 809–814 (2014)
5. A. Khan, A. Sohail, U. Zahoora, A.S. Qureshi, A survey of the recent architectures of deep convolutional neural networks. Artif. Intell. Rev. **53**(8), 5455–5516 (2020)
6. R. Girshick, J. Donahue, T. Darrell, J. Malik, Region-based convolutional networks for accurate object detection and segmentation. IEEE Trans. Pattern Anal. Mach. Intell. **38**(1), 142–158 (2015)
7. R. Girshick, Fast r-cnn, in *Proceedings of the IEEE International Conference on Computer Vision*, (2015), pp. 1440–1448
8. S. Ren, K. He, R. Girshick, J. Sun, Faster r-cnn: Towards real-time object detection with region proposal networks. Adv. Neural Inf. Proces. Syst, 91–99 (2015)
9. K. He, G. Gkioxari, P. Dollár, R. Girshick, Mask r-cnn, in *Proceedings of the IEEE International Conference on Computer Vision*, (2017), pp. 2961–2969
10. W. Liu, D. Anguelov, D. Erhan, C. Szegedy, S. Reed, C.Y. Fu, A.C. Berg, Ssd: Single shot multibox detector, in *European Conference on Computer Vision*, (Springer, Cham, 2016), pp. 21–37
11. M. Chen, X. Shi, Y. Zhang, D. Wu, M. Guizani, Deep feature learning for medical image analysis with convolutional autoencoder neural network. IEEE Transactions on Big Data. **7**(4), 750–758 (2017)
12. J. Long, E. Shelhamer, T. Darrell, Fully convolutional networks for semantic segmentation, in *Proceedings of the IEEE Conference on Computer Vision and Pattern Recognition*, (2015), pp. 3431–3440
13. V. Badrinarayanan, A. Kendall, R. Cipolla, Segnet: A deep convolutional encoder-decoder architecture for image segmentation. IEEE Trans. Pattern Anal. Mach. Intell. **39**(12), 2481–2495 (2017)
14. L.C. Chen, G. Papandreou, I. Kokkinos, K. Murphy, A.L. Yuille, Deeplab: Semantic image segmentation with deep convolutional nets, atrous convolution, and fully connected crfs. IEEE Trans. Pattern Anal. Mach. Intell. **40**(4), 834–848 (2017)

15. O. Ronneberger, P. Fischer, T. Brox, U-net: Convolutional networks for biomedical image segmentation, in *International Conference on Medical Image Computing and Computer-Assisted Intervention*, (Springer, Cham, 2015), pp. 234–241
16. M.Z. Alom, M. Hasan, C. Yakopcic, T.M. Taha, V.K. Asari, Recurrent residual convolutional neural network based on u-net (R2U-net) for medical image segmentation. arXiv preprint **arXiv**, 1802.06955 (2018)
17. N. Abraham, N.M. Khan, A novel focal tversky loss function with improved attention U-Net for lesion segmentation. arXiv preprint **arXiv**, 1810.07842 (2018)
18. Y. Yuan, Y.C. Lo, Improving dermscopic image segmentation with enhanced convolutional-deconvolutional networks. IEEE J. Biomed. Health Inform **23** (2017)
19. Y. Li, L. Shen, Skin lesion analysis towards melanoma detection using deep learning network. Sensors **18**(2), 556 (2018)
20. L. Bi, J. Kim, E. Ahn, D. Feng, Automatic skin lesion analysis using large-scale dermoscopy images and deep residual networks. arXiv preprint **arXiv**, 1703.04197 (2017)
21. M. Goyal, M.H. Yap, Multi-class semantic segmentation of skin lesions via fully convolutional networks. arXiv preprint **arXiv**, 1711.10449 (2017)
22. S. Vesal, N. Ravikumar, A. Maier, SkinNet: A deep learning framework for skin lesion segmentation. arXiv preprint **arXiv**, 1806.09 (2018)
23. H. Wen, II-FCN for skin lesion analysis towards melanoma detection. arXiv preprint **arXiv**, 1702.08699 (2017)
24. M. Attia, M. Hossny, S. Nahavandi, A. Yazdabadi, Skin melanoma segmentation using recurrent and convolutional neural networks, in *2017 IEEE 14th International Symposium on Biomedical Imaging (ISBI 2017)*, (IEEE, 2017), pp. 292–296
25. Y. Yuan, Y.C. Lo, Improving dermoscopic image segmentation with enhanced convolutional-deconvolutional networks. IEEE J. Biomed. Health Inform. **23**(2), 519–526 (2017)
26. S. Izadi, Z. Mirikharaji, J. Kawahara, G. Hamarneh, Generative adversarial networks to segment skin lesions, in *2018 IEEE 15th International Symposium on Biomedical Imaging (ISBI 2018)*, (IEEE, 2018), pp. 881–884
27. Y. Tang, F. Yang, S. Yuan, C.A. Zhan, A multi-stage framework with context information fusion structure for skin lesion segmentation, in *2019 IEEE 16th International Symposium on Biomedical Imaging (ISBI 2019)*, (IEEE, 2019), pp. 1407–1410
28. Y.K. Ch'ng, H. Nisar, V.V. Yap, K.H. Yeap, J.J. Tang, Segmentation and grading of eczema skin lesions, in *2014 8th International Conference on Signal Processing and Communication Systems (ICSPCS)*, (IEEE, 2014), pp. 1–5
29. Y.K. Ch'ng et al., A two level k-means segmentation technique for eczema skin lesion segmentation using class specific criteria, in *Biomedical Engineering and Sciences (IECBES), 2014 IEEE Conference on*, (IEEE, 2014)
30. H. Nisar, Y.K. Ch'ng, Y.K. Ho, Automatic segmentation and classification of eczema skin lesions using supervised learning, in *2020 IEEE Conference on Open Systems (ICOS)*, (IEEE, 2020), pp. 25–30
31. H. Nisar, Y.R. Tan, Y.K. Ho, Segmentation of eczema skin lesions using U-Net, in *2020 IEEE-EMBS Conference on Biomedical Engineering and Sciences (IECBES)*, (IEEE, 2021), pp. 362–366
32. Nisar et al., *Color Space Study for Segmentation of Eczema Skin Lesions* (ICCSA, Kuala Lumpur, 2013)
33. H. Nisar, Y. K. Ch'ng, K. H. Yeap, Non invasive automated approach for eczema lesions segmentation using color space normalization. J. Natl. Sci. Found of Srilanka. 50:705 (2022)

Chapter 11
Biomedical Signal Processing for Automated Detection of Sleep Arousals Based on Multi-Physiological Signals with Ensemble Learning Methods

Navabeh Sadat Jalili Shani and Mohammad Hasan Moradi

Abstract Sleep-related breathing disorders such as sleep apnea and hypopnea are potentially serious disorders and can be the cause of a wide range of physical and mental health problems and also reduce the quality of life. Therefore, sleep studies are essential for identifying and treating these sleep disorders. This study aims to detect arousal regions caused by sleep non-apnea and non-hypopnea in polysomnography signals by using ensemble techniques. The dataset used in this study is related to Polysomnography measurement channels of 100 patients provided in the 2018 Physionet challenge database. The data was split into small epochs with 50% overlap. Several different features were extracted from each epoch in the time and frequency domain. Wilcoxon rank-sum test and Genetic Algorithm optimization algorithm were used to find a set of features with the most discriminative information. A technique for data augmentation was used to tackle the unbalanced data problem. For final classification, linear discriminant analysis, logistic regression, bagged tree from the bagging technique, and LightGBM from the boosting method were applied. Based on the Physionet Challenge indices, the area under the receiver operating characteristic curve (AUROC), and the area under the precision-recall curve (AUPRC), we compared the performance of classifiers on this dataset. The highest performance on 20 test subjects was 0.497 for AUPRC and 0.878 for AUROC.

N. S. Jalili Shani · M. H. Moradi (✉)
Biomedical Engineering Department, Amirkabir University of Technology, Tehran, Iran
e-mail: nava.jalili@aut.ac.ir; mhmoradi@aut.ac.ir

© The Author(s), under exclusive license to Springer Nature Switzerland AG 2023
S. Mian Qaisar et al. (eds.), *Advances in Non-Invasive Biomedical Signal Sensing and Processing with Machine Learning*, https://doi.org/10.1007/978-3-031-23239-8_11

263

11.1 Introduction

The human body spends a third of its life sleeping, which is a complex process among living beings [1]. During sleep, fatigue is eliminated and mental and physical performance is restored [2]. During sleep, changes occur in many physiological functions of the body. There are also variations in these changes during different stages of sleep. The changes in physiological functions during sleep have led to associated variations in electrophysiological signals, which form the basis for research in sleep medicine [2].

Sleep disorders are a widespread problem in society today. Decreased consciousness due to sleep disorders has a negative impact on patients' lives [2]. Accurately diagnosing sleep disorders is difficult because of their clinical similarities. With the ability to record biosignals, the assessment of sleep quality became more accurate. To assess sleep quality, a variety of medical signals are used, including electroencephalogram (EEG), electrocardiogram (ECG), electromyogram (EMG), and electrooculogram (EOG), which the EEG signal is the most useful in evaluating sleep. These signals are called polysomnographic recordings [3, 4].

As defined by the American Sleep Disorders Association (ASDA) in 1992, arousal in sleep is a sudden increase in the frequency of the EEG signal that lasts at least 3 seconds and less than 15 seconds, and the person has been asleep for at least 10 seconds before it occurs [5]. A handbook of new sleep staging guidelines and respiratory, cardiac, and motor events was published in 2004 by the American Academy of Sleep Medicine (AASM). Accordingly, arousals can be defined as the transition between sleep and wakefulness, or the transition between REM and NREM stages. Brain arousals are defined as a sudden change in EEG frequency, including alpha, theta, or frequencies above 16 Hz, typically lasting between 3 and 15 seconds and at least 3 seconds. An important feature of arousal is unexpected changes in brainwave activity patterns. Arousals are usually observed in the second NREM stage or REM stage. Also, during the presence of arousals in the REM stage, the amplitude of the EMG signal increases further, which lasts at least 1 second [6, 7].

One of the leading causes of drowsiness during the day is the appearance of arousals that change the natural structure of sleep and cause sleep deprivation. This process is directly related to the development of sleep disorders in the individual [8]. As mentioned, these disorders can have significant effects on quality of life and daily cognitive function, including memory, learning, and concentration [9]. As a result, identifying EEG arousals in the polysomnographic recording is a good indicator for measuring sleep quality. The most important disorders that can cause arousals in sleep are sleep apnea, hypopnea, bruxism, snoring, and respiratory effort-related arousals (RERAs).

Visual examination of the signals recorded in polysomnography to diagnose the presence of arousals by physicians and specialists is a time-consuming and tedious task; in addition, Judging these events is also completely subjective and varies significantly from expert to expert [10]. Therefore, finding algorithms for automatic detection of these disorders based on signals helps physicians in diagnosing them [11].

Diagnosis of arousal can also affect sleep staging. Diagnosis of arousal can also affect sleep staging. According to AASM rules, once an arousal region is detected, it may mean that it is best to rank the next 30-second sleep window as another (lighter) sleep stage unless the next 30-second window features maintain the current sleep stage (for example, the presence of rapid eye movements in the REM stage or the presence of sleep spindles and k complex in the N2 stage) [12].

Two types of factors can cause sleep arousal. The first cause is apnea and hypopnea disorders such as obstructive and mixed apneas, central apneas, and hypopneas. Therefore, many studies have been performed to diagnose these arousals [3, 13–15]. Another is arousal related to disorders other than apnea and hypopnea, which include arousal caused by RERA, bruxism, snoring, etc. These arousals, which are very important to diagnose, are relatively hidden in polysomnography and are difficult to detect [16]. RERA is a respiratory disorder characterized by an obstructive decrease in airflow due to narrowing the upper airways and lasts for more than 10 seconds. RERA does not reach the threshold for apnea and hypopnea, i.e., it is associated with less reduction in airflow and little or no hypoxia. In plethysmography or polysomnography, respiratory cycles are recorded from a decrease or increase in respiratory effort, which leads to the continuous appearance of arousals on physiological signals and ends before the criteria for apnea or hypopnea are met [17, 18]. This disorder can lead to serious consequences, such as loss of attention while driving [19]. Diagnosing sleep apnea with disorders other than apnea and hypopnea is a challenge. Therefore, our aim in this study focused on the automatic detection of arousal regions due to non-apnea disorders, especially RERA, which is more common.

There have been many studies in the field of arousal detection. There have been three methods used to develop an algorithm for detecting sleep disorders automatically in these studies. Most of these studies have proposed neural network-based algorithms. A group of studies [20–24] first considered the raw data as input of a neural network after making the necessary preprocessing on them, and another group first extracted a set of valuable features from the data after the necessary preprocessing to reduce data dimension and then trained their designed deep neural network with the extracted features [3, 25]. Another group of studies has used basic machine learning algorithms such as logistic regression, linear differential analysis [26], and support vector machine.

The remainder of this chapter is organized as follows: Section 11.2 discusses polysomnography. Section 11.3 is dedicated to sleep stages. Section 11.4 will cover the method. Results are reported in Sect. 11.5. Finally, the last section is the conclusion.

11.2 Polysomnography

Polysomnography is a nocturnal test during several hours of sleep in which different measurement techniques are used to simultaneously and continuously record neurophysiological, cardio-respiratory, and other physiological and physical parameters [27].

This method uses mentioned medical signals, pulse oximetry, airflow, and respiratory effort to provide data on physiological changes in many different systems of the body that are affected by sleep and therefore may not be present at waking time to assess the essential causes of sleep-related disorders. Polysomnographic recordings are divided into 30-second segments and are interpreted based on expert opinion and published sleep guidelines. Fig. 11.1 shows a segment of airflow and SaO2 signals. The patient has an apnea disorder in the green portion of the signal. When apnea occurs, the amplitude of the SaO2 signal and the airflow are reduced by more than 90%. Both signals are characterized by this reduction when apnea occurs. The part of the signal marked in blue is related to RERA arousal, and the decrease in airflow is less severe than in apnea.

11.2.1 EEG

The EEG signal is the main basis of the objective diagnosis of awakening, arousals, and sleep stages during the sleep study. In most cases, the brain waves are irregular, and there is no general pattern, but specific patterns appear in some cases, such as epilepsy. The EEG also contains waves with various frequency ranges, the presence of which in different brain regions corresponds to a specific activity or state. Rhythms in the EEG signal that include Delta, Theta, Alpha, Beta, and Gamma waves, as well as particular patterns in this signal that include Vertex sharp wave or V-waves, slow waves, K-complexes, and sleep spindles, are used to distinguish between waking, sleeping, classifying stages and disorders of sleep [6]. Table 11.1 shows the rhythms in the EEG signal. Figure 11.2 also shows these rhythms.

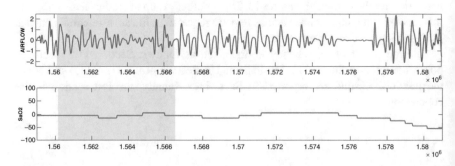

Fig. 11.1 A segment of airflow and SaO2 signals. The green parts are related to apnea arousal and the blue parts are related to RERA arousal

Table 11.1 The EEG rhythm specifications [28]

Delta	0.1–4 Hz	In adults, found in the frontal region
Theta	4–8 Hz	High amplitude waves in comparison to other EEG sub-bands
Alpha	8–12 Hz	Always seen in frontal and parietal
Beta	Above 12 Hz	During deep relaxation and while focusing

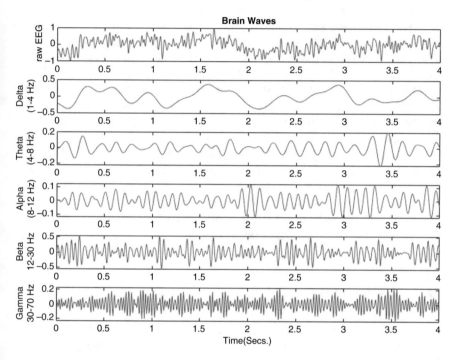

Fig. 11.2 Rhythms in EEG

11.2.1.1 Special Patterns in EEG

Identifying three specific patterns in sleep is very important in analyzing EEG recorded during sleep. Sharp vertex wave is one of the most important patterns of NREM sleep that are most often seen in stage N1 and sometimes in stage N2. They are seen in the EEG as quite distinctive, seven-shaped waves with peaks in the amplitude of about 100 to 200 microvolts [29]. Sleep spindles are a sequence of oscillations in the amplitude of the EEG signal, usually lasting between 0.5 and 3 seconds, and the frequency of these changes varies between 11 and 16 Hz [30]. K-complexes are complicated seven-shaped patterns of sleep waves that indicate the transition into a deeper stage of sleep. This pattern is seen as a sharp negative wave with a high amplitude followed by a low slope wave. K-complexes have a duration criterion that must at least last 0.5 seconds. K-complexes may include other events like periodic movements of the limbs in sleep, apnea, or appear with arousal (Alpha rhythm in EEG) [6].

11.3 Sleep Stage

REM and NREM are the two main stages of sleep. NREM sleep is also divided into four stages. Stages 1 and 2 are called the light stage of sleep, and stages 3 and 4 are called the deep stage or slow-wave sleep. There are four or five sleep cycles during each night, each consisting of one part of NREM sleep followed by REM sleep [31]. The first stage is wakefulness which may last 5 to 10 minutes. At this stage, the brain is between sleep and wake state. The predominant brain waves at this stage are Alpha waves. In the EOG signal at this stage, blinking and rapid movements are observed. Stage N1, or somnolence, is another stage of NREM sleep. At this stage, called light sleep, EEG activity is fast with low voltage. This stage is defined when Theta waves (4 to 7 Hz) form more than 15 seconds (more than half) of the epoch. The next stage is N2, also known as sigma, and the sleep spindle. This stage is in the middle of sleep and, at first, takes about 20 minutes. At this stage, sleep enters a deeper level, and heart rate and the body temperature decrease. Next is stage N3, which is also called deep sleep, sleep with slow waves, or delta. At this stage, muscle and brain activities decrease. The last stage is REM which is also called active or paradoxical sleep. At this stage, eyes are closed but have a rapid movement. In this state, the brain waves show an activity similar to the state of awakening. Dreaming is at this stage of sleep, and this stage occurs in adults between 90 and 120 minutes after the beginning of sleep [6, 32].

11.4 Methodology

In this section, we discussed the ensemble learning algorithms used in this study, the performance evaluation criteria, the dataset, their preprocessing process, extracted features, and methods for selecting the effective features.

11.4.1 Ensemble Learning

An ensemble learning algorithm is a machine learning method that incorporates a number of simple and weak algorithms to form a strong learning algorithm with higher accuracy. This type of learning is one of the best ways to maintain the balance between variance and bias. An effective model should be able to balance these two types of errors. Ensemble methods can be mainly divided into three groups: boosting, bagging, and stacking. In the present study, we use the random forest and XGboost algorithms, which apply "bagging" and "boosting" methods, respectively.

11.4.1.1 Bootstrap Aggregation (Bagging)

The bagging method creates algorithms parallel to one another. Several independent models are generated, and their predictions are averaged. The variance of the combined base models is reduced in proportion to the number of models or samples. In addition, the independence of the basic learning models significantly reduces the error through the application of averaging.

Bagging is used when the goal is to variance reduction of the decision tree classifier without impacting bias. The reduction of variance leads to increased accuracy and avoidance of overfitting, which is a major challenge in many predictive models. Multiple subsets of training instances are randomly created with replacement, and the data from each subset is used to learn the corresponding decision tree. In this way, a number of different models are eventually created. The average of all the predictions from the individual trees is the final result, which performs better than a single decision tree classifier.

11.4.1.1.1 Random Forest (RF)

RF is based on the ensemble learning algorithm and involves a large amount of classification and regression trees (CARTs). The core of the RF algorithm relies on the concept of 'bagging' and selecting features randomly. At the beginning of the RF algorithm, a bootstrap sample is taken from the training data. In each CART node, features are randomly selected, and feature subsets are searched to find the optimal split. An unpruned CART is formed when this process is repeated at each node. Additionally, for evaluating the model performance and estimating feature importance, bootstrap sample data - known as out-of-bag sample (OOB) – can be used as a test set. Repeating this process for each tree will result in a fully grown forest.

11.4.1.2 Boosting

Boosting is a sequential ensemble method in which the weight of each input is modified according to the latest classification. In boosting, when an input is misclassified by one hypothesis, its weight is increased, so the new hypothesis is more likely to be classified correctly. The goal at each step is to improve the prediction accuracy over the previous tree's performance. In boosting, like bagging, a single algorithm is used as the basic learning model, and in the process, weak learning models become a model with more robust performance. Boosting comes in many forms, including Adaboost, GBDT, XGBoost, and LightGBM. In this study, the LightGBM algorithm, the most recent one, is used, which is explained in the following.

11.4.1.2.1 Gradient Boosting Decision Tree (GBDT)

Another ensemble learning algorithm that uses several decision trees as base learners and a gradient descent optimization algorithm to calculate the error of its previous models is GBDT. Newly added decision trees increase the emphasis on samples misclassified by the previous decision tree.

In the GBDT algorithm, the residual of the previous decision tree is intended as input to the following decision trees. Then, the new decision tree adds to minimize the residual so that each time the iteration is repeated, the cost decreases as it progresses in the negative gradient direction. All decision tree results are then used to determine the prediction result.

Supposing the data samples are represented $(x_i, y_i)_{i=1}^m$.

Which x_i is data value and l_i is the predicted label. The GBDT algorithm is explained as the follows.

First the initial constant value θ is obtained from the eq. (11.2).

$$F(x, \theta) = \sum_m^{n=1} L(y_n, \theta) \tag{11.1}$$

$$F_0(x) = \min_\theta F(x, \theta) \tag{11.2}$$

Where $L(y_i, \theta)$ is the loss function.

Based on the gradient, the residual is calculated as follows:

$$\hat{y}_i = -\left[\frac{\partial L(l_i, F(x_i))}{\partial F(x_i)} \right]_{f(x)=f_{n-1}(x)} \tag{11.3}$$

Where $n = 1, 2, \ldots, N$ indicates the number of iterations.

The initial model $T(x_i; \alpha_n)$ is determined by using the sample data, and α_n is computed based on the least square method as follows:

$$a_n = \min_{\alpha, \theta} \sum_{i=1}^m (\hat{y}_i - \theta T(x_i; \alpha_n))^2 \tag{11.4}$$

Based on the loss function minimization, the weight of the model is computed as follows:

$$\theta_n = \min_\theta \sum_m^{i=1} L(y_i, F_{n-1}(x) + \theta T(x_i; \alpha_n)) \tag{11.5}$$

The model can be written as follows:

$$F_n(x) = F_{n-1}(x) + \theta_n T(x_i; \alpha_n) \tag{11.6}$$

This loop continues until the number of iterations is defined or until the convergence is [33].

11.4.1.2.2   Light Gradient Boosting Machine (LightGBM)

LightGBM is another ensemble algorithm that is designed by Microsoft using the GBDT framework. It is intended to improve computation performance and thus provide a more accurate solution to the problems associated with handling big data in prediction. To calculate the information gain of all possible split points, conventional GBDT implementations must examine all sample data for each feature, which takes much time when dealing with big data (both for the number of features and data size). Thus, computational complexions would be proportional to the number of features and samples. In LightGBM, a histogram-based algorithm and growth strategy through the leaves of trees are adopted with maximum depth size to enhance training speed and optimize memory utilization.

In order to address these limitations and further improvement of model efficiency, the LightGBM algorithm presents *Gradient-based One-Side Sampling (GOSS)* and *Exclusive Feature Bundling (EFB)*.

(a) *Gradient-based one-side sampling*

In Adaboost, a sample's weight works as a good indicator of the importance of data samples. However, in GBDT, there is no local weight for the samples, so the proposed sampling methods for Adaboost cannot be applied directly. Gradient for each sample in GBDT provides practical information for data sampling. In other words, a sample with a small gradient had a small training error and had been well trained. The simple idea is to put aside data samples with small gradients. Nevertheless, it changes the data distribution and negatively affects the accuracy of the trained model. The Gradient-based One-Side Sampling (GOSS) method was developed to minimize this problem and maintain the accuracy of trained decision trees while reducing data samples.

GOSS maintains all samples with large gradients and takes randomly the ones with small gradients. GOSS selects the top a × 100% samples after sorting the data samples based on the absolute value of their gradients. Then it randomly selects b × 100% of samples from the remaining data. Then, for amplifying the sampled data with small gradients, GOSS uses a constant $\frac{1-a}{b}$ for computing the information gain to compensate for the effect of data distribution. In this way, it is possible to focus more on the data that has not been trained yet, without any changes to the original data distribution. More details about the theory of GOSS can be found in [34].

(b) *Exclusive Feature Bundling*

The purpose of the EFB method is to effectively reduce the number of features. In general, high-dimensional data are sparse. By considering the sparse nature of the feature space, we can devise a method of reducing the number of features almost without losing any information. Particularly, many features in sparse feature space are mutually exclusive; that is, they cannot take nonzero values simultaneously. Exclusive features can be grouped into a single feature (an exclusive feature bundle). By a carefully designed feature scanning algorithm, identical feature histograms can be constructed from these feature bundles as the same histograms for single features. Thus, the histogram structure complexity from the number of features multiplied by the number of samples changes to the number of feature bundles multiplied by the number of samples, in which the number of feature bundles is much less than the number of features alone. In this way, the speed of GBDT training can be significantly increased without compromising accuracy. To do this by turning the ranking problem into a graph coloring process (adding edges for both non- exclusive features and features as vertices) and its solution is designed by another algorithm with a fixed approximation ratio of an effective algorithm.

Compared to the level-wise growth run in the XGBoost algorithm, the limited growth process through leaves used by the LightGBM algorithm is more efficient; because it is distributed only through a leaf with the highest information gain, and as a result, it achieves much better accuracy than other boosting algorithms, and the limited depth can effectively prevent overfitting. As mentioned, this algorithm is surprisingly fast; hence the word "light" is dedicated to it [34]. Studies have indicated that this algorithm can make the training process 20 times faster [35].

11.4.2 Evaluating Performance

For evaluating the performance of the implemented algorithms, we used two measurement criteria: the Area Under the Receiver Operating characteristic Curve (AUROC) and the Area Under the Precision-Recall Curves (AUPRC).

AUROC indicates the ability of a model to classify samples accurately. A ROC curve represents the exchange between true positive rate (TPR) and false positive rate (FPR) at a range of decision thresholds. In ROC curves, the decision threshold is implicit. There is no axis for decision thresholds, and AUROC is the area under the ROC curve. On the ROC curve, the x-axis represents the FPR, and the y-axis represents the TPR. AUROC for a specified curve is simply the area below it. The lowest AUROC value is 0.5, and the highest is 1.

The AUPRC criterion is used to evaluate model performance when classes are highly unbalanced and positive samples are essential. The precision-recall curve illustrates the relationship between precision and recall for different thresholds. Having a large area under the curve indicates high precision and recall of the model, where high precision is related to a low false positive rate (FPR) and high recall is related to a low false negative rate (FNR). A high value for both indicates that the classifier returns correct (high precision) and the most positive (high recall) results [36]. The area under the PR curve is known as the AUPRC. PR curves represent the tradeoff between accuracy and sensitivity over a range of decision thresholds. A recall is also known as a true positive rate (TPR). As a result, both AUPRC and AUROC use TPR.

Unlike the ROC curve where the y-axis represents recall, the x-axis represents the FPR, the x-axis represents the PR-recall curve, and the y-axis represents precision.

One of the features of the PR curve is that it does not use TNs in any way. According to the definitions of precision and recall, they are calculated as follows:

$$Recall = TPR = \frac{True\,Positives\,(TP)}{True\,Positives\,(TP) + False\,Negatives\,(FN)}$$

(11.7)

The recall of a classifier can be defined as the ability to correctly identify all positive samples.

$$Precision = \frac{True\,Positives\,(TP)}{True\,Positives\,(TP) + False\,Positives\,(FP)}$$

(11.8)

A classifier's precision is its ability to avoid mislabeling a negative sample as positive.

In PR curves, there are no TNs, so AUPRC will not be affected by TNs. If AUPRC is used for datasets with 95% negative and 5% positive samples, it focuses on how 5% of the samples are treated. If the model performs well in detecting positive samples, the AUPRC will be high; if not, it will be low. The AUPRC is therefore most useful when its baseline is the lowest because it focuses on the smallest fraction of positive samples possible across large datasets with large numbers of TNs [37].

11.4.3 Data Description

As mentioned earlier, the current study aimed to provide a method for automatic detection of arousals related to non-apnea sleep disorders using polysomnographic signals with ensemble learning. In this study, we used Physionet Challenge 2018 database [16].

A total of 1983 polysomnographic data were provided, which included 994 subjects for training and 989 subjects for the test. Polysomnography in these data is recorded according to the AASM standard. A total of 13 signals are provided, including:

- six EEG channels; F3-M2, F4-M1, C3-M2, C4-M1, O1-M2, and O2-M1, based on the international 10–20 system;
- one left eye EOG channel, referenced to the right ear EEG electrode (M2);
- Three EMG channels, one on the chin and two channels of breathing signal from the abdomen and chest;
- one airflow channel;
- one oxygen saturation channel (SaO2);
- And one ECG channel located below the right clavicle close to the sternum and across the left lateral chest wall

All signals were measured at a sampling frequency of 200 Hz except SaO2. SaO2 was upsampled to 200 Hz to synchronize samples using a sample and hold. Also, all signals are measured in microvolts.

The specialists labeled the training data in two different ways in the data source. In the first state, the samples were labeled into three classes −1, 0, and + 1. In these three classes:

- Label +1 is related to non-apnea and non-hypopnea arousals
- Label 0 is related to normal sleep
- Label −1 is related to apnea and hypopnea arousals

In the second state, the labeling has been done more precisely, and types of arousals related to each region are also determined. The sleep stages were labeled too.

According to the available data, arousals that were considered in this study are classified as spontaneous arousals, RERA, hypoventilation, bruxisms, hypopneas, snores, apneas (central, obstructive and mixed), vocalizations, periodic leg movements, Cheyne-Stokes breathing or partial airway obstructions.

The proposed method was evaluated using recordings belonging to 100 subjects from the training group. 80% of this data, which includes 80 subjects, have been considered for the training stage, and 20%, including 20 subjects, have been considered for the test stage [16].

11.4.4   Pre-Processing

Before extracting the features from the data, the signals were preprocessed to remove noise.

11.4.4.1   EEG and EOG Signals

Due to the non-invasive nature of EEG signals, the distance between the signal source and the recording electrode, as well as the low amplitude of this signal, adding unwanted signals can reduce the signal to noise ratio and cause many problems in the analysis of these signals; as a result, it is necessary to preprocess them before analyzing.

Both EEG and EOG signals are first preprocessed using a fourth-order low-pass Butterworth filter with a cut-off frequency of 42 Hz and then a fourth-order Butterworth high-pass filter with a cut-off frequency of 1 Hz.

Although EEGs are typically interpreted as recording brain activity, other electrical activities are also captured. Extra activities tend to be harmful artifacts, whether they are physiological, like EOG, EMG, or ECG, or extra artifacts like power line interference. Frontal electrodes are mainly responsible for recording EOG measurements, however they can also affect other electrodes [38]. Furthermore, due to the volume conduction effect, both effects of eye activity and EEG activity are diffused to the surface of the head and recorded by electrodes. EOGs usually have a greater amplitude than EEGs. However, due to its similar frequency to EEG signals, removing this artifact is one of the most critical problems in studying brain activity [39].

The power spectrum of some of these artifacts created during recording is different from the power spectrum of the EEG, making its removal easy with an IIR filter. Even so, ECG and EOG, whose power overlaps significantly with EEG, are not easily removed and require specialized algorithms [40].

For this purpose, we used the adaptive filter, which is a successful method in the non-stationary signals processing field. This method uses raw EEG signals as inputs and EOG and ECG artifacts as reference signals. Pure EEG can be obtained by reducing the filtered output. The ability to adapt the parameters of an adaptive filter based on the minimization of mean square error (MSE) is between the output signal of the system and the desired signal. The recursive least squares (RLS) and the least mean square (LMS) are commonly used algorithms of adaptive filter algorithms. The advantages of the RLS algorithm over the LMS are its stability and fast convergence speed. Therefore, we used the RLS algorithm to adjust the filter coefficients to ensure that the reference signal has the most appropriate specifications for these artifacts.

To do so, we used the method proposed in [38]. In order to detect the additional presence of EOG and ECG, the filtered EEG, EOG, and ECG signals after being divided into segments with 2048 samples, the cross-correlation between each EEG segment with the respective EOG and ECG sections has been calculated. Adaptive RLS filters are used when the cross-correlation coefficients between EEG-EOG or EEG-ECG are greater than two thresholds of 0.5 and 0.2, respectively. If the threshold values for the cross-correlation coefficients are not met, the corresponding EEG part is transferred without changing the output. In Fig. 11.3 More details can be found in [38].

11.4.4.2 EMG Signal

After preprocessing with a Butterworth low-pass filter with a cut-off frequency of 70 Hz, the EMG signals were then passed through a Butterworth high-pass filter with a cut-off frequency of 10 Hz. Then, an adaptive filter was applied to remove ECG artifacts.

11.4.4.3 ECG Signal

This signal is also passed through a fourth-order Butterworth low-pass filter, with a cut-off frequency of 25 Hz, and a high-pass filter with a cut-off frequency of 0.1 Hz with the same specifications. Fig. 11.4 shows the ECG signal before and after the filtering.

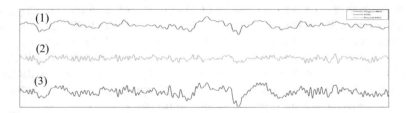

Fig. 11.3 One segment of (1) EOG signal, (2) EEG after the removal of EOG by RLS method and (3) EOG impregnated EEG

11.4.4.4 Airflow Signal

In order to preprocess this signal, in the first step, the DC value is removed from the signal. Thus, a window of 20,000 samples is considered. The median of the window is subtracted from the total in the length of the signal. In the next step, a fourth-order low-pass filter with a cut-off frequency of 5 Hz is applied to the signal. Fig. 11.5 shows one segment of the airflow signal before and after the filtering.

Any extra preprocessing step applied to SaO2 signal.

11.4.4.5 Signal Segmentation

One of the most critical early steps in biosignal processing is to segment the signals into smaller and relatively stationary segments. Each part must have nearly the same statistical characteristics, such as amplitude and frequency. In this study, first, the data are normalized using mean and standard deviation. Then, to divide the data into shorter epochs, we take some steps to choose the appropriate epoch size, and then labeling was done on each epoch.

Since arousals are the minority class, we first extracted the lengths of the signal intervals in which the arousal occurred continuously in those areas. First, the minimum and maximum arousal intervals were calculated for each individual to determine the most appropriate window size. About 95% of these intervals contain at least 1750 samples and in terms of time is 8.75 seconds. As a result of applying an adaptive filter after windowing, 149 samples were added to this range at the beginning and end to reduce distortion of the labeled signal. It will also be helpful for applying the hamming window to extract the frequency properties.

After analyzing the minimum arousal interval lengths of non-apnea among 994 patients, we realized that forty-nine patients had no non-apnea/hypopnea arousals, and no sample labeled +1 was observed in their data. We did not include these people in the training phase.

Therefore, each biosignal was segmented into an epoch with 2048 samples with 50% overlapping to eliminate sharp transitions between segments in such a way that 1750 samples in the middle of each segment must have the same label, and the whole window is considers to have that label.

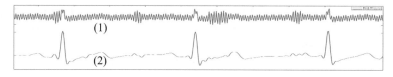

Fig. 11.4 A segment of (1) the noisy and (2) filtered ECG signal.

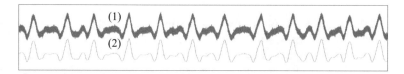

Fig. 11.5 A segment of (1) the noisy and (2) filtered airflow signal.

11.4.4.6   Labeling Epochs

The following were considered non-apnea arousals:

- In the period of two seconds before and ten seconds after a RERA arousal,
- A period of 2 seconds before a non-RERA, non-apnea arousal happens, up to 2 seconds after it ends [16].

In this study, we consider segmentation in the exact areas of arousal in the signals. In other words, the extra samples labeled at the beginning and end of arousal are not considered and are labeled 0 (Except for the 149 samples described above).

11.4.5   Feature Extraction

A detailed discussion of all the features that are extracted from signals is provided in this section.

11.4.5.1   Features Extracted from EEG Signals

EEG signals can provide helpful information about Sleep-related breathing disorders. This signal is, in fact, one of the most critical signals in diagnosing sleep-related breathing disorder [41]. Different features are extracted from each fragment of the preprocessed and segmented EEG signals, generally divided into the temporal, frequency, and time-scale domains.

Statistical features are some of the most common ones that can be extracted from the EEG. In this study we extracted median, mean, zero-crossing rate (ZCR), standard deviation (SD), variance, kurtosis, skewness, Root Mean Square (RMS), correlation between channels and three Hjorth parameters as time domain features.

The Activity parameter is the power of the signal (which is filtered wideband), the Mobility parameter is the mean frequency, and the Complexity parameter is the frequency change [42]. Studies show that changes in power along the EEG frequency bands provide information about arousal detection [43].

11.4.5.1.1 Frequency Features

As frequency features, the power spectral density estimate using the Welch Method with a hamming window with a length of about 2 seconds or 256 samples has been used to extract power from different EEG frequency bands. The relative and absolute power of the delta, theta, alpha, and beta bands are extracted from each segment. In addition, the power ratio of each sub-band relative to the others is also considered a feature.

11.4.5.1.2 Time-Frequency Features

Then the Deabeuchies order 8 Discrete Wavelet Transform (DWT) is used to decompose the signals into five stages. The coefficients obtained from this analysis include five detailed coefficients and an approximation coefficient. From these six coefficients, seven statistical features were extracted: Mean Absolute Value (MAV), variance, Average Power (AVP), standard deviation, entropy, mean, and skewness.

11.4.5.1.3 Nonlinear Features

Another category is nonlinear features. Because the EEG signal behaves erratically, entropy and fractal methods can provide a good indication of the irregularity of the signal. In other words, the more non-stationary the behavioral signal, the higher the entropy and fractal dimension. As entropy-based features, we extracted Renyi and relative spectral entropy that Renyi entropy provides information about the randomness of a system numerically and is the generalized Shannon entropy.

(a) *Features based on fractal dimension*

A new method for measuring the dimension of irregular shapes was first proposed by Mandelbrot [44]. The fractal dimension is a non-linear measure of irregularity. As a measure of self-similarity, fractal dimension describes the behavior of random signals [45]. In this study, the methods of Katz and Higuchi for calculating the fractal dimension were used. Two algorithms, Higuchi fractal dimension (HFD) and, Katz fractal dimension (KFD) are used in this study.

- *Katz fractal dimension*

Katz fractal dimensions are shown below for a signal of length n:

$$D = \frac{\log(n)}{\log(n) + \log\left(\dfrac{d}{T}\right)'}$$

(11.7)

Where T is the segment length (Euclidean distance between consecutive data points) and d indicates the maximum distance between the initial and other points [46].

- *Higuchi fractal dimension (HFD)*

The HFD is a fast, nonlinear method of measuring fractal dimension that gives more accurate results. Due to the shift in time series structure over a particular characteristic frequency, it is challenging to determine power law indices and a characteristic time scale based on the power spectrum. With very limited data points, the HFD method can still provide stable indices and time scales as a function of the characteristic frequency. Below are the equations of Higuchi's algorithm.

From a L-length one-dimensional time series x(1), x(2), ..., x(l) with equal intervals, form a new time series X_n^k:

$$X_n^r = \left\{ x(n), x(n+r), x(n+2r), \ldots, x\left(n + \left|\frac{L-n}{r}\right| . r\right) \right\}$$

(11.10)

Where r represents the distance between two consecutive time series and n = 1, 2, ..., r is the time value at the beginning of the sequence. For each x_n^r, the average length of each time series is calculated as follows:

$$L_n(r) = \sum_{[(n-L)/r]}^{i=1} \left| x(n+ir) - x(n+(i-1).r) \right| . \frac{(L-1)}{\left[(L-n)/r\right].r}$$

(11.11)

As a result, the average length of the whole series of discrete time signals is as follows:

$$L(r) = \frac{1}{r} \sum_{r}^{n=1} L_n(r).$$

(11.12)

The following result can be obtained using logarithmic transformation:

$$\ln(L(r)) \propto D_f . \ln\left(\frac{1}{r}\right).$$

(11.13)

The D_f slope is the Higuchi fractal dimension [47].

(b) *Detrended Fluctuation Analysis (DFA)*

The other feature extracted from the EEG signal is the Features of *detrended fluctuation analysis (DFA)*. DFA is one of the nonlinear methods used to determine the fractal scalability properties of the EEG signal that is a modified method of root mean square for the random walk. A function of scale parameter is used to calculate the mean square distance of a signal from a trend line. Usually, there is a power-law dependency, and the main parameter is power. The terms related to it are explained below.

The time series $s(i)$ represents the EEG signal contribution of N_s samples. In the DFA algorithm, first, time series are corrected and integrated. Afterward, the integrated time series $s(m)$ is divided into separate sections of the same length. The length of this section in this study is considered as 1024 samples. The local trend is calculated for each section. By subtraction of the local trend $s_n(m)$ in each section, this trend is removed from the EEG time series $s(m)$. After determining the variation of the root square mean of this non-trended time series F(n), it can be expressed as follows:

$$F(n) = \sqrt{\frac{1}{N_s} \sum_{N_s}^{m=1} \left(S(m) - S_n(m) \right)^2}$$

(11.14)

As a function of section size, F(n) is calculated throughout all time scales to identify its dependence on average variations. On a log-log plot, linear relationships demonstrate fractal scaling. Therefore, the fluctuation is proportional to n^α. The parameter α, which indicates the variation rate of a complex signal, is the self-similarity or autocorrelation parameter. It can be defined as

$$\alpha \propto \frac{\log F(n)}{\log n}$$

(11.15)

By finding the slope of log F(n) - log n line, this can be calculated [48]. The value of this parameter is considered a feature.

Similar features as EEG signals are also extracted from the EOG signal.

11.4.5.2 Features Extracted from EMG

From the EMG signal, features such as MAV, AVP, standard deviation, variance, 95th percentile, skewness, kurtosis, frequency band energy of each four Hz window (five frequency bands), waveform length (WL), ZCR, the derivative zero-crossing rate, amplitude, and root mean square, are extracted.

11.4.5.3 Features Extracted from SaO2

From the SaO2 signal, thirteen features are extracted, including mean, standard deviation, coefficient of variation, kurtosis, mean, variance, and range. Since arousals occur in a few seconds, power spectrum density is calculated using Yule-Walker autocorrelation estimation of order 5, and an average frequency range of 0.016–5 Hz is also considered a feature. In addition, the percentage of time when $SaO2 \geq 96$, $90 \leq SaO2 \leq 96$, $80 \leq SaO2 \leq 90$ and $SaO2 < 80$ in each window used to determine the duration of normal, mild, moderate, and severe oxygen saturation are also extracted as features.

11.4.5.4 Features Extracted from Airflow

Features extracted from airflow, similar to other signals, are in the time and frequency domain. These features include statistical features such as respiration rate, frequency band energy per 0.25 Hz, average, minimum, maximum, range, variance, coefficient of variation, skewness, and kurtosis, and also other features like integral of absolute value (IAV), MAV, ZCR, slope sign changes (SSC), WL, RMS. Since the airflow is also nonstationary, Welch's method is used to calculate power spectrum density as another feature.

11.4.5.5 Features Extracted from ECG

Features such as heart rate, heart rate variability, low-frequency band-power, and the ratio of low-frequency band-power (0.003 to 0.4 Hz) to high-frequency power (0.04 to 0.15 Hz) are extracted from ECG signals.

This study considers another set of features associated with signal variation over time. Due to the time intervals between the selected segments and their effect, it's necessary to effectively use the features of each segment adjacent. However, considering the purpose of this study of detecting non-apnea arousals and ineffective regions related to apnea, not all selected segments have adjacent necessarily. For this reason, we used the ratio between the first half of the segment and its second half as new features extracted from each segment in order to consider the course of change in each segment. In this way, each segment first is divided into two equal parts, and the features considered for each part are extracted separately. Then, the ratio of these extracted features in two parts is considered the new feature.

Also, the autocorrelation of the segments is considered. In this way, autocorrelation is calculated from all segments, and then time features are extracted from them.

A total of 1741 features were extracted from 13 channels. Table 11.2 shows the number of features extracted from each channel.

Table 11.2 The number of features that extracted

	EEG + EOG	Corr of EEGs	EMG	SaO2	Airflow	ECG	All
Initial features	1160	15	325	26	114	101	1741

11.4.6 Data Balancing

In order to improve the classifier learning performance and also to apply statistical analysis, the data in the two classes need to balance. Due to the significant imbalance, the class needs to choose a method for balancing the data. In this method, the classifier is trained each time by a random subset of data. The second approach is increasing the minority class by multiplying a little random noise of about 0.1% by the feature values of each part of the class labeled 1.

11.4.7 Feature Selection

There are two general types of feature selection methods: individual evaluation and subset evaluation. Feature ranking also known as individual evaluation measures the relevance of individual features by giving them a score. However, using this approach provides a subset of selected features according to a specific method of searching. This method compares each selected subset to the previous best by evaluating it based on a specific evaluation criterion.

Besides this category, three general feature selection approaches are filter, wrapper, and embedded. In this study, the first two approaches are used.

The filter method does the feature selection process as a preprocessing step without considering any specific classification algorithm and only by ranking features based on their importance in the dataset. The advantage of this method is its low computational cost and good generalization ability. In this study, we used two methods of correlation-based feature selection (CFS) and the Wilcoxon rank-sum test among the filtering methods [49, 50].

To determine the usefulness of a subset of features, the wrapper method uses a learning algorithm as a black box. In order to find practical features to improve the performance and reduce the speed of classification, the significance of the extracted features at the significance level of 0.01 was evaluated using Wilcoxon statistical test. This test was used as the first step in selecting better features, and features with were removed from the feature vector. Thus, 320 features out of a total of 1741 features did not reject the Wilcoxon null hypothesis of having samples of continuous distributions with different medians and so were removed from the feature vector.

Then, the 711 features with higher scores are selected by ranking the features using the CFS method, and then by using the genetic algorithm with KNN fitness function, which is one of the wrapper methods, the features have increased to 249. Table 11.3 shows the number of features selected in each step.

Based on this table, we can see which of these 13 signals contributes most to classifying target class or non-apnea arousals. Among the selected features, the relative power of different EEG frequency bands and their autocorrelation signals, the ratio of the first half spectrum power to the second half of the epoch related to EEG and EMG signals, 95th percentile autocorrelation of EEG signals can be named.

11.5 Classification Result

In this section, the results of the classifiers are reported in several steps. First, using the features obtained after the CFS, i.e., 711 features, the performance results of the two approaches of data reduction and data augmentation in order to balance. Tables 11.4, 11.5, and 11.6 shows the results of the RF algorithm with 50 trees in both steps. RF parameters are selected experimentally. According to the definition of the AUPRC criterion, it is necessary to calculate the baseline to compare the value of this criterion. The baseline in each step is equal to the total number of epochs with label 1 to the total available data. In Table 11.4, the baseline for the test data used is 0.114.

Data augmentation improves classification results because all zero-class data samples are included every time that model is trained, so the whole dataset is taken into account when used to train the model. For this reason, this method has been used to balance the data in the following.

In this section, the random forest algorithm is implemented separately on the extracted initial features of each of the 13 channels. The results are presented in Table 11.5 N is the number of features of each channel.

As a result of measuring the importance of each feature group for the detection of non-apnea arousal with the AUPRC criteria, it can be concluded that airflow with a score equal to 0.367 is the second most important feature after the EMG signal. The best result is related to the EMG signal with AUPRC equal to 0.375. This is understandable since more than 90% of the non-apnea arousal regions identified in the data include RERA, related to respiration. The best result is related to the EMG signal with AUPRC equal to 0.375. The reason for this is understandable since more than 90% of the non-apnea arousal regions identified include RERA, which is a breath-related disorder. Among the EEG signals, the features of the C3-M2 central channel were more important than the other channels, and this channel alone can be used to identify arousals.

Table 11.3 The number of features that selected in each stage of feature selection

Selected by	EEG + EOG	Corr of EEGs	EMG	SaO2	Airflow	ECG	Total
Wilcoxon	952	10	286	22	61	90	1421
CFS	496	2	163	4	22	24	711
GA	166	1	60	2	12	8	249

Table 11.4 Comparing the performance of two approaches of data reduction and data augmentation for balancing

Random Forest						
Data Reduction			Data Augmentation			
	Recall/ TPR	F1-score			Recall/ TPR	F1-score
Class 0	0.814	0.882	Class 0		0.834	0.894
Class 1	0.750	0.457	Class 1		0.793	0.487
Macro average	0.782	0.669	Macro average		0.801	0.685
Weighted average	0.807	0.834	Weighted average		0.829	0.848
Accuracy	0.806		Accuracy		0.811	
Baseline	0.114		Baseline		0.114	
AUPRC	0.378		AUPRC		0.436	
AUROC	0.834		AUROC		0.860	

Table 11.5 The result of applying random forest on each signal

AUROC	AUPRC	N		AUROC	AUPRC	N	
0.789	0.329	99	Chin EMG	0.751	0.277	136	F3-M2
0.740	0.265	92	Abdominal EMG	0.724	0.310	136	F4-M1
0.722	0.298	95	Chest EMG	0.766	0.321	136	C3-M2
0.815	0.375	286	All channels of EMG	0.748	0.309	136	C4-M1
0.802	0.367	61	Airflow	0.742	0.293	136	O1-M2
0.770	0.298	22	SaO2	0.752	0.305	136	O2-M1
0.791	0.252	90	ECG	0.814	0.332	816	All channels of EEG

Table 11.6 Comparison of results for two ensemble algorithms under the same condition

Bagged Tree (RF)				LightGBM			
		Predicted				Predicted	
		Class 0	Class 1			Class 0	Class 1
Actual	Class 0	85%	15%	Actual	Class 0	86%	14%
	Class 1	27%	73%		Class 1	26%	74%
		Recall TPR/	F1-score			Recall TPR/	F1-score
Class 0		0.847	0.900	Class 0		0.861	0.909
Class 1		0.724	0.497	Class 1		0.734	0.521
Accuracy		0.832		Accuracy		0.846	
Macro average		0.785	0.698	Macro average		0.797	0.715
Weighted average		0.833	0.854	Weighted average		0.847	0.865
AUPRC		0.466		AUPRC		0.496	
AUROC		0.865		AUROC		0.877	

Figure 11.6 shows the performance of the four classifiers using the AUPRC criteria on each feature category compared to each other. As it turns out, the respiratory properties performed best.

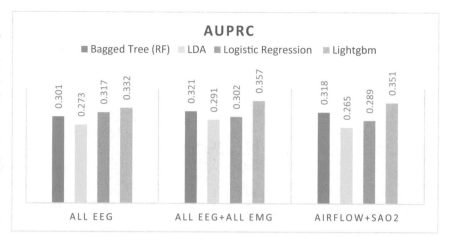

Fig. 11.6 The performance of classifier on different feature set

The mentioned algorithms are trained using 249 features obtained after applying the genetic algorithm with the five-fold cross-validation method, and the test results are given in Tables 11.6 and 11.7. The baseline here is about 0.18.

Figure 11.7 shows the diagrams for two main criteria for measuring performance in this study, AUPRC, and AUROC. As can be seen, in these diagrams and the results above, the ensemble algorithms, LightGBM of boosting category, and random forest of bagging category, in contrast to the individual algorithms, have a significant ability to identify arousal regions. The LightGBM algorithm performed better with much higher speeds than the other algorithms.

11.6 Conclusion

Studies show that detecting non-apnea arousal regions has less accuracy than identifying apnea arousals, and most of the studies have been done to identify apnea. The goal of the challenge held by Physionet in 2018, is to identify non-apnea arousal regions. In more than 90% of the models presented in this challenge, neural networks were used. The best results were obtained using deep neural networks with the area under the precision-recall and the area under the precision-recall scores of 0.93 and 0.54, respectively. However, intelligent feature extraction can still be promising, as only four papers in this challenge have applied pattern recognition methods using manual feature extraction and reached to the area under the precision-recall in the range of 0.21 to 0.29.

In this study, different features of all available signals have been extracted, and using ensemble algorithms that have received much attention today, results have been obtained that are relatively close to neural network-based methods.

Table 11.7 Comparison of results for two basic machine learning algorithms under the same condition

Linear discriminative Analysis			Logistic Regression			
Predicted					Predicted	
		Class 0	Class 1			Class 0	Class 1
Actual	Class 0	89%	11%	Actual	Class 0	90%	10%
	Class 1	53%	47%		Class 1	49%	51%
		Recall TPR/	F1-score			Recall TPR/	F1-score
Class 0		0.890	0.908	Class 0		0.903	0.891
Class 1		0.465	0.401	Class 1		0.506	0.448
Accuracy		0.841		Accuracy		0.857	
Macro average		0.678	0.654	Macro average		0.704	0.683
Weighted average		0.841	0.850	Weighted average		0.857	0.840
AUPRC		0.310		AUPRC		0.345	
AUROC		0.806		AUROC		0.824	

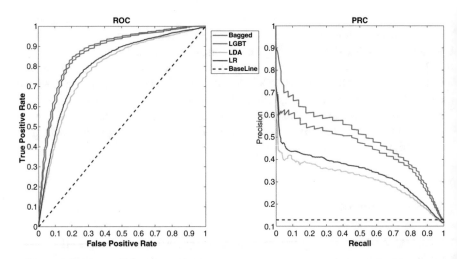

Fig. 11.7 Comparison of PRC and ROC curves

References

1. M.K. Pavlova, V. Latreille, Sleep disorders. Am. J. Med. **132**(3), 292–299 (2019)
2. W. Wen, Sleep quality detection based on EEG signals using transfer support vector machine algorithm, Front. Neurosci. 15, (2021)
3. H. Ragnarsdóttir, B. Marinósson, E. Finnsson, E. Gunnlaugsson, J. S. Ágústsson, H. Helgadóttir, Automatic detection of target regions of respiratory effort-related arousals using recurrent neural networks, in *2018 Computing in Cardiology Conference (CinC)*, (2018), vol. 45: IEEE, pp. 1–4
4. M. Diykh, Y. Li, Complex networks approach for EEG signal sleep stages classification. Expert Syst. Appl. **63**, 241–248 (2016)

5. E. Scoring, EEG arousals: Scoring rules and examples: A preliminary report from the sleep disorders atlas task force of the American sleep disorders association. Sleep **15**(2), 174–184 (1992)
6. R.K. Malhotra, A.Y. Avidan, Sleep stages and scoring technique. Atlas Sleep Med., 77–99 (2013)
7. T. Penzel, S. Canisius, Polysomnography, in *Sleep Apnea*, vol. 35: (Karger Publishers, 2006), pp. 51–60
8. D. Álvarez-Estévez, V. Moret-Bonillo, Identification of electroencephalographic arousals in multichannel sleep recordings. IEEE Trans. Biomed. Eng. **58**(1), 54–63 (2010)
9. S. Mariani, S. M. Purcell, S. Redline, Automated processing of big data in sleep medicine, in *Signal Processing and Machine Learning for Biomedical Big Data*, (CRC Press, 2018), pp. 443–463
10. R. Heinzer et al., Prevalence of sleep-disordered breathing in the general population: The HypnoLaus study. Lancet Respir. Med. **3**(4), 310–318 (2015)
11. S. Cho, J. Lee, H. Park, K. Lee, Detection of arousals in patients with respiratory sleep disorders using a single channel EEG, in *2005 IEEE Engineering in Medicine and Biology 27th Annual Conference*, (2006) IEEE, pp. 2733–2735
12. D. Chylinski et al., Validation of an automatic arousal detection algorithm for whole-night sleep EEG recordings. Clocks & sleep **2**(3), 258–272 (2020)
13. A.H. Khandoker, J. Gubbi, M. Palaniswami, Automated scoring of obstructive sleep apnea and hypopnea events using short-term electrocardiogram recordings. IEEE Trans. Inf. Technol. Biomed. **13**(6), 1057–1067 (2009)
14. R. Lazazzera et al., Detection and classification of sleep apnea and hypopnea using PPG and SpO $ _2 $ signals. IEEE Trans. Biomed. Eng. **68**(5), 1496–1506 (2020)
15. T. Sugi, F. Kawana, M. Nakamura, Automatic EEG arousal detection for sleep apnea syndrome. Biomed. Signal Proc. Control **4**(4), 329–337 (2009)
16. M.M. Ghassemi et al., You snooze, you win: the physionet/computing in cardiology challenge 2018," in *2018 Computing in Cardiology Conference (CinC)*, (2018), vol. 45: IEEE, pp. 1–4
17. V. Tsara, A. Amfilochiou, M. Papagrigorakis, D. Georgopoulos, E. Liolios, Guidelines for diagnosis and treatment of sleep-related breathing disorders in adults and children. Definition and classification of sleep related breathing disorders in adults: Different types and indications for sleep studies (part 1). Hippokratia **13**(3), 187–191 (2009)
18. E. J. Olson, W. R. Moore, T. I. Morgenthaler, P. C. Gay, B. A. Staats, Obstructive sleep apnea-hypopnea syndrome, in *Mayo Clinic Proceedings*, vol. 78, no. 12: Elsevier, 2003, pp. 1545–1552
19. J.F.M. Jiménez, M.R. González, L.J. Findley, Sleepy drivers have a high frequency of traffic accidents related to respiratory effort-related arousals. Archivos de bronconeumologia **39**(4), 153–158 (2003)
20. M. Howe-Patterson, B. Pourbabaee, F. Benard, Automated detection of sleep arousals from polysomnography data using a dense convolutional neural network, in *2018 Computing in Cardiology Conference (CinC)*, (2018), vol. 45: IEEE, pp. 1–4
21. R. He et al., Identification of arousals with deep neural networks (DNNs) using different physiological signals, in *2018 Computing in Cardiology Conference (CinC)* (2018), vol. 45: IEEE, pp. 1–4
22. A. Patane, S. Ghiasi, E. P. Scilingo, M. Kwiatkowska, Automated recognition of sleep arousal using multimodal and personalized deep ensembles of neural networks, in *2018 Computing in Cardiology Conference (CinC)*, (2018), vol. 45: IEEE, pp. 1–4
23. P. Warrick and M. N. Homsi, "Sleep arousal detection from polysomnography using the scattering transform and recurrent neural networks," in *2018 Computing in Cardiology Conference (CinC)*, 2018, vol. 45: IEEE, pp. 1–4
24. H. Li, Q. Cao, Y. Zhong, Y. Pan, Sleep arousal detection using end-to-end deep learning method based on multi-physiological signals, in *2018 Computing in Cardiology Conference (CinC)*, (2018), vol. 45: IEEE, pp. 1–4
25. B. Varga, M. Görög, P. Hajas, Using auxiliary loss to improve sleep arousal detection with neural network, in *2018 Computing in Cardiology Conference (CinC)*, (2018), vol. 45: IEEE, pp. 1–4

26. N. Sadr, P. de Chazal, Automatic scoring of non-apnoea arousals using the polysomnogram, in *2018 Computing in Cardiology Conference (CinC)*, (2018), vol. 45: IEEE, pp. 1–4
27. K.E. Bloch, Polysomnography: A systematic review. Technol. Health Care **5**(4), 285–305 (1997)
28. V.R. Badrakalimuthu, R. Swamiraju, H. de Waal, EEG in psychiatric practice: To do or not to do? Adv. Psychiatr. Treat. **17**(2), 114–121 (2011)
29. C.L. Drake, K.M. Mason, S.M. Bowyer, T. Roth, G.L. Barkley, N. Tepley, Vertex sharp waves during sleep localized by 2DII. Cortex **1**, 8 (2002)
30. M. Schönauer, D. Pöhlchen, Sleep spindles. Curr. Biol. **28**(19), R1129–R1130 (2018)
31. S. Tong and N. V. Thankor, Quantitative EEG Analysis Methods and Clinical Applications.. Artech House, 2009
32. M. Sharma, D. Goyal, P. Achuth, U.R. Acharya, An accurate sleep stages classification system using a new class of optimally time-frequency localized three-band wavelet filter bank. Comput. Biol. Med. **98**, 58–75 (2018)
33. H. Rao et al., Feature selection based on artificial bee colony and gradient boosting decision tree. Appl. Soft Comput. **74**, 634–642 (2019)
34. G. Ke et al., Lightgbm: A highly efficient gradient boosting decision tree. Adv. Neural Inf. Proces. Syst. **30**, 3146–3154 (2017)
35. J. Brownlee, how to Develop a Light Gradient Boosted Machine (LightGBM) Ensemble, ed (2020)
36. M. Thoma, Wikimedia Commons, the free media repository, Roc-draft-xkcd-style.svg, Ed., ed (June 2018)
37. Draelos. Measuring Performance: AUPRC and Average Precision. https://glassboxmedicine.com/2019/03/02/measuring-performance-auprc/. accessed
38. A. A. Gharbali, J. M. Fonseca, S. Najdi, and T. Y. Rezaii, "Automatic eog and emg artifact removal method for sleep stage classification," in *Doctoral Conference on Computing, Electrical and Industrial Systems*, 2016: Springer, pp. 142–150
39. P. Shooshtari, G. Mohammadi, B. Molaee Ardekani, M. B. Shamsollahi, Removing ocular artifacts from EEG signals using adaptive filtering and ARMAX modeling, in *Proceeding of World Academy of Science, Engineering and Technology*, vol. 11, no. CONF, (2006) pp. 277–280
40. X. Jiang, G.-B. Bian, Z. Tian, Removal of artifacts from EEG signals: a review. Sensors **19**(5), 987 (2019)
41. X. Li, S.H. Ling, S. Su, A hybrid feature selection and extraction methods for sleep apnea detection using bio-signals. Sensors **20**(15), 4323 (2020)
42. C. Vidaurre, N. Krämer, B. Blankertz, A. Schlögl, Time domain parameters as a feature for EEG-based brain–computer interfaces. Neural Netw. **22**(9), 1313–1319 (2009)
43. J.V. Liu, H.K. Yaggi, Characterization of Arousals in Polysomnography Using the Statistical Significance of Power Change, in *2018 IEEE Signal Processing in Medicine and Biology Symposium (SPMB)* (2018): IEEE, pp. 1–6
44. B. Mandelbrot, How long is the coast of Britain? Statistical self-similarity and fractional dimension. Science **156**(3775), 636–638 (1967)
45. E.B. Sadeghian, M.H. Moradi, Fractal dimension for detection of ERD/ERS patterns in asynchronous brain computer interface, in *2008 2nd International Conference on Bioinformatics and Biomedical Engineering*, (2008): IEEE, pp. 560–563
46. C.-T. Shi, Signal pattern recognition based on fractal features and machine learning. Appl. Sci. **8**(8), 1327 (2018)
47. A. Yilmaz, G. Unal, Multiscale Higuchi's fractal dimension method. Nonlinear Dynamics **101**(2), 1441–1455 (2020)
48. A. Adda, H. Benoudnine, Detrended fluctuation analysis of EEG recordings for epileptic seizure detection, in *2016 International Conference on Bio-engineering for Smart Technologies (BioSMART)*, (2016): IEEE, pp. 1–4
49. V. Bolón-Canedo, N. Sánchez-Maroño, A. Alonso-Betanzos, *Feature Selection for High-Dimensional Data* (Springer, 2015)
50. C.-j. Tian, J. Lv, X.-f. Xu, Evaluation of feature selection methods for mammographic breast cancer diagnosis in a unified framework. BioMed Res. Int. **2021**, 1–9 (2021)

Chapter 12
Deep Learning Assisted Biofeedback

Jorge J. Palacios-Venegas

Abstract After 60 years of brain waves biofeedback development, basic and applied research, therapeutics, and a variety of devices built, there are a well-defined set of applications both, in health and illness. During these years, advances in technology made big contributions to biofeedback therapeutic and training procedures development. Variability as a natural property in biological systems and a side effect of the limitations in actual biofeedback devices along with differences in treatments and training models, have placed regular practice in a landscape where outcome prediction is difficult, not always reliable, or replicable, and with lack of fundamentals for generalization. This chapter discusses the develop of Deep Learning (DL) solutions designed to control the biofeedback process. Aim is to substitute current devices and neurofeedback procedures with a robust set of DL options designed to reduce variability and deliver biofeedback process according to the natural brain waves relations and principles, proposing DL models oriented to fill the actual vacuum of precision in current neurofeedback (NFB) devices and practice.

12.1 Introduction

There is an increasing number of Machine Learning (ML) solutions and Deep Learning (DL) applications in biological sciences. It can be mentioned contributions in oncology [1], cardiology [2], neuroimage [3] and electroencephalography (EEG) [4] with a growing number of studies since 2018 [5]. Is not the case in NFB. There have only been described, design and tested Neural Networks (NN) and DL models for assessment the efficacy of one neurofeedback procedure [6] and the identification of the best NFB intervention [7]. Emerging field of DL models applied to analysis of peripheral biological signals has more reports, standardized

J. J. Palacios-Venegas (✉)
Biofeedback Center®. Computational Neurosciences Laboratory, Mexico City, Mexico
e-mail: jorgepalacios@biofeedbackcn.com

© The Author(s), under exclusive license to Springer Nature Switzerland AG 2023
S. Mian Qaisar et al. (eds.), *Advances in Non-Invasive Biomedical Signal Sensing and Processing with Machine Learning*, https://doi.org/10.1007/978-3-031-23239-8_12

procedures in cardiac electrophysiology [2], assessment of electrocardiogram (ECG) and blood pressure [8], development of prosthetic solutions for disabilities [9], decoding of motor intent in peripheral nerve signals [10], assessment of pain [11], treatment solutions for motor disfunctions [12], a biofeedback wearable device for movement rehabilitation [13], the assessment of accuracy in prediction models for augmented biofeedback training in precision shooting [14], among different types of Brain Computer Interfaces (BCI's), there are none for control and administration of the whole biofeedback and neurofeedback procedures.

Biofeedback (BFB) is particularly relevant in the study of control functions in biological systems. Feedback Loop (FL) has been clearly stablished [15] as the natural process for self-regulation, homeostasis and as a basic element in life support. The information a system is receiving about its interactions with other systems the environment and its current internal state is a key element for future actions to be organized as involuntary or voluntary reactions among other processes and biological functions during existence. In theoretical and experimental approaches to the study of FL processes, contributions of the Theory of Control [16, 17] opened a wide spectrum of research supporting the conclusion that FL processes should be considered as a crucial element for health and self-preservation in biological systems.

In this general context basic, applied, and clinical research in BFB began to grow after two mayor contributions took place in the second half of the last century, both based on the earlier studies of *interoception* as a specific sensory function [18], with a strong link with behavior [19]. Study of interoception became a milestone to the scientific context in which the first key experimental and clinical contributions of BFB emerged. The first one in the research of abnormal muscular contraction and coordination after neural lesion and how these functions could be restored using electromyographic information coming from the affected muscles and delivered to the patient by other sensory modalities. The objective was to provide the missing information from the neuromuscular spindle, element in the muscle that holds the FL process and was affeccted by the neural lesion. The flow of information to the brain was interrupted impeding the detection of the small potentials remaining and the machine could detect [20]. After a number of sessions using the machine, patients were able to control the affected muscles, feel its contractions, recover the function and the machine was no longer needed. These findings are now considered as first contributions of biofeedback applied research from where today's Peripheral Biofeedback (PB) procedures were born.

The second contribution arose in a different scenario, one of the most important laboratories of sleep neurophysiology in 1962. A researcher noticed alpha waves (8–12 Hz) distribution was interrupted after participants in sleep studies closed their eyes during EEG recordings preparation process. Happening frequently, even participants were with their eyes closed and awake the natural condition for the regular distribution of alpha waves in healthy human brain. Wondering if this phenomenon could be related to subjective experiences, cognitive processes or consciousness states taking place in that moment [21], adapted methodology developed for neuromuscular rehabilitation presuming mental activity will be different between the two

EEG states (alpha activity interrupted or not). Designed an experimental setting to deliver information to participants about the interruptions in its own alfa activity, using an analog auditory tone variations with changes in volume analog to voltage variations in alpha activity, using an arbitrary score to inform participants about their performance. He was developing the first brain waves biofeedback procedure years later called Neurofeedback [22, 23]. When the initial NFB works were published, contradicted reports regarding its replicability arose. First replication of alpha (8–12 Hz) biofeedback study result with contradictory findings [24] and the conclusions of the original author were that his study was not reproduced in the same conditions [25, 26]. Since then, variability and replicability issues in NFB studies have always been present.

With Electromyographic (EMG) biofeedback procedures, used to restore the muscular function loss, medical rehabilitation specialty was enriched, and EMG Biofeedback (EMGB) emerged as a powerful tool for recovery of function in patients suffering from different types of muscular palsies. Procedures were extended using a variety of biological signals as instant information delivered to patients, clients, or experiment participants to establish its control due to learning or conditioning, and later applied for treatment of specific conditions like tension type headache [27], migraine crisis [28] and anxiety and stress [29]. Due to nature of peripheral signals periodicity, stability, spatial and time resolution PB has been used regularly with predictable results and standard norms for assessment and non-invasive treatment of specific medical and neuropsychiatric conditions, relying in the excellent temporal and spacial resolution of the biological signals recorded for this purpose.

Initial NFB procedures out of the research laboratory were difficult to apply. EEG instrumentation was complicated and expensive resources needed for feedback procedures were rare or even inexistent and there was few information about EEG significance in cognitive, consciousness and emotional states. Regular EEG practice was reserved for clinical neurophysiologists to the study and diagnosis of epilepsy [30]. In the middle of 1970's decade a notable finding, the conditioning of sensorimotor rhythm (smr 13–15 Hz) [31, 32], changed NFB future. Results showed smr conditioning was effective to inhibit spikes and spontaneous seizures in cat [33] and monkey in experimental models of epilepsy [34]. These procedures were quickly adapted and applied to humans showing smr NFB effectiveness for attention deficit and hyperactivity disorder (ADH/D) management and non-invasive treatment [35]. Procedures for specific neurological and neuropsychiatric conditions emerged from the first standardized psychophysiological treatment protocol for Post-Traumatic Stress Disorder (PTSD) [36] initiating a new era around the 1990's decade. Scientists and clinicians in the field developed devices, software, and intervention procedures for alcoholism [37] depression [38–40], traumatic brain injury (TBI) [41], attention deficit disorder (ADD) [42, 43] and ADHD [44] among other protocols, leading to the professional NFB field definition [45]. BFB devices assisted by computers allowed contributions for therapeutic and training procedures and the evolution of clinical practice and research setups, from one channel analog devices to multichannel multimodal computer assisted interfaces.

Interventions became more complex arrangements with software capable to delivered feedback, according to clinical findings and normative databases opening a different type of practice with standard procedures based in statistical normative criteria [46, 47]. Develop in instrumentation and software made possible 19 EEG channels recording with online source biofeedback [48] with normative databases, developing brain mapping biofeedback procedure known as QEEG-Biofeedback [49] based in the low resolution tomography (LORETA) [50] environment [51, 52].

NFB expanded over the years, but replication of therapeutic findings and results frequently has been controversial, the so-called standardized treatment or training procedures have been subject to variability in individual conditions, specialist's decisions, or due to software preinstalled functions in the diversity of the today known as commercial NFB devices. Variability in the clinical and research results have made difficult the path for the field, nevertheless today there's a big number of professionals in the area all over the world, a substantial number of contributions published yearly and a growing interest in designing and developing more precise and reliable software interfaces.

NFB principle is to enhance through learning or conditioning the patient-trainee capability to "inhibit" specific EEG bands to induce the "predominance" of one in specific. This basic process was developed in the intent to replicate the natural organization of brain waves in health and specific consciousness states. EEG bands relations based in the power values were obtained from the clinical analog EEG recordings after simple statistical analysis. The purpose has been to achieve the resemblance of the general characteristics of normal or wellbeing EEG. This procedures until today frequently find obstacles due to the natural variability, the low spatial resolution of the EEG and the different standards in the fabrication of the commercial NFB devices [53].

The problem addressed in this chapter arises from the concern that after years of development in computational models and tools for the study and analysis of biological signals and the creation and use of ML and DL applications based in EEG recordings, none have reached regular NFB practice, nor the regular production of ML or DL based neurofeedback devices. The aim is to address the constant issue of variability in regular neurofeedback practice and the traditional paths taken to minimize its effects. The line of work discussed in this chapter is oriented to develop DL solutions capable to take care of the whole NFB process, with an architecture capable to substitute current devices and procedures preserving the basic noninvasive intervention principle.

12.2   Current Biofeedback and Neurofeedback Devices and Practice

EEG high temporal resolution property characterized NFB practice for years, beginning with the use of one scalp electrode hookups for ADHD management [47] and cephalic bipolar positions for depression [54]. Difficulties imposed to the traditional methods of analysis arise from EEG low spatial resolution that becomes evident as more channels are used in the recordings and that has always affected NFB research and practice initiated with the adaptation of devices engineered and built for a different purpose and practice [55]. At the time EEG devices were built to be used under specific conditions: restriction of movement, avoiding speech, laying with the eyes closed and were conducted inside a faraday chamber to avoid electrical and magnetic interference. Routine clinical EEG studies were conducted in such conditions and with two standard methods: hyperventilation and photo stimulation used for activation of the EEG to detect spontaneous epileptic activity [56]. Initial neurofeedback studies were instrumented using these types of devices and developing or adapting other instruments to perform approximate measures of the frequencies of interest. Feedback was delivered by auditive, or photo stimulators built for other type of studies, frequently applied manually and signals quantification in relation to feedback events were also taken manually. In such scenarios it was expected the recording contamination with many types and classes of artifacts. Consistent results began to appear encouraging professionals in the field to continue developing and standardizing procedures and techniques for conducting more studies. Devices built specially for these procedures made practice became more consistent, results replicable and due to research results with medical, neurological, and neuropsychiatric conditions clinical field finally emerged. NFB devices evolution can be synthetized as a journey from one channel analog stand-alone systems to multichannel multimodal (EEG and peripheral signals) computer assisted interfaces [57, 58]. NFB conditions requiring participants or patients to be seated with eyes opened, and not into a faraday chamber, lead to design procedures to reduce interference and artifacts. It must be recognized the hard work of the first professionals in the field for standardization of instrumentation, skin preparation techniques, basic room recordings characteristics design, adaptation and standardization of regular EEG techniques and procedures and the design of specific assessment and treatment intervention procedures that structured the specialty and its regulation by professional associations stablishing standards for training specialists and practitioners [59, 60].

Today's commercial NFB devices are built based in those initial procedures complying with federal agencies regulations and based in the same general principles with some research done to validate its reliability [61]. Many are manufactured with materials and components requiring less skin preparation and recording skills, relying in the structure of its software designed with basic elements to deliver feedback according to built-in protocols and applications. NFB software since the 1990's era is built into two different classes. One includes the *closed systems* with software with specific sets of prebuilt applications for specific training purposes and treatment procedures, users have to follow specific guides, montages, derivations and specific band configurations. The other class includes the *open systems* in which the user has more options to configure EEG and peripheral (ECG, EMG) signals acquisition and feedback, selecting different μV threshold settings, using monopolar or bipolar hookups with two or more recording channels to apply the same principle to deliver feedback procedures. Measures of μVs average values after gross separation of EEG frequency bands are showed in the screen every 3 seconds and treatment interventions rely in determined number of training hours in which the results resembling normal EEG are supposed to appear be stablished as a new normal EEG state expected to evolve during time promoting healthy neurological and neuropsychiatric states [62].

Occasionally some systems include impedance meter displays, more refined online impedance measures with standards indicating safe or poor recording conditions. Denoising is based in gross band filters conducted by differential amplifiers. The software is designed for a gross frequency decomposition and online management of the amplitude average and power measures [63]. Biological artifacts like ECG or eyeblinks are frequently ignored relying in basic and questionable principles like the derivations used in a given treatment intervention [64]. Off-line analysis is performed when the software is built with tools to export or convert files to common formats [65, 66] frequently, specific file formats are used, leaving the option to analyze data with built-in report features, with gross averages, fixed ratio comparisons and the same gross frequency decomposition used during the treatment session. These features have created a state where the NFB practice has been conducted during the last 30 years known as traditional neurofeedback (TN).

QEEG-Biofeedback based on the international 10/20 system [67, 68], is used by specialists to deliver feedback procedures using source localization [69] and inverse solution [70–72] principles, with normative databases as guidelines for more elaborated NFB arrangements. Interventions are conducted using more channels, z-scores norms of specific EEG frequencies and its relations, source localization procedures, and -as it is claimed by its creators and regular users-, online feedback of the brain functional connectivity with estimation of the cerebellar electrophysiological activity using only the 19 channels of the traditional 10/20 system [69, 73]. These procedures are not known and used by regular NFB practitioners nor common in the training for regular practice. Some EEG devices used for this specialty are built with clinical degree, safer and more precise, manufactured according to international regulations for clinical EEG practice, engineered with better quality and performance capabilities and some are manufactured by the same fabricants of the TN devices [74] in general do not match the standards of the EEG research grade instruments [75]. General principles for its use are the same that those in the TN and a lot must be done to reduce the effects of the sources of variability.

At the same time the reborn of the EEG has been taking place [76], academic software for EEG analysis have made enormous advances [77–79] and computational neuroscience and neuroinformatics are prolific fields for the study and understanding of brain electrophysiology.

12.3   Deep Learning Models
for Electroencephalography Analysis

EEG signals have good temporal resolution the clinical work is based in this property and in the band frequency graphic characteristics distinguishing "graphic elements" related to specific disfunctions or illnesses from normal EEG. Most of the time specialists work is based in two parameters: frequency and morphology with a minimal of spacial resolution. EEG practice requires advanced skills, lots of training and supervision, is time consuming and frequently offers conditions facilitating human error. Spatial resolution is poor due to the obstacles that electrical signals generated in the cerebral cortex face in its propagation to the scalp facing different type of tissues with different properties causing that original measures in millivolts (mV) reach the scalp in values within the microvolts (μV) range. It was assumed the sources of EEG signals were found beneath of each recording electrode, changes in technology and recordings techniques questioned this assumption opening the field for source localization based in the inverse solution model [80–82].

ML and DL solutions for EEG analysis began to appear since 2010 with communications for epilepsy analysis [83, 84] with a substantial number of studies of DL applications in EEG analysis in research and clinic.

Being raw EEG the basic element in NFB, it must be considered as the source in which DL models have to be applied. Contributions using DL models for end-to-end EEG analysis are encouraging. It was found the prediction of gender from brain rhythms using convolutional neural networks (CNN) for decoding and classification the EEG raw signal [85] showing CNNs potential to extract and classify very specific EEG "hidden" features. In a replication of this study designed to test CNN's precision in classification using the same data, it was found the model performs better with raw data than with spectral images [86]. These findings support the regular use of DL in neurofeedback, based in the fact that in both cases results were obtain from raw EEG data and the best performance was obtained with minimally processed raw data, basic conditions in NFB regular practice. Peculiarities of NFB settings suggest DL models should be applied as an end-to-end process with the raw data, performing online feature extraction, pre-classification and classification, filtering, pre-processing and processing, before the feedback process takes place. DL models used for offline EEG analysis, and some used in more complex scenarios with online recordings in invasive BCI's offer a basic platform for DL applications in NFB. An element in our current work is the use of CNNs in the EEG amplifiers processor's microcode to speed the process (Fig. 12.1). DL solutions have been used in EEG analysis, for signals classification [87, 88] online classification in BCI's with 84% of accuracy [89], and offline analysis in sleep scoring [90], epilepsy [91], and interictal monitoring [92] searching for accuracy in assessment and diagnosis [93]. A line of work for improving the processing tools has contributions with pipelines including feature learning and extraction [94], signal cleaning and denoising [95], artifact detection [96] classification and elimination [97], generation of data for developing hardware, simulations and DL solutions testing and development

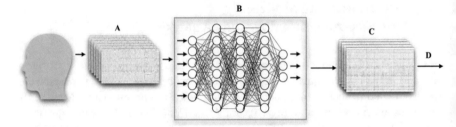

Fig. 12.1 Schematic overview of a NFB device processor with pretrained CNNs in the microcode. (**a**). Raw EEG recording samples. (**b**). NFB device processor with CNNs in microcode for online EEG preprocessing. (**c**). EEG samples selected for feedback. (**d**). To computer. (Source: Prof. Jorge J. Palacios-Venegas)

[98], and data handling models of EEG signal with lines of research in recordings generation [99] and augmentation [100].

Basic DL research in EEG analysis constitutes and strong line of research in BCI's develop [101], and cognitive and affective processes research [102]. From 2010 to 2018 a classification of the DL approaches to EEG analysis found lines of work that can be classified identifying: BCI's develop and testing [103], generation of data [100], and improvement of processing tools [104]. In this field DL strategies have generated information supporting fundamentals for its regular use in NFB, suggesting DL models could be the basic tools for neurofeedback research and practice since it has been successfully used in most of the stages of EEG analysis [105]. DL applications for denoising, artefact elimination, feature extraction and classification are mainly used in offline analysis [4, 106] and frequently used with BCI's in which analysis and decomposition methods are applied from raw data performing average, average adjusted, normalized, mean adjusted and spectral data analysis based in different methods: fast Fourier transform (FFT), power spectral density (PSD) and spectrogram with statistical analysis of signal parametric values (frequency and voltage) and very specific analysis like wavelet decomposition [107] all in an increasing number of studies in motor imagery [108. 109, 110], and emotion recognition [111–114] processes.

The efficacy of DL models under such specific conditions supports its regular use with online EEG raw data processing in NFB, in this area of application it must be noted that DL approaches are built with a variety of architectures CNNs [115–117], fully connected (FC) [118], long short-term memory (LSTM) [119, 120], auto-encoders (AE) [121], recurrent neural networks (RNN) [122, 123], support vector machines (SVM) [122], and generative adversarial networks (GAN) [123, 124]. All used successfully in EEG analysis in different conditions from resting-state task-negative and task-positive, emotion recognition tasks [113, 125], event related potential detection [127], motor functions induced from imagery [108, 128], and neurological and neuropsychiatric conditions [129, 130]. Prevalent DL architectures are CNNs with structures up to 30 layers with residual blocks and recurrent layers commonly with ranges between 2 to 16 or 18 layers [131]. A typical model of a CNN tested for EEG data analysis from end to end is usually built with a total of 21 layers [132]. Most frequently used structures can be synthetized in sets composed by a 2 Dimension Convolutional Layer (Conv2d) a Rectified Linear Unit (ReLU), a Max pooling operation for 2D spatial data (MaxPool2d), and a Dropout, repeating the sequence until the 28th layer followed then by a Flatten and two consecutives Linear layers [85]. EEG data are structured as 2D matrices representing time and channels, with real values of the negative and positive fluctuations of brain waves. These are the type of data to feed CNNs, Deep Belief Networks (DBN) and Recurrent Neural Networks (RNN) all prevalent in DL EEG processing and analysis [83], showing in some cases accuracies between 81% [133] to 89% [134] combined with analysis based in hybrid Neural Networks (NN) architectures combining CNNs and RNNs, RNNs and LSTM or DBN and 3 restricted Boltzmann machine (RBM) with one dense layer [135, 136]. DL neural, decoding and classification algorithms are the most advanced and precise methods used for these purposes, due to the success obtained in most of the cases [137] are becoming a frequent part of the routine pipeline analysis [138] along with a diversity of NNs, feed forward networks (FFN), CNNs and RNNs are also the most common due to the accuracy obtained in different studies [139]. There are three types of pipelines for EEG data analysis, usually the first composed by the preprocessing methods for cleaning the data and isolate the signals from those in the interference and artifacts spectrum, the second centered in feature extraction process, for decomposition analysis in time, frequency, time-frequency dimensions [140], and used for specific procedures in the spatial domain [141]. Performance of NNs discriminating biological characteristics like gender or individuals, identifying biometric properties of EEG [4], suggests DL models are sensitive to specific and distinctive features in EEG signal and that this sensibility could be extended to most of its regular uses, identifying new ones and implying the future design and use of more complex architectures based in NNs with more layers (beyond 30) designed specifically for every stage in the EEG data analysis and online processing. DL classification and feature extraction from EEG is applied with accuracy in different conditions where EEG was activated with cognitive, emotional, imagery and motor tasks for detection of clinical EEG key components in epilepsy, distinctive elements identification in neuropsychiatric conditions, neurologic disabilities and design and testing of EEG-based authentication technology [142]. Consistency of DL models accuracy obtained in a variety of studies from different conditions, procedures, and methodologies is a promising scenario to develop applications in NFB, based in stability in results using Artificial Neural Networks (ANNs) in a variety of conditions with a variety of procedures [143, 144].

From BCI's research there are interesting proposals for non-invasive applications [145–149], ML and DL algorithms have proved its best performance with EEG data processing and classification tasks obtained under conditions very similar of those in NFB regular practice, raw signals online analysis, several number of trials and sessions, constant audiovisual stimulation, long duration of the recording sessions, complex cognitive and motor tasks, noise and outliers, features with high dimensionality when converted as vectors and with amounts of information distributed in relatively short periods of time. Non-stationary properties of signals often increased in conditions that are task-related or caused by individual's reactions, traits, symptoms, or sequelae [149]. The amount of information distributed in time offers possibilities for analysis of concatenated features coming from different time segments and the combination of performing different classifications using dynamic procedures for feature extraction with immediate results used for communication with machines, the environment or the individual itself in NFB setups with processes performed using classification algorithms like generative, static, stable, and regularized. In this type of pipeline, classifiers are used for linear discriminant analysis (LDA) and data separation process prior to classification [151] and SVMs are applied for classes identification [152]. NNs have proved reliability in online EEG raw recording analysis and classification tasks, being the most used: Multi-Layer Perception (MLP) [153], Learning Vector Quantization (LVQ) [154], algorithm Fuzzy Logic, Adaptive Resonance Theory (ARTMAP), Finite Impulse Response (FIR), Time-Delay (TD), Gamma Dynamic Neural Networks (GDNN) [155], Radial Basis Function (RBF) [156], Bayesian Logistic Regression (BLR) [157], Adaptive Logic Network (AL) [158], and Probability Estimating Guarded Neural Classifier (PeGNC) [159]. Research in speech decoding from raw electro-corticographic (EcoG) online recordings with DL models, in a patient suffering from anarthria, reported the accuracy of the DL architecture called *natural language* performing without errors in an 80 to 150 trials sequence, using a display for communication [150].

12.4   Deep Learning Assisted Biofeedback (DLAB)

Our model is based in years of experience in research and clinical practice with traditional PB, NFB and QEEG-Biofeedback devices designed for all the stages in NFB process. Is built including previous contributions in the field, gathers the most relevant DL solutions used in biomedical signals analysis and processing and incorporates those designed specifically for NFB process. Is structured of a group of independent NN's running simultaneously and in sequence. Figure 12.2 shows the general diagram with model components. Named as Brain Computer Interface for Biofeedback (BCIB) and controlled by the Deep Learning Assisted Biofeedback Platform (DLABP) is a hybrid NNs design built to carry on with specific processing tasks designed to reduce variability by maintaining stability in the feedback process, working in task positive setups with individuals suffering from different type of conditions or sequelae and considering artifacts should be expected from different sources that can't be controlled. Our DL platform is conceived with the objective to obtain as final result a stable EEG recording during the NFB session. DLAB hybrid CNNs are built to control EEG stability correcting perturbances from environmental conditions, technical and instrumentation procedures, *natural perturbances* (fatigue, sleep, drowsiness, eye blinking) and *performance -task positive- perturbances* (movements, speech, emotional expressions, motor and movement sequelae).

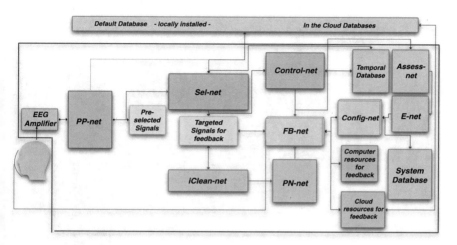

Fig. 12.2 Schematic overview of the DLAB model. (Source: Prof. Jorge J. Palacios-Venegas)

Model is based in a constant online database consultation in the cloud, or to a *default* basic database in the system, performing processes controlled by CNNs built to extract, features from databases and current recordings to select and "target" segments suitable to feedback. A set of NNs is designed to *supervise* the targeted segments performance during the feedback process with specific denoising functions identifying, classifying and removing artifacts with two different types of outputs *corrected* and not successfully cleaned. The next NN performs uncleaned segments quantification if results are above 5% feedback is interrupted until recording perturbations are absent. NNs for feedback delivery and administration control stability in targeted segments for feedback based on a predictive process for natural perturbances anticipation. Output of this NN is to interrupt the feedback action until perturbances are over. Three more NNs elements are built to independently measure and assess segments performance during the feedback process, classifying them by stability and types of deviations, the output will feed the group of NNs for quantification, assessment and selection functions, built to control the stability of the feedback process. Figure 12.3 is the schematic representation of the DLABP described in the following pages.

12.4.1   PP-net: EEG Online Preprocessing

PP.net (Fig. 12.3a) receives online raw EEG signals matrices input. Performs denoising, band pass filtering, artifacts rejection, identifies and reject bad channels and segments, performs independent component analysis (ICA) and classification (ICA labeling), frequency decomposition and classification functions for EEG spectrum definition including High Frequency Oscillations (HFOs). Table 12.1 contains

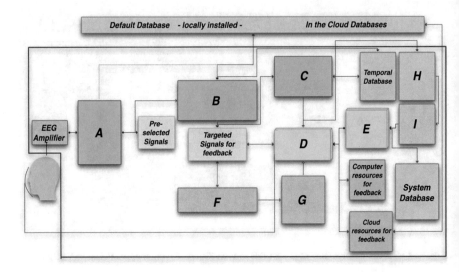

Fig. 12.3 Schematic overview of the DLABP. (Source: Prof. Jorge J. Palacios-Venegas)

Table 12.1 Frequency EEG bands in frequency decomposition. (Source: Prof. Jorge J. Palacios-Venegas)

Hz	EEG bands	Hz	EEG bands
0–0.3	Ultraslow	22 to 26	Beta4 β^4
0.3 to 4	Delta ∂	26 to 30	Beta5 β^5
4 to 8	Theta θ	30 to 80	Gamma γ
8 to 13	Alpha α	High Frequency Oscillations	
13 to 15	Beta1 β^1	80–250	Ripples
15 to 18	Beta2 β^2	250–500	Fast ripples
18 to 22	Beta3 β^3	>500–1000	Ultrafast ripples

the complete frequency bands selected for decomposition. Output are two sets of files one to be ignored (EEGI) and one selected for the feedback procedure organized in 5 seconds segments groups, identified as *pre-selected signals*. *PP-net* general structure is convolution layers (CL) for denoising, subsampling, band-pass filtering, CL for artifacts rejection, subsampling, CL for ICA, ICA labeling, subsampling, CL for frequency decomposition extraction and classification, flattening, FC layers for bad channels selection and extraction, output: EEGI segments and *preselected signals* to feed *Sel-net* (Fig. 12.3b). Results are stored in local database.

12.4.2   Sel-net: Classifying "Targeting" Signals for Feedback

Sel-net (Fig. 12.3b) identifies conditions: eyes closed (EC), eyes opened (EO), activity: task negative (TNg), task positive (TP) classifies the *neurophysiological markers* (NM) according to conditions: anxiety, depression, addiction or neural states: attention, inattention, drowsiness. Extracts and classifies neural markers matching them with correspondent features extracted from databases, *targeting* them for feedback. This process involves two types of bidirectional databases consultation. Depending on the resources available (machine capabilities, internet speed etc.) a consultation type is to a *small* basic *default* database with preprocessed EEG segments classified by gender, age and recording type and for conditions or state. The other type is a constant consultation to the international databases. Output are two types of files one identified for rejection and one *targeted* for modification through feedback. A temporal database will be stored for *Control-net* (Fig. 12.3c) consultation during control functions. *Sel-net* general structure is CL for condition, subsampling, CL for activity, subsampling, CL for matching to databases, CL for NM identification, subsampling, flattening, FC layers for NM classification. Output: predominant NM selected for feedback. Results are stored in the system database.

12.4.3   Control-net: Extracting and Classifying for Feedback

Control-net (Fig. 12.3c) is built of hybrid NNs with CNN, LSTM and recurrent neural network (RNN), to determine the best temporal sequences model, considering NM complex and nonlinear dynamics nature. Is design to *activate or not FB-net* (Fig. 12.3d) action based in the output obtained after processing. Is used as a predictive process built to control feedback online delivery. Predictions are made for the temporal stability of the targeted NM based in the stability of the correspondent EEG microstates. Stability is assessed in terms of recordings time permanence if predictions output is for 3 secs or more the feedback is allowed. *Control-net* general structure is CL, maxpooling, memory layers, flatten, FC. Output: stability NM sustentation in order to control *FB-net* action (Fig. 12.3d). Results are stored in system database.

12.4.4   FB-net: EEG Online Feedback

Feedback process is the output of a decision function controlled at the same time by two simultaneous NNs. *Control-net* (Fig. 12.3c) and *Config-net* (Fig. 12.3e). *FB-net* (Fig. 12.3d) runs a predictive process based on a hybrid CNNs and LSTMs design, built to assess signals stability runs decision processes based in NM current properties changes. Receives Config-net (Fig. 12.3e) output with estimated values of current NM that match feedback criteria. Its output refines rewarding or positive feedback to both the signals and the subject. Is designed to deliver feedback based in the current stability of NM expecting modifications in its properties (improvement in the general percentage of the performance, increment or decrement of μVs, ratios, asymmetry or synchrony). Implies a moment-to-moment stability measure of NM behavior with the last decision to interrupt the feedback. Is in direct responsibility of the FL control and administration. *FB-net* general structure is CL, maxpooling, memory layers, flatten, FC. Output: activation of locally stored audiovisual resources analogical to the variations in NM current measures simultaneously sent to *Assess-net* (Fig. 12.3h). Results are stored in local database.

12.4.5   Config-net: Predictive Maintenance and Feedback Modulation

Config-net (Fig. 12.3e) *modulates* with assessment and predictive functions current state in *FB-net* (Fig. 12.3d) performance and possible evolution anticipating faults. Receives *Asses-net* (Fig. 12.3h) and *E-net* (Fig. 12.3i) output, processing current NM values matching feedback criteria. *Tunes* de feedback operation, setting thresholds upon relations between performance in expected frequency μVs values and ratios, measuring general performance and difficulty level in terms of success/error rate during the last 30 seconds segments. *Config-net* structure is CL, maxpooling, memory layers, flatten, FC. Output: current NM values matching feedback criteria. Results are stored in local database.

12.4.6   iClean-net: Cleaning Performance Perturbances

iClean-net (Fig. 12.3f) is a parallel and independent NN. Feed with *current targeted signals for feedback* matrices built to extract perturbances consequence of performance during the feedback session. Process current measures performing denoising, artifact removing, identifying and classifying outliers and artifacts extraction. Runs predictive functions with bidirectional communication built to maintain stability in the signals during feedback process, maintaining NM stability cleaning them of interference. Its predictive capabilities are designed with functionality to anticipate stability deficiencies lasting more than 3 secs and performing *cleaning* process to ensure feedback. *iClean-net* general structure is CL for denoising, subsampling, CL for artifacts rejection, subsampling, CL for identifying and classifying outliers, CL for movements and artifacts extraction, subsampling, flattening, FC layers for bad channels selection and extraction, resulting in a rectified EEG with *clean* NM. Output: NM cleaned and corrected for feedback and uncleaned segments sent to *PN-net* (Fig. 12.3g). Results are stored in local database.

12.4.7   PN-net: Feedback Quality Control System and Interactive Database

PN-net (Fig. 12.3g) is a RNN modify from [159] and restructured to control feedback process based in the amount of perturbances generated during the task positive performance that could not be extracted by *iClean-net*. Receives online classified datasets performs quantification of identified and classified perturbations. Designed to interrupt the feedback process after 3 seconds of uncleaned segments accumulation. *PN-net* general structure is quantifiers, LSTM, last LSTM hidden state, FC layer, RELU, a smooth approximation to the hard maximum of the vector (SoftMax). Output: to *FB-net* for interruption of feedback action. Results are stored in the local database.

12.4.8   Assess-net: Feedback Modulation Control Database

Assess-net (Fig. 12.3h) built for feedback monitoring based in the performance curve of near in time sessions. Is an information central unit of general feedback performance. Exceptionally large deviations between predicted and current EEG signals are used as indicators of the near future or immediate performance. Has feedback process predictive, decision making and control capabilities. Is feed with wavelet transform, short time Fourier and spectral parameterization resolved in time (SPRINT) [160] scalogram images generated with databases information with the outcome of current session, has prediction capabilities based in previous and current performance and databases consultation. Controls the feedback intervention matching current session with performance history and resemblance to *default* and *control* data. Executes extraction, classification, quantification and qualification of targeted segments *once they have received feedback*. Its predictive capabilities anticipate segments probability to receive feedback. Predictive functions are used for preventing setbacks in current performance and treatment, predicting setbacks probability and classifying current data by selecting *feedback-performance ratio* of previous stages to enhance current preventing relapses or setbacks. Output is performance predicted classes and probabilities sent to the *E-net* (Fig. 12.3i). *Assess-net* general structure is input layer of three red, green and blue (RGB) channels, CL, pooling layer, flatten, FC, softmax (last three for classification). Results stored in the local database.

12.4.9   E-net

E-net (Fig. 12.3i) is built for EEG entropy assessment, measured in terms of the current stability in comparison with previous stable feedback periods during session(s) with databases consultation. This function is performed with the segments successfully rewarded with feedback action extracting, selecting and classifying them. Output generates the elements constituting EEG internal stability map, estimating coherence, synchrony, symmetry, stability permanence probability in time. Entropy is defined in terms of sample entropy or *SampEn* [162, 163]. *E-net* is built to evaluate whole brain activity (not only NFB derivations) during performance along feedback training session and treatment. *E-net* general structure is based in parallel SVMs with one class output to *Config-net* (Fig. 12.3e). Results are stored in local database.

12.5   Discussion

Current development in brain waves BFB leads to its overhauling and regular integration to Neurosciences basic and applied research field. NFB procedures need to be updated complementing them with the most recent advances in neuroinformatics and computational neurosciences, in order to take advantage of achievements in these fields that will make professional practice safer and more reliable and will incorporate NFB research as a regular specialty area in Neurosciences. Setbacks to NFB scientific development due to the issues discussed in this chapter could be overcome with the integration of current ML and DL solutions and the ones to be built, for the creation of an *Open Source neuroinformatic environment* specifically developed for biological signals acquisition and processing as end to end solutions design from online acquisition, preprocessing a processing to feedback intervention and offline analysis. Solution based in research grade 64 and on EEG channels systems including polygraphic recordings. Table 12.2 shows a comparison of some of the ML and DL key state of the art solutions mentioned in the chapter, to be considered in the development of such an *Open Source neuroinformatic* environment for NFB.

12.6   Conclusions

Our model is being built with applications for research and practice based in QEEG Biofeedback procedures. Advances and changes in EEG devices and affordability of more powerful computers will make possible to deploy it into a very different systems (recording devices and computers). Ideal solution is from 64 EEG with 5 polygraphic channels and on, with perspectives for addressing challenges in the

Table 12.2 ML and DL research in Biofeedback and EEG signals analysis. (Source: Prof. Jorge J. Palacios-Venegas)

References	Solution (s)	Publish year	Application
[134]	Sigmoid (AE) 20 individual AE's. Avg of AE's, 5 OUT	2016	Automatic sleep stage scoring
[114]	CNN, 1 conv (ReLU), 1 FC (Softmax), 4 OUT	2017	Bulling incidences identification
[136]	Hybrid CNN-RNN, 4 conv, 2 RNN layers, 1 FC, T OUT, ReLU (conv), Softmax (FC)	2017	Automatic sleep stage scoring from raw EEG
[95]	CNN Hilbert-Huang transform	2018	EEG signals preprocessing
[123]	Hybrid CNN-RNN, 4 conv, 2 RNN layers, 1 FC, 2 OUT. ReLU (conv), Softmax (FC)	2018	Sleep stage classification
[91]	Deep Convolutional Neural Network	2020	Epilepsy EEG diagnosis
[85]	Convolutional NN (6 layers), Pooling (4 layers), Dropout (4 layers), Dense Layer (Softmax), ReLU (conv)	2018	Biometric identification
[126]	Cross-correlation values and Mahalanobis distance	2018	Biometric identification
[124]	Entropy, SVM, K-Nearest Neighbors (KNN)	2019	Alzheimer's diagnosis
[113]	CNN (7 layers), Flatten, FC, Softmax,	2020	Speech emotion recognition
[109]	RNN-LSTM, 2 LSTM layers, 2 OUT,	2021	Motor imagery classification
[86]	CNN (6 layers), MaxPol (4 layers), Dropout (4 Layers), FC (2 layers), Softmax (1 layer)	2021	Biometric identification
[161]	Decision tree (DT), Naïve Bayes (NB), SVM, KNN, ANN,	2021	Evaluation of Neurofeedback training
[150]	Not specified,	2021	Neuroprosthesis for decoding speech

NFB spatial domain allowing a more precise work, overcoming some of the spacial resolution restrictions of the traditional NFB EEG recordings. Developing a new generation of integral solutions in temporal and spatial domains with NFB process, that could be used with magnetoencephalography (MEG) devices in the emerging field of MEG-Biofeedback (MEG-B). It also must be considered the developing for regular use of the minimally invasive NFB brain computer interfaces (subcutaneous) to be used with autonomy, for a constant neuromodulation with applications to prevalent neurologic and neuropsychiatric conditions: Alzheimer's, Parkinson's, Depression, Autistic Spectrum Disorders or Epilepsy. Conditions requiring constant attention. The aim of this line of work is to develop a less vulnerable, precise and diverse generation of neurofeedback and neuromodulation systems based in Deep Learning solutions.

References

1. J.N. Kather, A.T. Pearson, N. Halama, D. Jäger, J. Krause, S.H. Loosen, A. Marx, P. Boor, F. Tacke, U.P. Neumann, H.I. Grabsch, T. Yoshikawa, H. Brenner, J. Chang-Claude, M. Hoffmeister, C. Trautwein, T. Luedde, Deep learning can predict microsatellite instability directly from histology in gastrointestinal cancer. Nat. Med. **25**(7), 1054–1056 (2019). https://doi.org/10.1038/s41591-019-0462-y
2. R.G. Muthalaly, R.M. Evans, Applications of machine learning in cardiac electrophysiology. Arrhythmia Electrophysiol. Rev. **9**(2), 71–77 (2020). https://doi.org/10.15420/aer.2019.19
3. R. de Filippis, E.A. Carbone, R. Gaetano, A. Bruni, V. Pugliese, C. Segura-Garcia, P. De Fazio, Machine learning techniques in a structural and functional MRI diagnostic approach in schizophrenia: A systematic review. Neuropsychiatr. Dis. Treat. **15**, 1605–1627 (2019). https://doi.org/10.2147/ndt.s202418
4. S. Zhang, L. Sun, X. Mao, C. Hu, P. Liu, Review on EEG-based authentication technology. Comput. Intell. Neurosci. **2021**, 1–20 (2021). https://doi.org/10.1155/2021/5229576
5. Y. Roy, H. Banville, I. Albuquerque, A. Gramfort, T.H. Falk, J. Faubert, Deep learning-based electroencephalography analysis: A systematic review. J. Neural Eng. **16**(5), 10.1088/1741-2552/ab260c 6 (2019)
6. M.G.M. Saif, M.A. Hassan, A. Vuckovic, Efficacy evaluation of neurofeedback applied for treatment of central neuropathic pain using machine learning. *SN*. Appl. Sci. **3**(1), 1–11 (2021). https://doi.org/10.1007/s42452-020-04035-9
7. S.A. Plotnikov, M. Lipkovich, D.M. Semenov, A.L. Fradkov, Artificial intelligence-based neurofeedback. Cybernetics Phys. **8**(4), 287–291 (2019). https://doi.org/10.35470/2226-411 6-2019-8-4-287-291
8. M. Seera, C.P. Lim, W.S. Liew, E. Lim, C.K. Loo, Classification of electrocardiogram and auscultatory blood pressure signals using machine learning models. Expert Syst. Appl. **42**(7), 3643–3652 (2015)
9. H. Wang, Q. Su, Z. Yan, F. Lu, Q. Zhao, Z. Liu, F. Zhou, Rehabilitation treatment of motor dysfunction patients based on deep learning brain–computer Interface technology. Front. Neurosci. **14**(October), 595084 (2020). https://doi.org/10.3389/fnins.2020.595084
10. D.K. Luu, A.T. Nguyen, M. Jiang, J. Xu, M.W. Drealan, J. Cheng, E.W. Keefer, Q. Zhao, Z. Yang, Deep learning-based approaches for decoding motor intent from peripheral nerve signals. Front. Neurosci. **15**(June), 1–12 (2021). https://doi.org/10.3389/fnins.2021.667907
11. Y. Zhao, F. Ly, Q. Hong, Z. Cheng, T. Santander, H.T. Yang, P.K. Hansma, L. Petzold, How much does it hurt: A deep learning framework for chronic pain score assessment. IEEE International Conference on Data Mining Workshops, ICDMW, 2020-November, (2020) pp. 651–660. https://doi.org/10.1109/ICDMW51313.2020.00092
12. R. Argent, A. Bevilacqua, A. Keogh, A. Daly, B. Caulfield, The importance of real-world validation of machine learning systems in wearable exercise biofeedback platforms: A case study. Sensors **21**(7) (2021). https://doi.org/10.3390/s21072346
13. B.J. Stetter, F.C. Krafft, S. Ringhof, T. Stein, S. Sell, A machine learning and wearable sensor based approach to estimate external knee flexion and abduction moments during various locomotion tasks. Front. Bioeng. Biotechnol. **8**(January) (2020). https://doi.org/10.3389/fbioe.2020.00009
14. L. Yang, J. Guo, R. Bie, A. Umek, A. Kos, Machine learning based accuracy prediction model for augmented biofeedback in precision shooting. Procedia Comp. Sci. **174**(2019), 358–363 (2020). https://doi.org/10.1016/j.procs.2020.06.099
15. N. Wiener, J.P. Schade, *Cybernetics of the Nervous System* (Elsevier, 1965)
16. N. Wiener, *Cybernetics or Control and Communication in the Animal and the Machine* (MIT press, 2019)
17. O. Mayr, *The origins of feedback control*, vol 223 (MIT Press, Cambridge, MA, 1970), pp. 110–118

18. G. Razran, The observable and the inferable conscious in current soviet psychophysiology: Interoceptive conditioning, semantic conditioning, and the orienting reflex. Psychol. Rev. **68**(2), 81–147 (1961)
19. G. Adam, Visceroception, awareness, and behavior, in *Consciousness and Self-Regulation*, ed. by G. E. Schwartz, D. Shapiro, (Springer, Boston, MA, 1978). https://doi.org/10.1007/978-1-4684-2571-0_5
20. J.V. Basmajian, *Biofeedback: Principles and Practice for Clinicians* (Williams & Wilkins, 1979)
21. J. Kamiya, Behavioral, subjective, and physiological aspects of drowsiness and sleep, in *Functions of Varied Experience*, ed. by D. W. Fiske, S. R. Maddi, (Dorsey Press, Homewood, IL, 1961), pp. 145–174
22. J. Kamiya, Conscious control of brain waves. Psychol. Today **1**, 57–60 (1968)
23. J. Kamiya, Operant control of the EEG alpha rhythm and some of its reported effects on consciousness, in *Altered States of Consciousness*, ed. by C. T. Tart, (Wiley, New York, 1969), pp. 507–517
24. W.B. Plotkin, On the self-regulation of the occipital alpha rhythm: Control strategies, states of consciousness, and the role of physiological feedback. J. Exp. Psychol. Gen. **105**(1), 66–99 (1976)
25. S. Ancoli, J. Kamiya, Methodological issues in alpha biofeedback training. Biofeedback Self Regul. **3**(2), 159–183 (1978)
26. J. Hardt, J. Kamiya, Some comments on Plotkin's self-regulation of the electroencephalographic alpha. J. Exp. Psychol. Gen. **105**(1), 100–108 (1976)
27. T. Budzynski, J. Stoyva, C. Adler, Feedback-induced muscle relaxation: Application to tension headache. J. Behav. Ther. Exp. Psychiatry **1**(3), 205–211 (1970). https://doi.org/10.1016/0005-7916(70)90004-2
28. J.D. Sargent, E.D. Walters, E.E. Green, Psychosomatic self-regulation of migraine headaches. Semin. Psychiatry **5**(4), 415–428 (1973)
29. T.H. Budzynski, J.M. Stoyva, Biofeedback methods in the treatment of anxiety and stress, in *Principles and Practice of Stress Management*, ed. by R. L. Woolfolk, P. M. Lehrer, (Guilford Press, New York, 1984)
30. O. Mecarelli, *Clinical Electroencephalography. Springer Nature Switzerland*, vol 1, Issue 1, 1st edn. (Springer, Cham, 2019). https://doi.org/10.1007/978-3-030-04573-9
31. M.B. Sterman, Sensorimotor EEG operant conditioning: Experimental and clinical effects. Pavlovian J. Biol. Sci. **12**(2), 63–92 (1977)
32. W. Wyrwicka, M.B. Sterman, Instrumental conditioning of sensory motor cortex EEG spindles in the waking cat. Physiol. Behav. **3**, 703–707 (1968)
33. M.B. Sterman, The role of sensorimotor rhythmic EEG activity in the etiology and treatment of generalized motor seizures, in *Self-Regulation of the Brain and Behavior*, (Springer, Berlin, Heidelberg, 1984), pp. 95–106
34. M.B. Sterman, EEG biofeedback: Physiological behavior modification. Neurosci. Biobehav. Rev. **5**(3), 405–412 (1981)
35. M.N. Shouse, J.F. Lubar, Operant conditioning of EEG rhythms and ritalin in the treatment of hyperkinesis. Biofeedback Self Regul. **4**(4), 299–312 (1979)
36. E.G. Peniston, P.J. Kulkosky, Alpha-theta brain wave neuro-feedback therapy for Vietnam veterans with combat-related post-traumatic stress disorder. Med. Psychother. **4**, 47–60 (1991)
37. E.G. Peniston, P.J. Kulkosky, Alpha-theta EEG biofeedback training in alcoholism & post-traumatic stress disorder. Newsletter Int. Soc Study Subtle **2**(4), 5–7 (1991)
38. J.P. Rosenfeld, EEG biofeedback of frontal alpha asymmetry in affective disorders. Biofeedback **25**(1), 8–25 (1997)
39. J.P. Rosenfeld, G. Cha, T. Blair, I. Gotlib, Operant biofeedback control of left- right frontal alpha power differences. Biofeedback Self-Regulation **20**, 241–258 (1995)

40. J.P. Rosenfeld, E. Baehr, R. Baehr, I. Gotlib, C. Ranganath, Preliminary evidence that daily changes in frontal alpha asymmetry correlate with changes in affect in therapy sessions. Int. J. Psychophysiol. **23**, 241–258 (1996)

41. R.W. Thatcher, Electroencephalography and mild traumatic brain injury. Foundations of Sport-Related Brain Injuries, 241–265 (2006). https://doi.org/10.1007/0-387-32565-4_11

42. J.F. Lubar, Neocortical dynamics: Implications for understanding the role of neurofeedback and related techniques for the enhancement of attention. Appl. Psychophysiol. Biofeedback **22**, 11–126 (1997)

43. J.O. Lubar, J.F. Lubar, Electroencephalographic biofeedback of SMR and beta for treatment of attention deficit disorders in a clinical setting. Biofeedback Self-Regulation **2**, 1–23 (1984)

44. J.F. Lubar, Discourse on the development of EEG diagnostics and biofeedback treatment for attention-deficit/hyperactivity disorders. Biofeedback Self-Regulation **16**, 201–225 (1991)

45. T. Budzynski, H. Kogan, B.H. Evans, A. Abarbanel. Introduction to Quantitative EEG and Neurofeedback (n.d.)

46. R. W. Thatcher, J. F. Lubar, History of the scientific standards of QEEG normative databases. In *Introduction to Quantitative EEG and Neurofeedback* (2009). https://doi.org/10.1016/b978-0-12-374534-7.00002-2

47. J.F. Lubar, J.O. Lubar, Neurofeedback assessment and treatment for attention deficit/hyperactivity disorders, in *Introduction to Quantitative EEG and Neurofeedback*, (Academic, 1999), pp. 103–143

48. M. Congedo, J.F. Lubar, D. Joffe, Low-resolution electromagnetic tomography neurofeedback. IEEE Trans. Neural Syst. Rehabil. Eng. **12**(4), 387–397 (2004)

49. R.W. Thatcher, Handbook of quantitative electroencephalography and EEG biofeedback. Scientif. Foundations Pract. Appl. **1**, 1–117 (2012). http://www.anipublishing.com

50. R.D. Pascual Marqui, C.M. Michel, D. Lehmann, Low resolution electromagnetic tomography: A new method for localizing electrical activity in the brain. Int. J. Psychophysiol. **18**(1), 49 65–49 65 (1994)

51. L. Sherlin, T. Budzynski, H. Kogan Budzynski, M. Congedo, M.E. Fischer, D. Buchwald, Low resolution electromagnetic brain tomography (LORETA) of monozygotic twins discordant for chronic fatigue syndrome. NeuroImage **34**(4), 1438–1442 (2007)

52. L. Sherlin, M. Congedo, Obsessive compulsive dimension localized using low resolution electromagnetic tomography (LORETA). Neurosci. Lett. **387**(2), 72 74–72 74 (2005)

53. M.E. Ayers, M.W. Sams, M.B. Sterman, J. Lubar, When to inhibit EEG activity instead of reinforcing and inhibiting simultaneously. J. Neurother. **4**(1), 83–90 (2000)

54. E. Baehr, J.P. Rosenfeld, R. Baehr, C. Earnest, Clinical use of an alpha asymmetry neurofeedback protocol in the treatment of mood disorders, in *Introduction to Quantitative EEG and Neurofeedback*, (Academic, 1999), pp. 181–201

55. L. Fehmi, T.F. Collura, The effects of electrode placement upon EEG biofeedback training: The monopolar/bipolar controversy. J. Neurother. **11**(2), 45–63 (2007)

56. J.M. Stern, *Atlas of EEG patterns*, vol 65 (Lippincott Williams & Wilkins, 2005), p. E6. https://doi.org/10.1212/01.wnl.0000174180.41994.39

57. T.F. Collura, History and evolution of computerized electroencephalography. J. Clin. Neurophysiol. **12**(3), 214–229 (1995)

58. N. Birbaumer, Coming of age, brain-computer interface research, in *Annual Conference*, (International Society of Neurofeedback and Research, San Diego, CA, 2007)

59. D.C. Hammond, G. Bodenhamer-Davis, G. Gluck, D. Stokes, S.H. Harper, D. Trudeau, L. Kirk, Standards of practice for neurofeedback and neurotherapy: A position paper of the International Society for Neurofeedback & research. J. Neurother. **15**(1), 54–64 (2011)

60. B.C.I.A. Board, *Professional Standards and Ethical Principles of Biofeedback* (BCIA, Wheat Ridge, CO, 2015)

61. N.A. Badcock, P. Mousikou, Y. Mahajan, P. De Lissa, J. Thie, G. McArthur, Validation of the Emotiv EPOC® EEG gaming system for measuring research quality auditory ERPs. Peer J **1**, e38 (2013)

62. E. Niedermeyer, da Silva, F. L. (Eds.)., *Electroencephalography: Basic Principles, Clinical Applications, and Related Fields* (Lippincott Williams & Wilkins, 2005)
63. Atlantis II Series Brainmaster neurofeedback system. https://brainmaster.com/product/atlantis-ii-series/
64. Atlantis I Series Brainmaster neurofeedback system. https://brainmaster.com/product/atlantis/
65. Nexus 32 QEEG system. https://www.biofeedback-tech.com/nexus-32
66. Deymed TruScan QEEG system. https://deymed.com/truscan-qeeg-neurofeedback
67. R. Coben, J.R. Evans, Neurofeedback and neuromodulation techniques and applications, in *Neurofeedback and Neuromodulation Techniques and Applications*, (2011). https://doi.org/10.1016/C2009-0-64101-5
68. J. Kropotov, *Quantitative EEG, Event-Related Potentials and Neurotherapy* (Academic, 2010)
69. R.W. Thatcher, D. North, C. Biver, Evaluation and validity of a LORETA normative EEG database. Clin. EEG Neurosci **36**(2), 116–122 (2005)
70. L.H. Sherlin, Diagnosing and treating brain function through the use of low resolution brain electromagnetic tomography (LORETA), in *Introduction to Quantitative EEG and Neurofeedback: Advanced Theory and Applications*, (2009), pp. 83–102
71. L.H. Sherlin, Diagnosing and treating brain function through the use of low resolution brain electromagnetic tomography (LORETA), in *Introduction to Quantitative EEG and Neurofeedback*, ed. by T. Budzynski, H. K. Budzynski, J. R. Evans, A. Abarbanel, (2009)
72. M. Congedo Recent advances in minimum norm inverse solutions: model-driven and data-driven sLORETA and eLORETA. First trimestral advancement meeting of the Open-ViBE project. France (2008)
73. R.W. Thatcher, D. North, C. Biver, EEG inverse solutions and parametric vs. non-parametric statistics of low resolution electromagnetic tomography (LORETA). Clin. EEG Neurosci. **36**(1), 1–9 (2005)
74. Discovery 24 Neurofeedback Brainmaster system. https://brainmaster.com/product/discovery-24/
75. Neuroscan EEG/ERP/EP Amplifiers. https://compumedicsneuroscan.com/neuroscan-eeg-erp-amplifiers/
76. J. Duun-Henriksen, M. Baud, M.P. Richardson, M. Cook, G. Kouvas, J.M. Heasman, et al., A new era in electroencephalographic monitoring? Subscalp devices for ultra–long-term recordings. Epilepsia **61**(9), 1805–1817 (2020)
77. F. Tadel, S. Baillet, J.C. Mosher, D. Pantazis, R.M. Leahy, Brainstorm: A user-friendly application for MEG/EEG analysis. Comput. Intell. Neurosci. **2011**, 1–13 (2011). https://doi.org/10.1155/2011/879716
78. A. Delorme, S. Makeig, EEGLAB: An open source toolbox for analysis of single-trial EEG dynamics. J. Neurosci. Methods **134**(1), 9–21 (2004)
79. D. Brunet, M.M. Murray, C.M. Michel, Spatiotemporal analysis of multichannel EEG: CARTOOL. Comput. Intell. Neurosci. **2011**, 1–15 (2011)
80. V. Jurcak, D. Tsuzuki, I. Dan, 10/20, 10/10, and 10/5 systems revisited: Their validity as relative head-surface-based positioning systems. NeuroImage **34**(4), 1600–1611 (2007). https://doi.org/10.1016/j.neuroimage.2006.09.024
81. S. Sadaghiani, M.J. Brookes, S. Baillet, Connectomics of human electrophysiology. NeuroImage **247**, 118788 (2022). https://doi.org/10.1016/J.NEUROIMAGE.2021.118788
82. T. Hinault, S. Baillet, Courtney, †, Age-related changes of deep-brain neurophysiological activity (2022). https://doi.org/10.1101/2022.04.27.489652
83. A. Craik, Y. He, J.L. Contreras-Vidal, Deep learning for electroencephalogram (EEG) classification tasks: A review. J. Neural Eng. **16**(3), 031001 (2019). https://doi.org/10.1088/1741-2552/AB0AB5
84. M.A. Naderi, H. Mahdavi-Nasab, Analysis and classification of EEG signals using spectral analysis and recurrent neural networks 17th Iranian conference of biomedical engineering (IEEE), pp 1–4. (2010)

85. M.J.A.M. Van Putten, S. Olbrich, M. Arns, Predicting sex from brain rhythms with deep learning. Sci. Rep. **8**(1), 1–7 (2018). https://doi.org/10.1038/s41598-018-21495-7

86. D. Truong, M. Milham, S. Makeig, A. Delorme, Deep convolutional neural network applied to electroencephalography: Raw data vs spectral features. Proceedings of the Annual International Conference of the IEEE Engineering in Medicine and Biology Society, EMBS (2021) pp. 1039–1042. https://doi.org/10.1109/EMBC46164.2021.9630708, 1039, 1042

87. An J. and Cho S. (2016). Hand motion identification of grasp-and-lift task from electroencephalography recordings using recurrent neural networks International Conference on Big Data and Smart Computing, Big Comp. (2016), pp. 427–429

88. M.A. Moinnereau, T. Brienne, S. Brodeur, J. Rouat, K. Whittingstall, E. Plourde, Classification of auditory stimuli from EEG signals with a regulated recurrent neural network reservoir. arXiv preprint arXiv:1804.10322 (2018)

89. Z. Tayeb, J. Fedjaev, N. Ghaboosi, C. Richter, L. Everding, X. Qu, Y. Wu, G. Cheng, & J. Conradt Validating deep neural networks for online decoding of motor imagery movements from EEG signals (2019). https://doi.org/10.3390/s19010210

90. M. Längkvist, L. Karlsson, A. Loutfi, Sleep stage classification using unsupervised feature learning. *Advances in Artificial Neural Systems* (2012)

91. Y. Gao, B. Gao, Q. Chen, J. Liu, Y. Zhang, Deep convolutional neural network-based epileptic electroencephalogram (EEG) signal classification. Front. Neurol. **11**, 375 (2020). https://doi.org/10.3389/FNEUR.2020.00375

92. C. da Silva Lourenço, M.C. Tjepkema-Cloostermans, M.J.A.M. van Putten, Machine learning for detection of interictal epileptiform discharges. Clin. Neurophysiol. **132**(7), 1433–1443 (2021). https://doi.org/10.1016/j.clinph.2021.02.403

93. N.D. Truong, A.D. Nguyen, L. Kuhlmann, M.R. Bonyadi, J. Yang, S. Ippolito, O. Kavehei, Convolutional neural networks for seizure prediction using intracranial and scalp electroencephalogram. Neural Netw. **105**, 104–111 (2018)

94. T. Wen, Z. Zhang, Deep convolution neural network and autoencoders-based unsupervised feature learning of EEG signals IEEE. Access **6**, 25399–25410 (2018)

95. S. Wang, B. Guo, C. Zhang, X. Bai, Z. Wang, EEG detection and de-noising based on convolution neural network and Hilbert-Huang transform Proc. (2017). 10ᵗʰ International Congress on Image and Signal Processing, BioMedical Engineering and Informatics (2018), pp 1–6

96. B. Yang, K. Duan, T. Zhang, Removal of EOG artifacts from EEG using a cascade of sparse autoencoder and recursive least squares adaptive filter. Neurocomputing **214**, 1053–1060 (2016)

97. S. Wang, B. Guo, C. Zhang, X. Bai, Z. Wang, EEG detection and de-noising based on convolution neural network and Hilbert-Huang transform proceedings 2017 10th international congress on image and signal processing. Bio Med. Eng. Informat., 1–6 (2018)

98. F. Wang, S.H. Zhong, J. Peng, J. Jiang, Y. Liu, Data augmentation for eeg-based emotion recognition with deep convolutional neural networks lecture notes computational science. LNCS **10705**, 82–93 (2018)

99. J.T.C. Schwabedal, J.C. Snyder, A. Cakmak, S. Nemati, G.D. Clifford. Addressing class imbalance in classification problems of noisy signals by using fourier transform surrogates (arXiv:1806.08675) (2018)

100. Hartmann K.G., Schirrmeister R.T., T. Ball, EEG-GAN: Generative adversarial networks for electroencephalograhic (EEG) brain signals (arXiv:1806.01875) (2018)

101. Q. Zhang. Y. Liu, Improving Brain Computer Interface Performance by Data Augmentation with Conditional Deep Convolutional Generative Adversarial Networks (arXiv:1806.07108) (2018)

102. H. Wang, Q. Su, Z. Yan, F. Lu, Q. Zhao, Z. Liu, F. Zhou, Rehabilitation treatment of motor dysfunction patients based on deep learning brain–computer interface Technology. Front. Neurosci. (2020) https://doi.org/10.3389/fnins.2020.595084

103. P. Bashivan, I. Rish, S. Heisig, Mental state recognition via wearable EEG. (arXiv:1602.00985) (2016)

104. F. Lotte, M. Congedo, A. Lécuyer, F. Lamarche, B. Arnaldi, A review of classification algorithms for EEG-based brain–computer interfaces. Journal of Neural Engineering, IOP Publishing, 2007, 4, (2007). pp.24. HAL Id: inria-0013495. https://hal.inria.fr/inria-00134950

105. J. Pardede, M. Turnip, D.R. Manalu, A. Turnip, Adaptive recurrent neural network for reduction of noise and estimation of source from recorded EEG signals ARPN. J. Eng. Appl. Sci. **10**, 993–997 (2015)

106. P.K. Johal; N. Jain, Artifact removal from EEG: A comparison of techniques. In Proceedings of the International Conference on Electrical, Electronics, and Optimization Techniques (ICEEOT), Chennai, India, 3–5 March 2016 (2016).

107. P. Jahankhani, V. Kodogiannis, K. Revett, EEG signal classification using wavelet feature extraction and neural networks, in *IEEE John Vincent Atanasoff 2006 International Symposium on Modern Computing (JVA'06)*, (IEEE, 2006, October), pp. 120–124

108. Y.R. Tabar, U. Halici, A novel deep learning approach for classification of EEG motor imagery signals. J. Neural Eng. **14**, 016003 (2017)

109. X. Liu, L. Lv, Y. Shen, P. Xiong, J. Yang, J. Liu, Multiscale space-time-frequency feature-guided multitask learning CNN for motor imagery EEG classification. J. Neural Eng. **18**(2), 026003 (2021)

110. W. Abbas, N.A. Khan, DeepMI : Deep learning for multiclass motor imagery classification 40th Annu. Int. Conf. IEEE Eng. Med. Biol. Soc. (EMBC) (2018)

111. H. Xu, K.N. Plataniotis, Affective States Classification Using EEG and Semi-Supervised Deep Learning Approaches 2016 IEEE 18th Int. Workshop Multimedia Signal Processing (2016)

112. J. Huang, X. Xu, T. Zhang, L. Chen, Emotion Classification Using Deep Neural Networks and Emotional Patches 2017 IEEE International Conference on Bioinformatics Biomedicine (2017)

113. Mustaqeem, S. Kwon. A CNN-assisted enhanced audio signal processing for speech emotion recognition. *Sensors. Switzerland)*, **20**. (2020). https://doi.org/10.3390/S20010183

114. V. Baltatzis, K.-M. Bintsi, G.K. Apostolidis, L.J. Hadjileontiadis, Bullying incidences identification within an immersive environment using HD EEG-based analysis: A swarm decomposition and deep learning approach. Sci. Rep. **7**, 17292 (2017)

115. A. Pereira, D. Padden, J. Jay, K. Lin, Cross-Subject EEG Event-Related Potential Classification for Brain–Computer Interfaces Using Residual Networks Preprint (HAL-id:hal-01878227) (2018).

116. X. Wei, L. Zhou, Z. Chen, L. Zhang, Y. Zhou, Automatic seizure detection using three-dimensional CNN based on multi-channel EEG 18: 133 (2018)

117. J. Shamwell, H. Lee, H. Kwon, A.R. Marathe, V. Lawhern, W. Nothwang, Single-trial EEG RSVP classification using convolutional neural networks proc. SPIE **9836**, 983622 (2016)

118. R. Hefron, B. Borghetti, C. Schubert Kabban, J. Christensen, J. Estepp, Cross-participant EEG-based assessment of cognitive workload using multi-path convolutional recurrent neural networks Sensors 18: 133 (2018)

119. X. Ma, S. Qiu, C. Du, J. Xing, H. He, Improving EEG-based motor imagery classification via spatial and temporal recurrent neural networks 2018 40th Annu. Int. Conf. IEEE Eng. Med. Biol. Soc. (EMBC) (2018)

120. S. Hochreiter, J. Schmidhuber, Long short-term memory. Neural Comput. **9**, 1735–1780 (1997)

121. L. Vareka, *Application of Stacked Autoencoders to P300 Experimental Data (Int. Conf. On Artificial Intelligence and Soft Computing)* (Springer, Cham, 2017)

122. P. Bashivan, I. Rish, M. Yeasin, N. Codella, Learning Representations from eeg with Deep Recurrent- Convolutional Neural Networks (arXiv:1511.06448) (2015)

123. H. Dong, A. Supratak, W. Pan, C. Wu, P.M. Matthews, Y. Guo, Mixed Neural Network Approach for Temporal Sleep Stage Classification, IEEE Trans. Neural Syst. Rehabil. Eng (2018)

124. N. Kulkarni, EEG Signal Analysis for Mild Alzheimer's Disease Diagnosis by Means of Spectral-and Complexity-Based Features and Machine Learning Techniques, in *Proceedings*

of the 2nd International Conference on Data Engineering and Communication Technology, (Springer, Berlin/Heidelberg, 2019), pp. 395–403

125. I.A. Corley, Y. Huang, Deep EEG super-resolution: Upsampling EEG spatial resolution with generative adversarial networks IEEE EMBS Int. Conf. on Biomedical & Health Informatics (2018) pp. 4–7

126. K.P. Thomas, A.P. Vinod, EEG-based biometric authentication using gamma band power during rest state. Circ. Syst. Signal Proc. **37**(1), 277–289 (2018)

127. L. Vă, Stacked Autoencoders for the P300 Component Detection. Frontiers Neuroscience **11**, 302 (2017)

128. Z. Wang, Z. Zhang, X. Gong, Y. Sun, H. Wang, Short time Fourier transformation and deep neural networks for motor imagery brain computer interface recognition Concurrency and Computation: Practice and Experience. 30: e4413 (2018)

129. I. Ullah, M. Hussain, E. Qazi, H. Aboalsamh, An automated system for epilepsy detection using EEG brain signals based on deep learning approach expert. Syst. Appl **107**, 61–71 (2018)

130. U.R. Acharya, S. Lih, Y. Hagiwara, J. Hong, H. Adeli, D.P. Subha, Automated EEG-based screening of depression using deep convolutional neural network Comput. Methods Progr. Biomed. **161**, 103–113 (2018)

131. J. Zhang, S. Li, R. Wang, Pattern recognition of momentary mental workload based on multi-channel electrophysiological data and ensemble convolutional neural networks. Frontiers Neurosci **11**, 1–16 (2017)

132. S.R. Tibor, S.J. Tobias, F.L.D. Josef, G. Martin, E. Katharina, T. Michael, H. Frank, B. Wolfram, B. Tonio, Deep learning with convolutional neural networks for EEG decoding and visualization hum. Brain Mapping **38**, 5391–5420 (2017)

133. A. Bablani, D.R. Edla, V. Kuppili, Deceit identification test on EEG data using deep belief network 2018 9th Int. Conf. Computing Communication Networking Technologies, 1–6 (2018)

134. O. Tsinalis, P.M. Matthews, Y. Guo, Automatic sleep stage scoring using time-frequency analysis and stacked sparse autoencoders annuals. Biomed. Eng. **44**, 1587–1597 (2016)

135. X. Li, D. Song, P. Zhang, G. Yu, Y. Hou, B. Hu, Emotion recognition from multi-channel EEG data through convolutional recurrent neural network (2016). IEEE international conference of bioinformatics biomedicine. (2016), pp. 352–9

136. A. Supratak, H. Dong, C. Wu, Y. Guo, DeepSleepNet: A model for automatic sleep stage scoring based on raw single-channel EEG IEEE trans. Neural Syst. Rehabil. Eng. **25**, 1998–2008 (2017)

137. S. Kuanar, V. Athitsos, N. Pradhan, A. Mishra and K.R. Rao, Cognitive analysis of working memory load from EEG, by a deep recurrent neural network (2018). IEEE International Conference on Acoustics, Speech and Signal Processing (ICASSP), pp 352–5

138. A. Delorme, T. Sejnowski, S. Makeig, Enhanced detection of artifacts in EEG data using higher-order statistics and independent component analysis. NeuroImage **34**, 1443–1449 (2007)

139. Roy, S., Kiral-kornek, I. and Harrer, S., Deep learning enabled automatic abnormal EEG identification 40th Annu. Int. Conf. IEEE Eng. Med. Biol. Soc. (EMBC), (2018). pp. 2756–2759

140. A.H. Phan, A. Cichocki, Tensor decompositions for feature extraction and classification of high dimensional datasets. Nonlinear Theory Appl **1**, 37–68 (2010)

141. S-E. Moon., S. Jang, J-S. Lee. Convolutional Neural Network Approach for Eeg-Based Emotion Recognition Using Brain Connectivity and its Spatial Information (2018). IEEE Int. Conf. on Acoustics, Speech and Signal Processing (ICASSP) 2018

142. S.B. Salem, Z. Lachiri, CNN-SVM approach for EEG-based person identification using emotional dataset, in *In 2019 International Conference on Signal, Control and Communication (SCC)*, (IEEE, 2019, December), pp. 241–245

143. F. Lotte, L. Bougrain, A. Cichocki, M. Clerc, M. Congedo, A. Rakotomamonjy, F. Yger, A review of classification algorithms for EEG-based brain–computer interfaces: A 10 year update. J. Neural Eng. **15**(3), 031005 (2018)

144. M. Saeidi, W. Karwowski, F.V. Farahani, K. Fiok, R. Taiar, P.A. Hancock, A. Al-Juaid, Neural decoding of EEG signals with machine learning: A systematic review. Brain Sci. **11**(11), 1525 (2021)

145. V. Salari, S. Rodrigues, E. Saglamyurek, C. Simon, D. Oblak, Are brain–computer interfaces feasible with integrated photonic chips? Front. Neurosci. **15**(January), 1–16 (2022). https:// doi.org/10.3389/fnins.2021.780344
146. A. Lau-Zhu, M.P.H. Lau, G. McLoughlin, Mobile EEG in research on neurodevelopmental disorders: Opportunities and challenges. Dev. Cogn. Neurosci. **36**, 100635 (2019). https:// doi.org/10.1016/J.DCN.2019.100635
147. R. Maskeliunas, R. Damasevicius, I. Martisius, M. Vasiljevas, Consumer-grade EEG devices: Are they usable for control tasks? Peer J **2016**(3), 1–27 (2016). https://doi.org/10.7717/ peerj.1746
148. Y. Muhammad, D. Vaino, Controlling electronic devices with brain rhythms/electrical activity using artificial neural network (ANN). Bioengineering **6**(2), 46 (2019)
149. F.R. Willett, D.T. Avansino, L.R. Hochberg, J.M. Henderson, K.V. Shenoy, High-performance brain-to-text communication via handwriting. Nature **593**(7858), 249–254 (2021)
150. D.A. Moses, S.L. Metzger, J.R. Liu, G.K. Anumanchipalli, J.G. Makin, P.F. Sun, J. Chartier, M.E. Dougherty, P.M. Liu, G.M. Abrams, A. Tu-Chan, K. Ganguly, E.F. Chang, Neuroprosthesis for decoding speech in a paralyzed person with anarthria. N. Engl. J. Med. **385**(3), 217–227 (2021). https://doi.org/10.1056/nejmoa202754
151. S.N.A. Seha, D. Hatzinakos, EEG-based human recognition using steady-state AEPs and subject-unique spatial filters. IEEE Trans. Inf. Foren. Security **15**, 3901–3910 (2020)
152. K. Brigham, B.V. Kumar, Subject identification from electroencephalogram (EEG) signals during imagined speech. In *2010 Fourth IEEE International Conference on Biometrics: Theory, Applications and Systems (BTAS)* (2010, September) (pp. 1–8). IEEE
153. F. Lotte, L. Bougrain, M. Clerc, Electroencephalography (EEG)-Based Brain-Computer Interfaces (2015)
154. A. Singandhupe, H.M. La, D. Feil-Seifer, P. Huang, L. Guo, M. Li, Securing a uav using individual characteristics from an eeg signal, in *In 2017 IEEE International Conference on Systems, Man, and Cybernetics (SMC)*, (IEEE, 2017, October), pp. 2748–2753
155. T. Hoya, G. Hori, H. Bakardjian, T. Ni shimura, T. Suzuki, Y. Miyawaki, J. Cao, Classification of single trial EEG signals by a combined principal+ independent component analysis and probabilistic neural network approach. In *Proc. ICA2003* (Vol. 197) (2003, January)
156. T. Verhoeven, D. Hübner, M. Tangermann, K.R. Müller, J. Dambre, P.J. Kindermans, True zero-training brain–computer interfacing an online study. J. Neural Eng. **14**, 036021 (2017)
157. A. Kostov, M. Polak, Parallel man-machine training in development of EEG-based cursor control. IEEE Trans. Rehabil. Eng. **8**(2), 203–205 (2000)
158. T. Felzer, B. Freisieben, Analyzing EEG signals using the probability estimating guarded neural classifier. IEEE Trans. Neural Syst. Rehabil. Eng. **11**(4), 361–371 (2003)
159. A. Esuli, A. Moreo Fernandez, F. Sebastiani, A recurrent neural network for sentiment quantification. Int. Conf. Info. Knowl. Manag. Proc. **3**, 1775–1778 (2018). https://doi. org/10.1145/3269206.3269287
160. L.E. Wilson, J. da Silva Castanheira, S. Baillet, Time-resolved parameterization of aperiodic and periodic brain activity. *bioRxiv*, 2022.2001.2021.477243. (2022). https://doi. org/10.1101/2022.01.21.477243
161. M.G.M. Saif, M.A. Hasan, A. Vuckovic, M. Fraser, S.A. Qazi, Correction to: Efficacy evaluation of neurofeedback applied for treatment of central neuropathic pain using machine learning. SN Appl. Sci. **3**(8), 1 (2021). https://doi.org/10.1007/s42452-021-04714-1
162. U.R. Acharya, F. Molinari, S.V. Sree, S. Chattopadhyay, K.H. Ng, J.S. Suri, Automated diagnosis of epileptic EEG using entropies. Biomed. Signal Proc. Control **7**(4), 401–408 (2012). https://doi.org/10.1016/j.bspc.2011.07.007
163. J.S. Richman, J.R. Moorman, Physiological time-series analysis using approximate entropy and sample entropy maturity in premature infants physiological time-series analysis using approximate entropy and sample entropy. Am. J. Phys. Heart Circ. Phys. **278**, H2039–H2049 (2000)

Chapter 13
Estimations of Emotional Synchronization Indices for Brain Regions Using Electroencephalogram Signal Analysis

Noor Kamal Al-Qazzaz, Reda Jasim Lafta, and Maimonah Akram Khudhair

Abstract Recognizing emotions based on brain activity has become crucial for understanding diverse human behavior in daily life. The electroencephalogram (EEG) has been proven to help gather information regarding the distribution of waveforms across the scalp. This project serves two goals. Firstly is to examine the synchronization and connectivity indices for emotion recognition. Secondly is to develop a framework to study the relationship between emotional state and brain activity based on synchronization and functional connectivity. The EEGs of 23 healthy volunteers were recorded while they viewed 18 film clips. To investigate the synchronization between various brain regions, a hybrid technique combining empirical mode decomposition with wavelet transform ($EMD - WT$) was employed. Linear features like cross-correlation ($xCorr$), coherence (Coh), and phase lag index (PLI) as well as nonlinear features like cross fuzzy entropy ($CFuzzEn$) and joint permutation entropy (JPE) were computed to capture various dynamical properties from emotion-based multi-channel EEG signals. Then, in order to increase the classification *accuracy* of various emotional states, choose features based on statistical analysis. At the end, the classifying process was utilized using the k-nearest neighbours (kNN) classifier. The classification results demonstrated the impact of the combination of $CFuzzEn$ and JPE features as a remarkable synchronization index for analyzing emotions derived from an EEG-based data set. As a result, EEG indices enable a more thorough knowledge of the varied impacts of brain therapies on behavioral outcomes in humans.

N. K. Al-Qazzaz (✉) · R. J. Lafta · M. A. Khudhair
Department of Biomedical Engineering, Al-Khwarizmi College of Engineering, University of Baghdad, Baghdad, Iraq
e-mail: noorbme@kecbu.uobaghdad.edu.iq

13.1 Introduction

It is acknowledged that emotions are the manifestation of mental and psychophysiological states. Human-computer interaction (HCI) systems reveal hidden information from the brain and control peripheral devices [1]. It is difficult to create trustworthy emotion recognition algorithms that are accurate enough and flexible enough for use in practical applications [2].

Emotional state is believed to be a complex phenomenon comprised of biological, social, and cognitive components due to its modulating effects on physiological and behavioral processes. In brain-computer interface (BCI) applications and cognitive neuroscience research, two distinct models for characterizing the emotional state have been studied: In emotion recognition application mapping, the Circumplex model is a cognitive-emotional state model. The two measurements used to depict emotions on a two-dimensional coordinate plane are valance and arousal. Valence indicates the positive and negative intensity of an emotion, whilst arousal measures the intensity of an emotion, ranging from ecstatic to tranquil [3]. The Circumplex Model of emotion serves as an example of how this model graphs all emotions to a valance-arousal graph [4]. Researchers [5, 6] have added a third dimension that accounts the attention-rejection characteristic.

Visual and auditory inputs influence the amplitude of the sensorimotor rhythm [7]. It is believed that these inputs are the two most prevalent approaches for humans to trigger different emotional states [8] in order to reveal distinctive characteristics that would be useful for accurately determining an individual's emotion in daily life. Recent research suggests that the optimal setting for automatic emotion recognition requires both stimulants of visual and acoustic inputs [9] to evoke a particular emotional condition. Typically, audible and visual elicitation employing short video clips is used to evoke different emotional states more effectively than other techniques [2, 7, 10]. Therefore, in this work, short audio-visual video segments were used to elicited emotion.

Numerous study investigations on the identification of human emotions have been carried out over the last few decades utilizing a range of approaches, including facial expressions [11]., peripheral physiological signs for identifying individuals based on emotional shifts are obtained using many biological measurements, such as Electrocardiogram (ECG) [12] and Electroencephalogram (EEG) [13–17].

Throughout this study, the EEG dataset was preprocessed with conventional filters and the hybrid empirical mode decomposition with wavelet transform ($EMD - WT$) technique. Linear features such as cross-correlation ($xCorr$), coherence (Coh), and phase lage index (PLI) as well as nonlinear features such as cross fuzzy entropy ($CFuzzEn$) and joint permutation entropy (JPE) were computed to capture various dynamical properties from emotion-based multi-channel EEG signals. A two independent variables analysis of variance (ANOVA) of these features is evaluated to determine the significant features that enhance the *accuracy* of classification of nine short emotional video clips (excitement, sadness, happiness, calmness, disgust, fear, anger, amusement and surprise). *k*-Nearest Neighbours (*k*NN) classifier was used for classification in its final step.

This work has focused on the role of emotion synchronization in the brain-emotion relationship. The paper novelty is therefore twofold. This is to be the first study to use the hybrid *EMD − WT* technique with the aforementioned features to evaluate emotions using EEG-based functional connectivity patterns to assess changes in brain network activity. Second, it is the first study to combine linear and nonlinear features to capture the changes in connectivity between brain lobes as measured by EEGs based on emotional states. Therefore, EEG indices allow for a more comprehensive understanding of the various effects of brain interventions on human behavior.

13.2 Related Works

In the past decade, EEG has been considered as a non-surgical clinical tool capable of monitoring neuronal activity in the brain with millisecond precision and a high level of temporal resolution [18]. Using EEG, numerous channels are recorded and analyzed for neurophysiology applications [18, 19] responsible for detecting and differentiating various brain diseases, such as epilepsy and sleep disorders. EEG signals have been used to classify mental tasks and sleep stages as well as to diagnose a number of brain disorders, such as *epilepsy*, *ADHD*, Alzheimer's disease (*AD*), and vascular dementia (*VaD*) [20, 21]. A viable indication for assessing various affective reactions may be an EEG dataset with many channels spanning different brain areas [22]. Similarly, in [23] in order to identify current affective moods based on neural feedback and personalized modification of treatment, an integrated music therapy was developed using instantaneous techniques of affect recognition based on EEG.

The most challenging part of brain activity recognition is the low *accuracy* of recognition because of the significant noise compared to the EEG signal. EEG signals are subject to various types of artifacts, including physiological artifacts such as pulse, blinking eyes, and muscular activity [24–27] and sweat and other non-physiological phenomena like power line interference noise [27, 28]. Artifacts have a direct effect on EEG signals due to their frequency overlap with EEG signals. Therefore, a variety of denoising methods must be used to get over these problems and retrieve valuable data from the EEG dataset. Consequently, the most popular denoising techniques are wavelet transform (*WT*) [29, 30], independent component analysis (*ICA*) [31], empirical mode decomposition (*EMD*) [32], *Savitzky − Golay* (*SG*) [33] which can eliminate EEG artifacts. Numerous studies [34–37] have used hybrid techniques based on the combined use of *ICA* and *WT* to denoise EEG signals.

EMD and *WT* approaches were often used in ECG and EEG studies, either separately or in combination, depending on the data and the analysis's objectives [38, 39].

EMD is frequently used with biological data that are nonlinear and non-stationarity sequence, like heart rate variability (*HRV*), electromyography (*EMG*), and *EEG*. This is because of its characteristics and qualities. In a similar way, wavelet transforms have found extensive usage in BCI systems because to their ability to retain details in the time and frequency domain with a broad range of scale and translation functions. Both approaches were successfully used as a foundation for filtering or further feature extraction to successfully obtain higher *accuracy* in classification.

To distinguish between focal and unfocal EEG data taken from epileptic patients, Das and Bhuiyan [40] employed *EMD* followed by wavelet. In the combination *EMD − DWT*, they used entropy-based characteristics to achieve excellent classification *accuracy*. For the elimination of EEG artifacts in [41], wavelet packet transform was used before wavelet packet transform after *EMD*. Generally speaking, *EMD* performed better than WT while denoising EEG data and getting ready for feature extraction [42].

Earlier emotional states of EEG-based studies used linear features such as correlation (Corr), coherence (*Coh*), and phase lag indices (*PLI*) between pairs of EEG sensors to estimate functional brain connectivity [43]. Coherence is a metric that has worked in a number of research fields, including physiology [44] and neurological disease [45]. Phase synchronization among the contributing neurological groups is one more technique for determining the functional connectivity of the EEG between different locations of the brain. This method is based on how two signals change in phase with one another. Neurological illnesses are studied using measures of EEG synchronization in phases [46].

Even so, using linear features, the complexity of the brain structure necessitates needs highly informative methods to inform about brain connectivity; thus, EEG signals are very effective bio-indicator of brain linear and nonlinear activity [29, 47–50].

The Hurst exponent (*Hur*) [51] and fractal dimension (*FD*) [52] are a well-known nonlinear algorithm used to examine the complex dynamic data produced by the cerebral cortex and reflect complex emotive tasks [53, 54].

The integration of entropy to EEG signals have improved the study of mental and sleep states, with techniques for identifying emotion levels. In [55], for instance, the emotions elicited by short clips were analyzed using *sample entropy* (*SampEn*), *approximate entropy* (*ApEn*), and *permutation entropy* (*PerEn*), as these techniques are unaffected by noise and capable of accurately measuring time sequence complexity. In a dissimilar study, clinical assessments of *EEG* signals based on symbolic transfer entropy and *PerEn* entropy were conducted, demonstrating that the EEG entropy investigation to relate to clinical cases of countless cognitive conditions [56]. *Fuzzy entropy* (*FuzzEn*), which substitutes fuzzy membership functions for Heaviside functions [57, 58], is also suggested for EEG examination. Existing research indicates that *FuzzEn* mitigates the issue of entropy mutation; however, when using such entropy approaches, pertinent information is lost since they need single-scale analysis. Compared to *SampEn*, *FuzzEn* exhibits more consistency and less dependency on data length [59]., despite the fact that *SampEn* is somewhat faster. The present research focuses on EEG-synchronization derived markers to categorize the gender variances in EEG signals based on emotion across the brain.

Artificial neural networks (ANNs), support-vector networks (SVNs), the $k - nearest neighbours$ (kNN) classifier, and *hidden Markov models* (HMM) have all been closely examined as machine learning algorithms for a gender classification system [60, 61]. In [62], a gender and age classification system based on EEG signals was created using the SVM classifier, whereas in [55], resting-state EEG data served as the foundation for a model for automatic gender detection. An automated system for estimating age and gender was developed by combining EEG sensors with wavelet transform frequency break-down as feature extraction and random forest classifier [63, 64].

Emotional reactivity is the main focus of investigations on EEG-based emotion identification [65–67]. emphasized the use of spectral relative powers in linear analysis. Nevertheless, many researchers have exploited nonlinear properties to study the complexity of the brain [17, 68, 69]. In the present research, we intend to estimate the synchronization based on the EEG role for recognition using both the linear and nonlinear features to classify the emotional-based signals by analyzing the behavior of coactivated and communicating brain regions during audiovisual video clips. Additionally, the particularity of emotion Functional connectivity-based EEG research have demonstrated the ability to distinguish between diverse emotional states; however, none of these investigations have directly evaluated these multiple synchronization indices within a single study. This study subject is important because various connection measures are sensitive to various EEG signal properties.

Therefore, the goal of the current work was to revisit the problem of EEG-based emotional specificity using the linear and nonlinear synchronization indices and discover which of the indices is more effective at identifying various affective states using pattern classification analyses. Correlation, cross coherence, and synchronization indices are examples of connectivity indicators that might potentially reveal important information, given that emotion processing is a complicated activity that is not limited to a small number of brain areas. Nine distinct emotional states were elicited through the use of emotive video clips.

13.3   Materials and Methods

The proposed study is depicted in Fig. 13.1 as a block diagram.

13.3.1   Subjects and Experimental Procedure

Electroencephalogram (EEG) and electrocardiogram (ECG) signals recorded in response to audio-visual stimuli comprise the multi-modal 'DREAMER' dataset [70]. The emotions of 23 participants were elicited and recorded alongside the

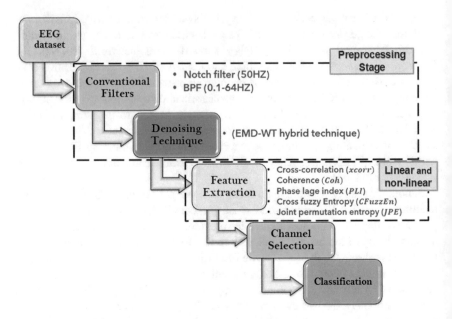

Fig. 13.1 Schematic representation of the proposed system

participants' self-assessments of their affective state in terms of valence, arousal, and dominance following each stimulus. There were 11 females and 14 males, with a mean age of 26.6 ± 2.7 years and a standard deviation of 2.7 years. 16 contact-sensors with plated gold connected to the flexible arms of a wireless headset and positioned in the Universal 10 – 20 system's locations: $AF3$, $F7$, $F3$, $FC5$, $T7$, $P7$, $O1$, $O2$, $P8$, $T8$, $FC6$, $F4$, $F8$, $AF4$, $M1$ and $M2$. Mastoid sensor $M1$ served as a ground reference point for comparing the voltage of all other sensors.

The EEG dataset consisted of 18 movie scenes chosen and analyzed by Gabert-Quillen et al. [71]. These movie clips include scenes from several movies that have been demonstrated to induce a variety of emotions. The duration of the movie clips ranged from 65 *to* 393 seconds (M = 199 seconds), which is deemed adequate because, according to psychologists, video stimuli between 1 – 10 minutes can trigger single emotions. However, an individual's emotional state may change over time, especially when longer video stimuli are employed. To prevent multiple emotions from contaminating data recordings, only the final thirty seconds of each movie clip were further analyzed. To prevent external influences, the experiments were conducted in an isolated setting with regulated lighting. The room was completely darkened by an electric curtain, and the video clips played back on a 45 – *inch* TV panel.

13.3.2   Preprocessing Stage

The majority of artifacts that emerge in EEG wave frequency bands, where there is a potential for overlap with brain processes, necessitate the removal of noise while processing EEG signals.

13.3.2.1   Conventional Filtering

In the cerebral cortex's scalp region, **14** channels of EEG data were recorded. Every channel of the recorded EEG dataset was initially treated using standard filtering methods. A band pass filter with a *frequency range* of (**0.5 – 64**) *Hz* was used to isolate the band of the recorded *EEG* signals, and a *notch* filter at **50** *Hz* was suggested to remove *power line interference* noise [72].

13.3.2.2   Empirical Mode Decomposition with Wavelet (*EMD – WT*) Hybrid Denoising Technique

In this study, *EMD* and DWT were used in a two-stage filtering process. It is proposed and discussed that *EMD – WT* is an automatic hybrid method for combining the benefits of *EMD* with WT and to mitigate their weaknesses. Consequently, the *EMD – WT* technique has been implemented as in the following sessions. In the initial stage, *EMD* decomposed the EEG dataset into Intrinsic Modal Functions (*IMF*) levels with a residue. Each *IMF* consists of limited-frequency bands that permit a more accurate representation of the EEG dataset and have the following properties [73]:

(i) Baseline crossings and Extermas are identical or differ by no more than one.
(ii) The envelopes average formed by extremes is equal zero. *EMD* can represent a raw EEG signal **y[n]** in terms of *IMF*s as [73]

$$y[n] = \sum_{m=1}^{M} I_m[n] + r_M[n]$$

(13.1)

where M, $I_m[n]$, and $r_M[n]$ indicate number of *IMF*s, m^{th} *IMF*, and residue, respectively. *IMF*s are parts of the original EEG signal, which may be either contain noise or information. Compared to informative components, it has been observed in [74] that noisy *IMF*s are poorly correlated with the original signal. The optimal threshold point of correlation C^{th} for removal of noisy components can be calculated as follows: [74],

$$C_{Th} = \frac{\max(C_i)}{10 \times \max(C_i) - 3}, i = 1, 2, \dots, M$$

(13.2)

C_i: the *IMF* correlation coefficient (CC) of the *i*th *IMF* with the original signal.
Max(C_i): maximum *CC* among *M IMF*s
The removal of noisy components algorithm is given as [73]:

1. Initialize denoised EEG signal, $S[n]_D = 0$
2. for $i = 1 : M$ do
3. if $C_i < C_{Th}$ then
4. *IMF_i* is a Noisy- *IMF*
5. else
6. $S[n]_D = S[n]_D + IMF_i$
7. end if
8. end for
9. Get → $S[n]_D$

Due to the *WT*'s ability to resolve EEG into distinct time and frequency components, discrete (*DWT*) was applied to each *IMF* in the second stage to gain a better understanding of the *WT*'s advantages for high frequencies, there is an excellent time resolution but a low frequency resolution and at low frequencies there's a good *frequency resolution* and a poor *time resolution*. *DWT* transform can be obtained as a set of decomposition functions of the *correlation* between the signal $f(t)$ and the shifting and dilation of a particular function known as the mother wavelet function $\psi(t)$. According to Eq. 13.1, the *mother wavelet* ($\psi \_ (a, b) (t)$) is shifted along the original signal by the position *parameter* (*b*) and stretched or compressed by the frequency scaling *parameter* (*a*) [29, 75–80]:

$$DWT_{m,n}(f) = a_0^{-m/2} \int f(t)\psi\left(a_0^{-m}t - nb_0\right)dt \tag{13.3}$$

a_0 and b_0 *values* are set to 2 and 1, respectively.

$$\psi_{a,b}(t) = \frac{1}{\sqrt{a}}\psi\left(\frac{t-b}{a}\right), a \in \mathbb{R}^+, b \in \mathbb{R} \tag{13.4}$$

This study indicated that '*sym9*' from the *Symlets* family of *order* 9 with four levels of decomposition is suitable for automatically removing artifacts and reducing computational time and complexity. *SURE* threshold is an adaptive *soft thresholding* technique that seeks to identify the threshold limit for every level based on *Stein's unbiased risk* estimation [81] and commonly employed values in [82–85]. To obtain EEG signals devoid of artifacts, the inverse *DWT* (*IDWT*) is applied at the conclusion.

13.3.3   Features Extraction Stage

In order to determine which approach is best for predicting emotions from multi-channel EEG signals evaluation, features from the temporal domain have been used with linear and nonlinear interdependence analysis to examine functional connectivity in various brain areas.

13.3.3.1   Linear Features

A. Cross-correlation (*xCorr*)
    Taking into account two separate time series x_n and y_n, $n = 1, ..., N$. The most often used linear synchronization method is the cross-correlation function c_{xy}, which is defined as [86]:

$$C_{xy}(\tau) = \frac{1}{N-\tau} \sum_{i=1}^{N-\tau} \left(\frac{x_i - \bar{x}}{\sigma_x} \right) \left(\frac{y_{i+\tau} - \bar{y}}{\sigma_y} \right)$$

(13.5)

where $\bar{x}$ and σ_x denote **mean** and **variance**, and τ is the time lag.

B. Coherence (*Coh*)
    The *cross − spectral density* function $C_{xy}(\omega)$, which is derived as the *Fourier* transform of the *cross correlation*, is called magnitude squared *coherence* or simply *coherence*. The normalization of the cross spectrum is therefore defined as the *coherence* function (γ_{xy}) [86]:

$$\gamma_{xy}(\omega) = \frac{|C_{xy}(\omega)|}{\sqrt{C_{xx}(\omega)C_{yy}(\omega)}}$$

(13.6)

Cross − correlation is a *time − lag − dependent* measure, whereas *coherence* is a *frequency − dependent* linear measure. For each pair of electrodes, we found peaks in coherence and *cross − correlation* and used these peak values to calculate the two-connectivity metrics.

C. Phase lag index (*PLI*)
    Even though the amplitudes of two linked nonlinear systems are not correlated, empirical tests have demonstrated that their phase can synchronize. The analytical signal for a real-valued signal $x(t)$ is defined as [86]:

$$Z_x(t) = x(t) + ix_H(t) = A_x^H(t)e^{i\varnothing_x^H(t)}$$

(13.7)

Where $x_H(t)$ is the **Hilbert transform** of **x(t)**. Then **similarly** for another signal **y(t)**, we define A_y^H and $\varnothing_y^H$. If we let the **synchronization** between **x(t)** and **y(t)** is

$n : m$, we define the (n, m) **phase difference** of their analytic signal as $\varnothing_{xy}^{H}(t) = n\varnothing_{x}^{H}(t) - m\varnothing_{y}^{H}(t)$, where n and m are integers. Then the **PLI** is defined as,

$$PLI = \left| e^{i\varnothing_{x}^{H}(t)} \right|_{t} = \sqrt{\cos\varnothing_{x}^{H}(t)_{t}^{2} + \sin\varnothing_{x}^{H}(t)_{t}^{2}} \tag{13.8}$$

When the phases are not synchronized, the **PLI** is zero, and when they are perfectly synchronized, it is one.

13.3.3.2 Nonlinear Features

A. Cross fuzzy entropy (*CFuzzyEn*)

The synchronization or similarity of patterns between two signals is measured using *cross − fuzzy entropy* (*CFuzzyEn*). *CFuzzyEn* is a cross- *SampEn* enhancement that is better suited to short time series and more noise resistant. *CFuzzyEn* is computed as for two times series of length N [87]:

$$CFuzzyEn(m,n,r,N) = \ln\varnothing^{m}(n,r) - \ln\varnothing^{m+1}(n,r) \tag{13.9}$$

where $\varnothing^{m}(n,r) = \dfrac{1}{N-m}\sum_{i=1}^{N-m}\left(\dfrac{1}{N-m}\sum_{j=1}^{N-m}D_{ij}^{m} \right)$ for vector X_{i}^{m}, and

$\varnothing^{m+1}(n,r) = \dfrac{1}{N-m}\sum_{i=1}^{N-m}\left(\dfrac{1}{N-m}\sum_{j=1}^{N-m}D_{ij}^{m+1} \right)$ for vector X_{i}^{m+1}, D_{ij}^{m} measures the

synchrony or similarity degree. Each **CFuzzyEn** computation requires the determination of three parameters. The first parameter, m, is the length of the sequences to be compared, or the dimension of the vector to be compared. The remaining two parameters, r and n, control the width and gradient of the exponential function's boundary, respectively. Setting the tolerance r between **0.1 *and* 0.3** and choosing small integers for the selection of n works well in practice.

B. Joint permutation entropy (*JPE*)

Yin et al. introduced the joint permutation entropy (*JPE*), which is used to measure the synchronism between two time series [88]. It is based on permutation entropy, which compares neighboring values of each point and converts them into ordinal patterns to quantify the complexity of a signal. *JPE* is calculated as the Shannon entropy of the $d! \times d!$ unique motif combinations ($\pi_{i}^{d,t}$, $\pi_{j}^{d,t}$) for two signals u and v [88]:

$$JPE(d,t) = -\sum_{i,j:\left(\pi_{i}^{d,t},\pi_{j}^{d,t}\right)} p\left(\pi_{i}^{d,t},\pi_{j}^{d,t}\right).\ln\left(\pi_{i}^{d,t},\pi_{j}^{d,t}\right) \tag{13.10}$$

where $p\left(\pi_i^{d,t},.\right)$ means the probability that the first time series has the ith pattern regardless of the second, and $p\left(.,\pi_j^{d,t}\right)$ denotes the chance that the second time series has the ith motif regardless of the first.

13.3.4 Features Selection Using Statistical Analysis

The emotional task channels were chosen using the ANOVA test as inputs for the classifiers. The significant p value of the EEG feature was a key factor in the selection of features for events. p values of less than 0.05 show a 95% significant difference between classes. Selected channels were determined by the Statistical Package for Social Sciences (SPSS) version 22's ANOVA test with a significance level of ($p < 0.05$).

As a result, the goal of this study is to examine the linear and nonlinear characteristics' most efficient channels. The *Kolmogorov − Smirnov* test was used to judge the normality of the tests. The relevant channels among the emotions (i.e. amusement, excitement, happiness, calmness, anger, disgust, fear, sadness and surprise) were chosen using two sessions of *two − way* ANOVA.

In the first session of ANOVA, linear features including *xCorr*, *Coh* and *PLI* were applied as *dependent variables* and the group factor (emotions and brain regions) were the *independent variable*. Moreover, in the second session of ANOVA, nonlinear features like *CFuzzEn* and *JPE* features and the group factor (emotions and brain regions) were the *independent variable*. The *significance* was set at $p < 0.05$.

Then, the feature reduction method was implemented to reduce the irrelevant daughter features (pair of channels) the method is as follows:

For each symmetric functional *connectivity matrix*, 14 diagonal elements were removed, and the upper triangle elements of the *connectivity matrix* were extracted as classification features, i.e., the feature space for classification was constituted by the $14 \times (14 − 1)/2 = 91$ dimensional feature vectors (pair of channels or connections).

The abnormal functional *connectivity* patterns associated with emotional states are mainly represented by the highly discriminating functional connections, and 91 dimensional feature vectors including all the differences caused by noise. Highly discriminatory features were selected from the original 128 features space, further reducing the number of features, accelerating computation and diminishing noise.

Therefore, the feature selection method was used to reduce the dimension for classification through retaining the most discriminative functional connections and eliminating the remaining indistinctive features. The discriminative power of a feature can be quantitatively measured by the importance of its degree of relevance to classification.

Based on how dependent each feature was on its corresponding class, features were rated. The features that are most reliant on the class were chosen, and this procedure provides those features a higher rank than other features. Based on each sample, these feature frequencies are calculated.

13.3.5 Emotion Classification Stage

Linear and nonlinear features had (91 connections without reduction) which were calculated for the last 30 second of each video clip recording with an epoch length of Fs×5 = 128×5 = 640 samples. Meaning 6 epochs for each video clip (emotion) and since we have 9 emotions and 23 subject the number of instances is 23×9×6 = 1242 for each pair connection.

In this section, *k nearest neighbors* (*k*NN) was used. One of the most often used non-parametric classification methods is *k*NN; when *k* > 1, in particular to lessen the impacted noisy points in the training set, it is more resilient. The Euclidean distance was used in this work as a similarity metric to categorize each trial using *k*NN.

13.4 Results and Discussions

13.4.1 Results of Preprocessing Stage

Datasets of EEG signals were filtered using traditional filters and then denoised using *EMD* − *WT* hybrid technique. The frontal brain region when anger is produced is shown by the data from *Channel* 7 in Fig. 13.2. Artifactual signal elements (red line) in the raw EEG data were successfully eliminated during signal denoising, leaving a clear EEG signal (blue line).

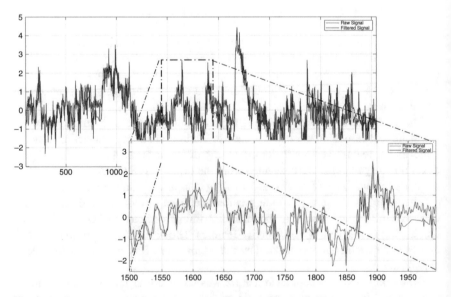

Fig. 13.2 The denoising results after preprocessing stage for *channel* 7 from *subject* 9

13.4.2 Results of Features Extraction Stage

To characterize the emotion synchronization of EEGs, linear features including *xCorr*, *Coh* and *PLI* and nonlinear features like *CFuzzEn* and *JPE* were computed for the EEGs. Features were estimated for each channel with a total length of 3,840 samples divided into 6 epochs; the length of each epoch was 640 data points (1 segment represents 5 *s*) of EEGs.

13.4.2.1 Results of Linear Features

The outcome demonstrates that particular brain areas have higher levels of connection during emotional reactions. These findings were revealed from linear features, which could be used to identify a synchronization diagnostic index that would be able to distinguish emotions from EEG-based signals. *Statistical analysis* of network parameters revealed these features from the two groups were *significantly different*.

A. Results of Cross-correlation (*xCorr*)

The calculated comparative plot of *xCorr* is shown in Fig. 13.3 to discriminate among nine different emotional states based on EEG signals. The matrix presents the topographical map of the nine emotions using linear bivariate features in all channel.

Figure 13.4 shows the *xCorr* ranking and the connection importance score of the feature of all channels in the EEG signals. Features that are strongly influenced by the emotional category and are ranked higher than other features.

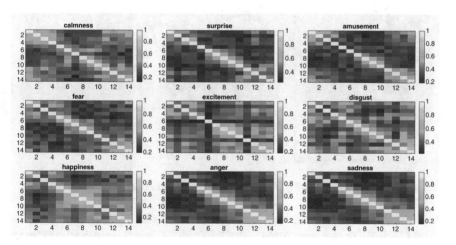

Fig. 13.3. Comparative plot of the functional connectivity matrices for the nine tested emotional states using linear *xCorr*

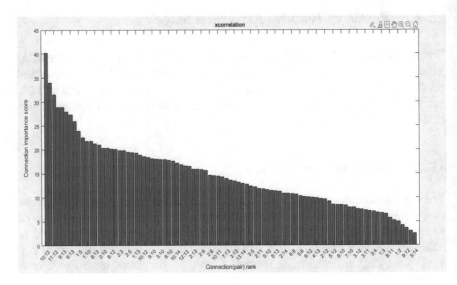

Fig. 13.4 Comparative plot of the *xCorr* rank of channels

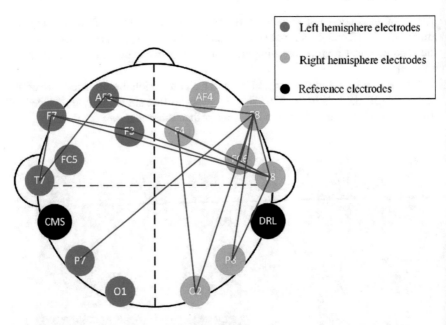

Fig. 13.5 Electrodes Connectivity plot of the *xCorr* first 15 ranked pairs

Plotting the first 15 ranked pairs of *xCorr* electrodes in Fig. 13.5 reveals that the most efficient pairs are conjugated with the F7 and F8 electrodes in the frontal lobe.

B. Results of Coherence (*Coh*)

Figure 13.6 illustrates the comparative plot of *Coh* which was shown to discriminate among nine different emotional states based on EEG signals. The matrix presents the topographical map of the nine emotions using linear bivariate features in all channel.

Figure 13.7 shows the *Coh* ranking and the connection importance score of the feature of all channels in the EEG signals. Features that are strongly influenced by the emotional category and are ranked higher than other features.

The most efficient pairs are conjugated with the O1 and O2 electrodes in the occipital lobe, as seen in Fig. 13.8, which plots the first 15 ranked pair of electrodes of the *Coh*.

C. Results of phase lag index (*PLI*)

Figure 13.9 illustrates the comparative plot of *PLI* which was illustrated to discriminate among nine different emotional states based on EEG signals. The matrix presents the topographical map of the nine emotions using linear bivariate features in all channel.

Figure 13.10 shows the *PLI* ranking and the connection importance score of the feature of all channels in the EEG signals. Features that are strongly influenced by the emotional category and are ranked higher than other features.

Plotting the first 15 ranked pairs of electrodes from the *PLI* in Fig. 13.11 reveals that the most efficient pairs are centered in the frontal right lobe.

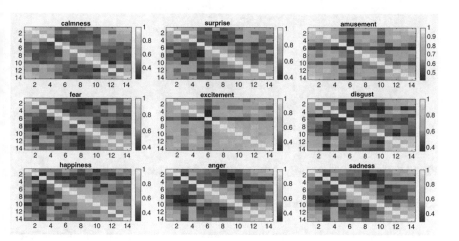

Fig. 13.6 Comparative plot of the functional connectivity matrices for the nine tested emotional states using linear *Coh*.

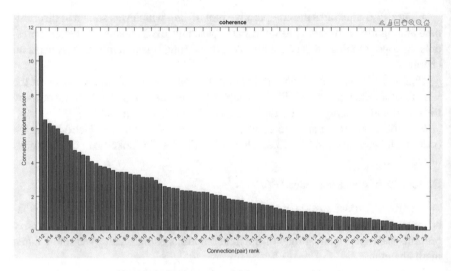

Fig. 13.7 Comparative plot of the *Coh* of channels

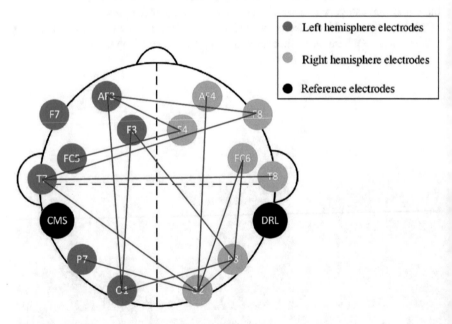

Fig. 13.8 Electrodes Connectivity plot of the *Coh*. first 15 ranked pairs

13.4.2.2 Results of Nonlinear Features

The results demonstrate that emotional responses are associated with higher levels of connection in specific brain locations. These findings were disclosed using nonlinear features that could be utilized to develop a synchronization diagnostic index

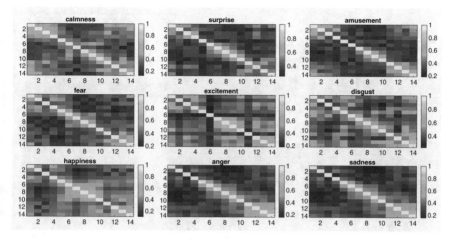

Fig. 13.9 Comparative plot of the functional connectivity matrices for the nine tested emotional states using linear *PLI*.

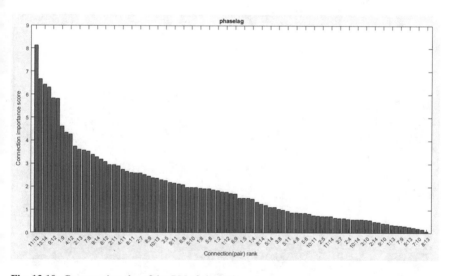

Fig. 13.10 Comparative plot of the *PLI* of channels

that could differentiate emotions from EEG-based signals, according to statistical analysis of network parameters.

A. Results of cross-fuzzy entropy (*CFuzzEn*)

Figure 13.12 illustrates the comparative plot of *CFuzzEn* which was computed to discriminate among nine different emotional states based on EEG signals. The matrix presents the topographical map of the nine emotions using nonlinear bivariate features in all channel.

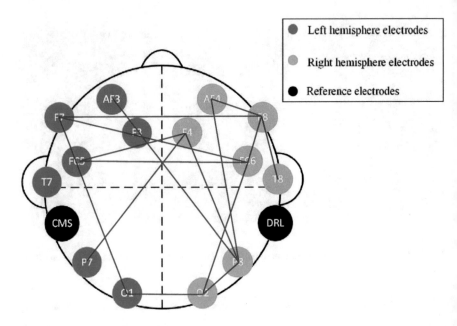

Fig. 13.11 Electrodes Connectivity plot of the *PLI* first 15 ranked pairs

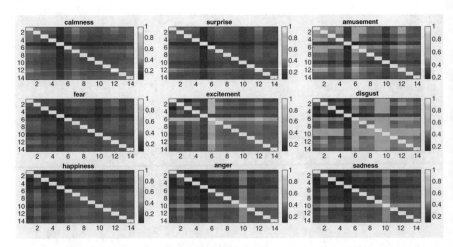

Fig. 13.12 Comparative plot of the functional connectivity matrices for the nine tested emotional states using nonlinear *CFuzzEn*

Figure 13.13 shows the *CFuzzEn* ranking and the connection importance score of the feature of all channels in the EEG signals. Features that are strongly influenced by the emotional category and are ranked higher than other features.

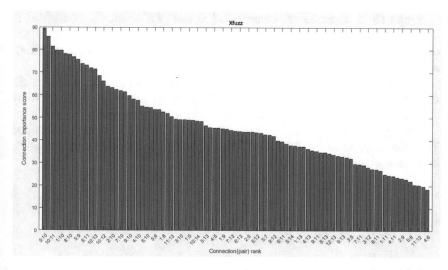

Fig. 13.13 Comparative plot of the *CFuzzEn* of channels

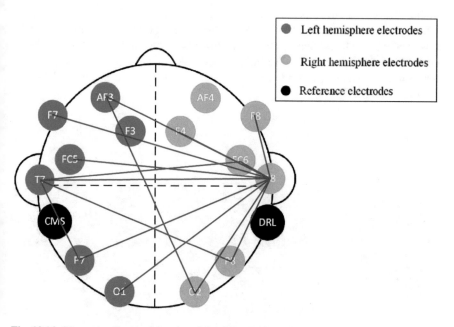

Fig. 13.14 Electrodes Connectivity plot of the *CFuzzEn* first 15 ranked pairs

Plotting the first 15 ranked pair of electrodes of the *CFuzzEn* in Fig. 13.14 reveals that the Temporal lobe electrodes T7 and T8 are related to the majority of the effective pairings (features).

B. Results of Joint Permutation Entropy (*JPE*)

Figure 13.15 illustrates the comparative plot of *JPE* which was considered to discriminate among nine different emotional states based on EEG signals. The matrix presents the topographical map of the nine emotions using nonlinear bivariate features in all channel.

Figure 13.16 shows the *JPE* ranking and the connection importance score of the feature of all channels in the EEG signals. Features that are strongly influenced by the emotional category and are ranked higher than other features.

The top 15 ranked pairings of the *JPE*, which are conjugated with the T7 and T8 in the temporal lobe and P8 and P7 in the parietal lobe, are the most successful in the categorization, as shown in Fig. 13.17.

13.4.3   Results of Features Selection and Emotion Classification Stages

13.4.3.1   Classification Results of Linear Features

Table 13.1 shows the *k*NN classification accuracies for full feature set of 91 attributes and the accuracies after applying the feature selection method. It can be observed that the linear features were fells to classify the emotions from EEG-based signals and that's may related to the brain complexity structure. Therefore, in the next stage this study was used nonlinear dynamical features to be compatible with the brain complexity.

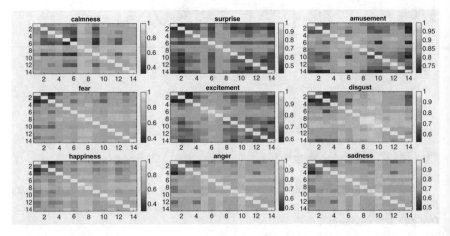

Fig. 13.15 Comparative plot of the functional connectivity matrices for the nine tested emotional states using nonlinear *JPE*.

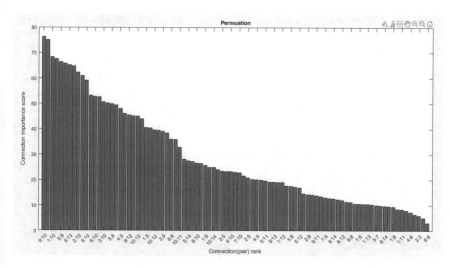

Fig. 13.16 Comparative plot of the *JPE* of channels

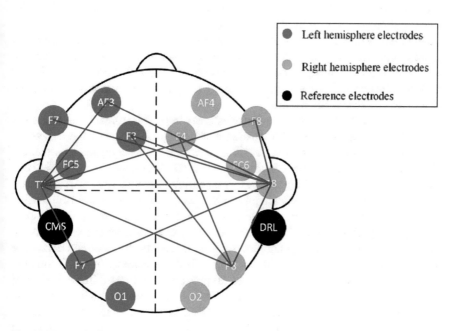

Fig. 13.17 Electrodes Connectivity plot of the *JPE* first 15 ranked pairs

13.4.3.2   Classification Results of Nonlinear Features

Table 13.2 shows the *k*NN classification accuracies for full feature set of 91 attributes and the accuracies after applying the feature selection method. It can be
observed that the nonlinear have better scores particularly for the *JPE* compared to

Table 13.1 kNN classification accuracies of full features set and after selection of linear features

Linear features	Accuracy (%)	Selected features	Accuracy (%)
xCorr	24.8	70 attributes	23.5
Coh	20.1	89 attributes	21.1
PLI	21.3	70 attributes	22.4
Linear features	Accuracy (%)	Selected features	Accuracy (%)
xCorr	24.8	70 attributes	23.5

Table 13.2 Classification accuracies of full features set and after selection of nonlinear features

Nonlinear features	Accuracy (%)	Selected features	Accuracy (%)
CFuzzEn	73.8	85 attributes	74.5
JPE	82.9	85 attributes	83.3

the linear features.

Moreover, the combination of *CFuzzEn* and *JPE* nonlinear entropy features increase the classification *accuracy* to 84.9%. The classification results illustrated the effect of *CFuzzEn* and *JPE* features as remarkable synchronization index for investigating emotions from EEG-based data set.

Figures 13.18 and 13.19 display the confusion matrices for linear and nonlinear features computed from emotional-based EEG signals in which correct recognition is shown on the diagonal; substitution errors are off-diagonal. According to the last confusion matrix of both data sets, sadness (Class 9) had the least misclassification due to its very low valance score.

Based on the studies that attempted to estimate the best features, Table 13.3 compares the proposed method with existing methodologies. However, these methods were obtained with reduction in detection *accuracy* due to complicated computational calculations due to the redundant features. The experimental results show that our approach achieves a high *accuracy* comparing to competitive state-of-the-art methods, indicating its potential in promoting future research on multi-person EEG recognition. Thus, this study presents an automatic emotion recognition model employing synchronization indices to extract features with the highest quality to enhance the ability of emotional-based EEGs to identify different emotions. The suggested technique improves the kNN classification *accuracy* by a fair amount. Moreover, these methods have been used to study emotional-based EEGs, but in this work, automatic emotion detection from synchronization indices utilizing emotional-based EEG is the first to be observed in order to choose the optimum quality of features that improved the *accuracy* of classification of emotions from amusement, excitement, happiness, calmness, anger, disgust, fear, sadness and surprise emotional-based EEGs. Additionally, the previous studies have used already existing public dataset datasets (*MAHNOB*, *DEAP*) with mainly linear features while in this investigation the EEG dataset was investigated and examined using linear and nonlinear features particularly bivariate *CFuzzEn* and *JPE* entropy features therefore, Since the EEG estimate technique has never been used to secure emotional information, emotion contrasts may be better expressed.

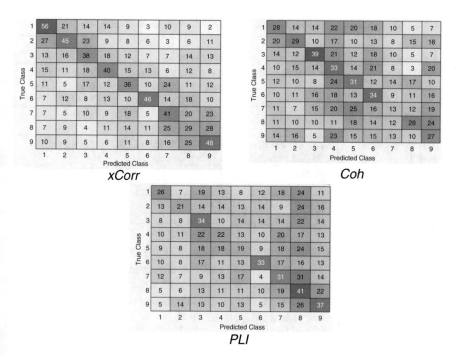

Fig. 13.18 The confusion matrix calculations for emotional-based EEGs classification using linear features

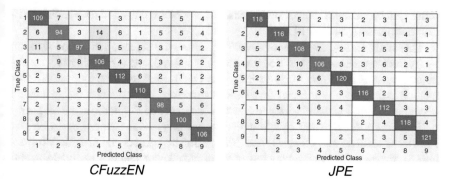

Fig. 13.19 The confusion matrix configuration for emotional-based EEGs classification using nonlinear features

There are some disadvantages, nevertheless, that should be taken into account. For instance, the suggested method made use of a regularized dimensionality reduction stage rather than including small sample size, and the future work will need to use a larger data source. This work compared only 3 linear and 2 nonlinear entropy feature sets, however, wavelet entropy, dispersion entropy, and multi-scale entropy are also worth looking into to see if they have the ability to detect emotional

Table 13.3 Qualitative comparison of the proposed method to the state-of-the-art

References	Denoising technique	Feature extraction	Classifier Accuracy (%)
A. M. Bhatti et al. [89]	bandpass filter (0.1 to 50) Hz	Time domain, Frequency domain, STFT, PSD	MLP (78.11), K-NN (72.80), SVM (75.62)
N. Jatupaiboon et al. [90]	notch at 50 Hz	Wavelet, PSD	SVM (65.12)
T. F. Bastos-Filho et al. [91]	bandpass filter (0.4 to 45) Hz	Statistical (STD, MAV), PSD, High Order Crossings	k-NN (69.5)
U. Wijeratne et al. [92]	Wavelet	PSD	ANN (75)
V. H. Anh et al. [93]	bandpass filter (1–30) Hz	HFD	SVM (70.5)

synchronization using EEG data. Nevertheless, the suggested EEG-based method does have a limitation, in this study. The EEG datasets were examined offline and data from examinations was gathered. However, in order to corroborate the findings, further research utilizing real-time online experiments is necessary due to the differences between offline and online categorizations.

Despite these limitations, the results from this study and those of past studies, which supported the potential of EEG signals to identify the majority of emotional disparities, are in accord and those discrepancies were reflected in the EEG bands as well [94]. Hence, when coupled with nonlinear feature sets and kNN classifier, the proposed method can provide valuable insight for automatic emotion estimation using synchronization indices on the basis of key biomarkers and dependable indicators for affective-based EEG.

This study adds to the body of knowledge about the detection of affective mood by its findings. However, additional research is needed, and combining other techniques, such as EEG and MEG or EEG and fMRI, may improve the results. This method is justified by the fact that various emotions do not affect the metabolic behavior of blood in capillaries and neuron electrical activity in the same manner.

To sum up, *EMD − WT* hybrid denoising technique was used, *xCorr*, *Coh* and *PLI* linear features and *CFuzzEn* and *JPE* nonlinear features can provide information to improve the synchronization of emotions. These features can yield useful information to characterize and identify the relation between brain lobes when the emotion changes. The former features have been used for further analysis including channels selection using ANOVA test. The results have been reported to extract the valuable EEG synchronization markers associated with emotions. This result implies that the denoising technique combined mainly with nonlinear entropy features may automatically detect and provide reliable synchronization markers to identify state of emotion of individuals. Indeed, the results emphasize the crucial role played by the novel proposed framework in the EEG signal processing chain particularly in the classification results.

13.5 Conclusion

Conventional filters and WT technique were used in the preprocessing stage to denoise the Dreamer EEG datasets of 23 subjects while watching 18 short emotional video clips with (amusement, excitement, happiness, calmness, anger, disgust, fear, sadness and surprise) audio-visual stimuli. In the second stage, linear features including *xCorr*, *Coh*, *PLI* and nonlinear features like *CFuzzEn* and *JPE* features were computed to capture different dynamical properties from emotional-based multi-channel emotional-based EEGs. Moreover, ANOVA has been used to statistically examined the individual performance of the used features. Finally, *k*NN classification technique has been used for automatic emotion recognition from EEG-based dataset. These Results shows increased emotion classification *accuracy* for the features that included high synchronization of certain lobe with the rest of the brain regions. The nonlinear features such as *JPE* and *CFuzzEn* had one lobe (Temporal lobe) synchronized with the rest of brain lobes (electrodes) thus providing the highest classification *accuracy* among the other features that are in the contrarily didn't have any specific lobe connected to the others.

References

1. N.K. Al-Qazzaz, Z.A.A. Alyasseri, K.H. Abdulkareem, N.S. Ali, M.N. Al-Mhiqani, C. Guger, EEG feature fusion for motor imagery: A new robust framework towards stroke patients rehabilitation. Comput. Biol. Med. **137**, 104799 (2021)
2. R. Nawaz, K.H. Cheah, H. Nisar, V.V. Yap, Comparison of different feature extraction methods for EEG-based emotion recognition. Biocybernet. Biomed. Eng. **40**, 910–926 (2020)
3. W. Tao, C. Li, R. Song, J. Cheng, Y. Liu, F. Wan, et al., EEG-based emotion recognition via channel-wise attention and self attention. IEEE Trans. Affect. Comput. (2020)
4. J. Cheng, M. Chen, C. Li, Y. Liu, R. Song, A. Liu, et al., Emotion recognition from multichannel eeg via deep forest. IEEE J. Biomed. Health Inform. **25**, 453–464 (2020)
5. J.A. Gaxiola-Tirado, R. Salazar-Varas, D. Gutiérrez, Using the partial directed coherence to assess functional connectivity in electroencephalography data for brain–computer interfaces. IEEE Trans. Cognit. Develop. Syst. **10**, 776–783 (2017)
6. M.A. Ferdek, C.M. van Rijn, M. Wyczesany, Depressive rumination and the emotional control circuit: An EEG localization and effective connectivity study. Cogn. Affect. Behav. Neurosci. **16**, 1099–1113 (2016)
7. O. Sporns, C.J. Honey, Small worlds inside big brains. Proc. Natl. Acad. Sci. **103**, 19219–19220 (2006)
8. M.J. Farah, J.B. Hutchinson, E.A. Phelps, A.D. Wagner, Functional MRI-based lie detection: Scientific and societal challenges. Nat. Rev. Neurosci. **15**, 123–131 (2014)
9. D.S. Bassett, N.F. Wymbs, M.A. Porter, P.J. Mucha, J.M. Carlson, S.T. Grafton, Dynamic reconfiguration of human brain networks during learning. Proc. Natl. Acad. Sci. **108**, 7641–7646 (2011)
10. M.G. Kitzbichler, R.N. Henson, M.L. Smith, P.J. Nathan, E.T. Bullmore, Cognitive effort drives workspace configuration of human brain functional networks. J. Neurosci. **31**, 8259–8270 (2011)

11. R. Ramirez-Melendez, E. Matamoros, D. Hernandez, J. Mirabel, E. Sanchez, N. Escude, Music-enhanced emotion identification of facial emotions in autistic Spectrum disorder children: A pilot EEG study. Brain Sci. **12**, 704 (2022)

12. S.T. Pan, W.C. Li, Fuzzy-HMM modeling for emotion detection using electrocardiogram signals. Asian J. Control **22**, 2206–2216 (2020)

13. N.K. Al-Qazzaz, M.K. Sabir, A.H. Al-Timemy, K. Grammer, An integrated entropy-spatial framework for automatic gender recognition enhancement of emotion-based EEGs. Med. Biol. Eng. Comput., 1–20 (2022)

14. N.K. Al-Qazzaz, M.K. Sabir, S.H.B.M. Ali, S.A. Ahmad, K. Grammer, Complexity and entropy analysis to improve gender identification from emotional-based EEGs. J. Healthc. Eng **2021** (8537000, 2021)

15. N. K. Al-Qazzaz, M. K. Sabir, S. H. M. Ali, S. A. Ahmad, and K. Grammer, The Role of Spectral Power Ratio in Characterizing Emotional EEG for Gender Identification," in 2020 IEEE-EMBS Conference on Biomedical Engineering and Sciences (IECBES) (2021), pp. 334–338

16. N.K. Al-Qazzaz, M.K. Sabir, S.H.B.M. Ali, S.A. Ahmad, K. Grammer, Multichannel optimization with hybrid spectral-entropy markers for gender identification enhancement of emotional-based EEGs. IEEE Access **9**, 107059–107078 (2021)

17. N.K. Al-Qazzaz, M.K. Sabir, S.H.B.M. Ali, S.A. Ahmad, K. Grammer, Electroencephalogram profiles for emotion identification over the brain regions using spectral, entropy and temporal biomarkers. Sensors **20**, 59 (2020)

18. P.R. Davidson, R.D. Jones, M.T. Peiris, EEG-based lapse detecti on with high temporal resolution. IEEE Trans. Biomed. Eng. **54**, 832–839 (2007)

19. F. Vecchio, C. Babiloni, R. Lizio, F.V. Fallani, K. Blinowska, G. Verrienti, et al., Resting state cortical EEG rhythms in Alzheimer's disease: Toward EEG markers for clinical applications: A review. Suppl. Clin. Neurophysiol. **62**, 223–236 (2012)

20. I. Hussain, M.A. Hossain, R. Jany, M.A. Bari, M. Uddin, A.R.M. Kamal, et al., Quantitative evaluation of EEG-biomarkers for prediction of sleep stages. Sensors **22**, 3079 (2022)

21. J.S. Sachadev, R. Bhatnagar, A comprehensive review on brain disease mapping—The underlying technologies and AI based techniques for feature extraction and classification using EEG signals. Med. Inf. Bioimag. Artif. Intel., 73–91 (2022)

22. N.K. Al-Qazzaz, S.H.B. Ali, S.A. Ahmad, K. Chellappan, M.S. Islam, J. Escudero, Role of EEG as biomarker in the early detection and classification of dementia. Scientif. World J. **2014**, 1–16 (2014)

23. O. Sourina, Y. Liu, M.K. Nguyen, Real-time EEG-based emotion recognition for music therapy. J. Multimodal User Interf. **5**, 27–35 (2012)

24. T.-P. Jung, S. Makeig, M. Westerfield, J. Townsend, E. Courchesne, T.J. Sejnowski, Removal of eye activity artifacts from visual event-related potentials in normal and clinical subjects. Clin. Neurophysiol. **111**, 1745–1758 (2000)

25. M. Habl, C. Bauer, C. Ziegaus, E. Lang, F. Schulmeyer, Can ICA help identify brain tumor related EEG signals, in Proceedings of ICA (2000), pp. 609–614

26. C. Guerrero-Mosquera, A.M. Trigueros, A.A. Navia-Vazquez, EEG Signal Processing for Epilepsy (2012)

27. I.M.B. Núñez, EEG Artifact Detection (2010)

28. G.N.G. Molina, Direct brain-computer communication through Scalp Recorded EEG signals., ÉCOLE POLYTECHNIQUE FÉDÉRALE DE LAUSANNE (2004)

29. N.K. Al-Qazzaz, S. Ali, S. Islam, S. Ahmad, J. Escudero, EEG wavelet spectral analysis during a working memory tasks in stroke-related mild cognitive impairment patients, in International Conference for Innovation in Biomedical Engineering and Life Sciences (2016), pp. 82–85

30. N.K. Al-Qazzaz, S. Ali, S.A. Ahmad, M.S. Islam, J. Escudero, Entropy-based markers of EEG background activity of stroke-related mild cognitive impairment and vascular dementia patients, in Sensors and electronic instrumentation advances: proceedings of the 2nd international conference on sensors and electronic instrumentation advances (2016), pp. 22–23

31. A. Mert, A. Akan, Emotion recognition based on time–frequency distribution of EEG signals using multivariate synchrosqueezing transform. Dig. Signal Proc. **81**, 106–115 (2018)
32. H. Ali, M. Hariharan, S. Yaacob, A.H. Adom, Facial emotion recognition using empirical mode decomposition. Expert Syst. Appl. **42**, 1261–1277 (2015)
33. N.K. Al-Qazzaz, S.H.M. Ali, S.A. Ahmad, Differential evolution based channel selection algorithm on EEG signal for early detection of vascular dementia among stroke survivors, in 2018 IEEE-EMBS Conference on Biomedical Engineering and Sciences (IECBES) (2018), pp. 239–244
34. N. Al-Qazzaz, S. Hamid Bin Mohd Ali, S. Ahmad, M. Islam, J. Escudero, Automatic artifact removal in EEG of normal and demented individuals using ICA–WT during working memory tasks, Sensors, vol. 17, p. 1326, 2017
35. N.K. Al-Qazzaz, S.H.B.M. Ali, S.A. Ahmad, M.S. Islam, J. Escudero, Discrimination of stroke-related mild cognitive impairment and vascular dementia using EEG signal analysis. Med. Biol. Eng. Comput. **56**, 1–21 (2017)
36. N. Mammone, F. La Foresta, F.C. Morabito, Automatic artifact rejection from multichannel scalp EEG by wavelet ICA. Sensors J. IEEE **12**, 533–542 (2012)
37. G. Inuso, F. La Foresta, N. Mammone, and F. C. Morabito, Wavelet-ICA methodology for efficient artifact removal from Electroencephalographic recordings, in Neural Networks, 2007. IJCNN 2007. International Joint Conference on, (2007), pp. 1524–1529
38. Z. Huang, B.W.-K. Ling, Joint ensemble empirical mode decomposition and tunable Q factor wavelet transform based sleep stage classifications. Biomed. Signal Proc. Control **77**, 103760 (2022)
39. B.K. Pradhan, M. Jarzębski, A. Gramza-Michałowska, K. Pal, Automated detection of caffeinated coffee-induced short-term effects on ECG signals using EMD, DWT, and WPD. Nutrients **14**, 885 (2022)
40. A.B. Das M.I.H. Bhuiyan, Discrimination and classification of focal and non-focal EEG signals using entropy-based features in the *EMD–DWT* domain, Biomed. Signal Proc. Control, vol. 29, pp. 11–21, 2016
41. V. Bono, S. Das, W. Jamal, K. Maharatna, Hybrid wavelet and EMD/ICA approach for artifact suppression in pervasive EEG. J. Neurosci. Methods **267**, 89–107 (2016)
42. A. Babiker, I. Faye, A hybrid EMD-wavelet EEG feature extraction method for the classification of students' interest in the mathematics classroom. Comput. Intel, Neurosci. **2021**, 6617462 (2021)
43. M.A. Brazier, J.U. Casby, Crosscorrelation and autocorrelation studies of electroencephalographic potentials. Electroencephalogr. Clin. Neurophysiol. **4**, 201–211 (1952)
44. J.L. Cantero, M. Atienza, R.M. Salas, C.M. Gómez, Alpha EEG coherence in different brain states: An electrophysiological index of the arousal level in human subjects. Neurosci. Lett. **271**, 167–170 (1999)
45. N.K. Al-Qazzaz, S.H.B. Ali, S.A. Ahmad, K. Chellappan, M. Islam, J. Escudero, Role of EEG as biomarker in the early detection and classification of dementia. Scientif. World J. **2014**, 906038 (2014)
46. P.J. Franaszczuk, G.K. Bergey, An autoregressive method for the measurement of synchronization of interictal and ictal EEG signals. Biol. Cybern. **81**, 3–9 (1999)
47. S. Xie, S. Krishnan, Wavelet-based sparse functional linear model with applications to EEGs seizure detection and epilepsy diagnosis. Med. Biol. Eng. Comput. **51**, 49–60 (2013)
48. D. Abásolo, R. Hornero, P. Espino, D. Alvarez, J. Poza, Entropy analysis of the EEG background activity in Alzheimer's disease patients. Physiol. Meas. **27**, 241–253 (2006)
49. N.K. Al-Qazzaz, S. Ali, M.S. Islam, S.A. Ahmad, J. Escudero, EEG markers for early detection and characterization of vascular dementia during working memory tasks, in Biomedical Engineering and Sciences (IECBES), 2016 IEEE EMBS Conference on, (2016), pp. 347–351
50. N.K. Al-Qazzaz, S. Ali, S.A. Ahmad, M.S. Islam, J. Escudero, Entropy-based markers of EEG background activity of stroke-related mild cognitive impairment and vascular dementia

patients, in 2nd International Conference on Sensors Engineering and Electronics Instrumental Advances (SEIA 2016), Barcelona, Spain (2016)
51. J. Selvaraj, M. Murugappan, K. Wan, S. Yaacob, Classification of emotional states from electrocardiogram signals: A nonlinear approach based on Hurst. Biomed. Eng. Online **12**, 44 (2013)
52. O. Sourina, Y. Liu, A Fractal-based Algorithm of Emotion Recognition from EEG using Arousal-Valence Model," in Biosignals (2011), pp. 209–214
53. B. García-Martínez, A. Martínez-Rodrigo, R. Zangróniz Cantabrana, J. Pastor García, R. Alcaraz, Application of entropy-based metrics to identify emotional distress from electroencephalographic recordings. Entropy **18**, 221 (2016)
54. N. Thammasan, K. Moriyama, K.-i. Fukui, M. Numao, Continuous music-emotion recognition based on electroencephalogram. IEICE Trans. Inf. Syst. **99**, 1234–1241 (2016)
55. P. Wang, J. Hu, A hybrid model for EEG-based gender recognition. Cogn. Neurodyn. **13**, 541–554 (2019)
56. A. Thul, J. Lechinger, J. Donis, G. Michitsch, G. Pichler, E.F. Kochs, et al., EEG entropy measures indicate decrease of cortical information processing in disorders of consciousness. Clin. Neurophysiol. **127**, 1419–1427 (2016)
57. J. Tian, Z. Luo, Motor imagery EEG feature extraction based on fuzzy entropy. J. Huazhong Univ. Sci. Technol **41**, 92–95 (2013)
58. Y. Cao, L. Cai, J. Wang, R. Wang, H. Yu, Y. Cao, et al., Characterization of complexity in the electroencephalograph activity of Alzheimer's disease based on fuzzy entropy. Chaos Interdisciplinary J. Nonlinear Sci. **25**, 083116 (2015)
59. H. Azami, A. Fernández, J. Escudero, Refined multiscale fuzzy entropy based on standard deviation for biomedical signal analysis. Med. Biol. Eng. Comput. **55**, 2037–2052 (2017)
60. P. Shen, Z. Changjun, X. Chen, Automatic speech emotion recognition using support vector machine, in Electronic and Mechanical Engineering and Information Technology (EMEIT), 2011 International Conference on (2011), pp. 621–625
61. Y. Pan, P. Shen, L. Shen, Speech emotion recognition using support vector machine. Int. J. Smart Home **6**, 101–108 (2012)
62. P. Nguyen, D. Tran, X. Huang, W. Ma, Age and gender classification using EEG paralinguistic features, in 2013 6th International IEEE/EMBS Conference on Neural Engineering (NER), (2013), pp. 1295–1298
63. B. Kaur, D. Singh, P.P. Roy, Age and gender classification using brain–computer interface. Neural Comput. & Applic. **31**, 5887–5900 (2019)
64. H. Shahabi, S. Moghimi, Toward automatic detection of brain responses to emotional music through analysis of EEG effective connectivity. Comput. Hum. Behav. **58**, 231–239 (2016)
65. K.-E. Ko, H.-C. Yang, K.-B. Sim, Emotion recognition using EEG signals with relative power values and Bayesian network. Int. J. Control, Autom. Syst. **7**, 865–870 (2009)
66. M. Murugappan, N. Ramachandran, Y. Sazali, Classification of human emotion from EEG using discrete wavelet transform. J. Biomed. Sci. Eng. **3**, 390–396 (2010)
67. M. Murugappan, R. Nagarajan, S. Yaacob, Combining spatial filtering and wavelet transform for classifying human emotions using EEG signals. J. Med. Biol. Eng. **31**, 45–51 (2011)
68. E. Bullmore, O. Sporns, Complex brain networks: Graph theoretical analysis of structural and functional systems. Nat. Rev. Neurosci. **10**, 186–198 (2009)
69. X. Jie, R. Cao, L. Li, Emotion recognition based on the sample entropy of EEG. Biomed. Mater. Eng. **24**, 1185–1192 (2014)
70. S. Katsigiannis, N. Ramzan, DREAMER: A database for emotion recognition through EEG and ECG signals from wireless low-cost off-the-shelf devices. IEEE J. Biomed. Health Inform. **22**, 98–107 (2017)
71. C.A. Gabert-Quillen, E.E. Bartolini, B.T. Abravanel, C.A. Sanislow, Ratings for emotion film clips. Behav. Res. Methods **47**, 773–787 (2015)

72. D. Abásolo, J. Escudero, R. Hornero, C. Gómez, P. Espino, Approximate entropy and auto mutual information analysis of the electroencephalogram in Alzheimer's disease patients. Med. Biol. Eng. Comput. **46**, 1019–1028 (2008)
73. S. Taran, V. Bajaj, Emotion recognition from single-channel EEG signals using a two-stage correlation and instantaneous frequency-based filtering method. Comput. Methods Prog. Biomed. **173**, 157–165 (2019)
74. A. Ayenu-Prah, N. Attoh-Okine, A criterion for selecting relevant intrinsic mode functions in empirical mode decomposition. Adv. Adapt. Data Anal. **2**, 1–24 (2010)
75. Z. German-Sallo and C. Ciufudean, Waveform-adapted wavelet denoising of ECG signals
76. A. Shoeb, G. Cliord, Chapter 16 - Wavelets; Multiscale Activity in Physiological Signals, in Biomedical Signal and Image Processing, Ed (2005)
77. N.K. Al-Qazzaz, M.K. Sabir, K. Grammer, Gender Differences identification from Brain Regions using Spectral Relative Powers of Emotional EEG, in Proceedings of the 2019 7th International work-conference on Bioinformatics and biomedical engineering, (2019), pp. 38–42
78. N.K. Al-Qazzaz, M.K. Sabir, K. Grammer, Correlation Indices of Electroencephalogram-Based Relative Powers during Human Emotion Processing, in Proceedings of the 2019 9th International Conference on Biomedical Engineering and Technology, (2019), pp. 64–70
79. N.K. Al-Qazzaz, M.K. Sabir, S. Ali, S.A. Ahmad, K. Grammer, Effective EEG channels for emotion identification over the brain regions using differential evolution algorithm," in 2019 41th Annual International Conference of the IEEE Engineering in Medicine and Biology Society (EMBC) (2019)
80. N. Al-Qazzaz, S.H.B.M. Ali, S. Ahmad, M. Islam, J. Escudero, Selection of mother wavelet functions for multi-channel EEG signal analysis during a working memory task. Sensors **15**, 29015–29035 (2015)
81. C.M. Stein, Estimation of the mean of a multivariate normal distribution. Ann. Stat., 1135–1151 (1981)
82. R. Romo-Vazquez, R. Ranta, V. Louis-Dorr, D. Maquin, EEG ocular artefacts and noise removal, in Engineering in Medicine and Biology Society, 2007. EMBS 2007. 29th Annual International Conference of the IEEE (2007), pp. 5445–5448
83. E. Estrada, H. Nazeran, G. Sierra, F. Ebrahimi, S. K. Setarehdan, Wavelet-based EEG denoising for automatic sleep stage classification, in Electrical Communications and Computers (CONIELECOMP), 2011 21st International Conference on, (2011), pp. 295–298
84. N.K. Al-Qazzaz, S. Ali, S.A. Ahmad, M.S. Islam, M.I. Ariff, Selection of mother wavelets thresholding methods in denoising multi-channel EEG signals during working memory task, in Biomedical Engineering and Sciences (IECBES), 2014 IEEE Conference on, (2014), pp. 214–219
85. N.K. Al-Qazzaz, S. Ali, S.A. Ahmad, M.S. Islam, M.I. Ariff, Selection of mother wavelets thresholding methods in denoising multi-channel EEG signals during working memory task, in 2014 IEEE conference on biomedical engineering and sciences (IECBES), (2014), pp. 214–219
86. W. Chang, H. Wang, C. Hua, Q. Wang, Y. Yuan, Comparison of different functional connectives based on EEG during concealed information test. Biomed. Signal Proc. Control **49**, 149–159 (2019)
87. H.-B. Xie, Y.-P. Zheng, J.-Y. Guo, X. Chen, Cross-fuzzy entropy: A new method to test pattern synchrony of bivariate time series. Inf. Sci. **180**, 1715–1724 (2010)
88. Y. Yin, P. Shang, A.C. Ahn, C.-K. Peng, Multiscale joint permutation entropy for complex time series. Physica A: Statist. Mech. Appl. **515**, 388–402 (2019)
89. A.M. Bhatti, M. Majid, S.M. Anwar, B. Khan, Human emotion recognition and analysis in response to audio music using brain signals. Comput. Hum. Behav. **65**, 267–275 (2016)
90. N. Jatupaiboon, S. Pan-Ngum, P. Israsena, Real-time EEG-based happiness detection system. Scientif. World J. **2013** (2013)

91. T.F. Bastos-Filho, A. Ferreira, A.C. Atencio, S.Arjunan, D.Kumar, "Evaluation of feature extraction techniques in emotional state recognition," in 2012 4th International conference on intelligent human computer interaction (IHCI), 2012, pp. 1–6
92. U. Wijeratne, U. Perera, Intelligent emotion recognition system using electroencephalography and active shape models, in 2012 IEEE-EMBS conference on biomedical engineering and sciences (2012), pp. 636–641
93. V.H. Anh, M.N. Van, B.B. Ha, T.H. Quyet, A real-time model based support vector machine for emotion recognition through EEG, in 2012 International conference on control, automation and information sciences (ICCAIS), (2012), pp. 191–196
94. A. Goshvarpour, A. Goshvarpour, EEG spectral powers and source localization in depressing, sad, and fun music videos focusing on gender differences. Cogn. Neurodyn. **13**, 161–173 (2019)

Chapter 14
Recognition Enhancement of Dementia Patients' Working Memory Using Entropy-Based Features and Local Tangent Space Alignment Algorithm

Noor Kamal Al-Qazzaz, Sawal Hamid Bin Mohd Ali, and Siti Anom Ahmad

Abstract Detecting dementia presents a barrier to advancing individualized healthcare. Electroencephalographic (EEG) signals' nonlinear nature has been characterized using entropies. While a working memory (*WM*), the EEGs of 5 patients suffering vascular dementia (*VD*), 15 patients had stroke-related mild cognitive impairment (*SMCI*), and 15 healthy normal control (*NC*) participants were evaluated in this study. A four-step framework for the automatic identification of dementia is provided, with the first stage employing the newly developed automatic independent component analysis and wavelet (AICA-WT) method. In the second stage, nonlinear entropy features using fuzzy entropy (*FuzzEn*), fluctuation-based dispersion entropy (*FDispEn*), and bubble entropy (*BubbEn*) were utilized to extract various dynamical properties from multi-channel EEG signals derived from patients with dementia. A statistical examination of the individual performance was conducted using analysis of variance (ANOVA) to determine the degree of EEG complexity across brain regions. Afterwards, the nonlinear local tangent space alignment (LSTA) dimensionality reduction approach was utilized to enhance the automatic

N. K. Al-Qazzaz (✉)
Department of Biomedical Engineering, Al-Khwarizmi College of Engineering, University of Baghdad, Baghdad, Iraq
e-mail: noorbme@kecbu.uobaghdad.edu.iq

Sawal Hamid Bin Mohd Ali
Department of Electrical, Electronic & Systems Engineering, Faculty of Engineering & Built Environment, Universiti Kebangsaan Malaysia, UKM Bangi, Bangi, Selangor, Malaysia
e-mail: sawal@ukm.edu.my

S. A. Ahmad
Department of Electrical and Electronic Engineering, Faculty of Engineering, Universiti Putra Malaysia, UPM Serdang, Serdang, Selangor, Malaysia

Malaysian Research Institute of Ageing (MyAgeing™), Universiti Putra Malaysia, Serdang, Serdang, Selangor, Malaysia
e-mail: sanom@upm.edu.my

© The Author(s), under exclusive license to Springer Nature Switzerland AG 2023   345
S. Mian Qaisar et al. (eds.), *Advances in Non-Invasive Biomedical Signal Sensing and Processing with Machine Learning*, https://doi.org/10.1007/978-3-031-23239-8_14

diagnosis of dementia patients'. Using *k*-nearest neighbors (*k*NN), support vector machine (*SVM*), and decision tree (*DT*) classifiers, the impairment of post-stroke patients was finally identified. BubbEn is chosen to develop a new *BubbEn*-LTSA mapping process for creating the innovative AICA-WT-*BubbEn*-LTSA dementia recognition framework, which is the basis for an automated VD detection.

14.1 Introduction

Cognitive impairment and dementia are progressive impairments of mental function that are frequent following a stroke and inevitably lead to limitations in independent life. It was estimated that 50 million individuals were affected globally in 2018, and by 2050, that number is anticipated to triple [1]. After Alzheimer's disease (*AD*), vascular dementia (*VD*) is the second most prevalent type of dementia, and its prevalence doubles every 5–10 years after age 65 [2–4]. The majority of people with vascular dementia are elderly adults over the age of 65. Clinically speaking, a reduction in mental ability that is higher than would be predicted given the people's age and education level but does not severely affect everyday activities is known as mild cognitive impairment (*MCI*) [5]. It's frequently thought of as being in the middle of the spectrum between early-on-normal brain cognition and late-on-severe dementia. Following a stroke diagnosis, the cognitive function most impacted by dementia and cognitive loss is memory [6, 7].

Better therapeutic therapy prior to brain damage from dementia would require earlier diagnosis. Early dementia diagnosis will help dementia patients start symptom-based treatment as quickly as possible. Recent years have seen significant advancements in the use of biomarkers to detect dementia in its earliest stages [8–11].

The use of magnetoencephalography (MEG) to record the brain activity of Alzheimer's disease (AD) patients has gained significant research interest over the past 20 years [12–15]. EEG is a therapeutic tool that has a high level of temporal resolution and can monitor brain activity in milliseconds [16]. Therefore, it is frequently used to establish a thorough study of a time-sensitive neurodynamic marker that assists in monitoring the brain for irregularities linked to cognitive decline and dementia [16, 17]. It can be used in neurophysiology to recognize and classify changes in the brain [18]. It is essential to develop a mechanism for detecting dementia in its early stages so that an ideal diagnostic index can be derived.

In this study, 15 healthy normal control (*NC*) volunteers, 15 patients with mild cognitive impairment (*SMCI*) following a stroke, and 5 patients with vascular dementia (*VD*) were used as *NC* to measure the background EEG activity during a working memory (WM) test. In the first step of a four-stage framework for the automatic identification of dementia, conventional filters with, a revolutionary automatic independent component analysis and wavelet (AICA-WT) approach was used. In the second stage, nonlinear entropy features such as fuzzy entropy (*FuzzEn*), fluctuation-based dispersion entropy (*FDispEn*), and bubble entropy (*BubbEn*) were utilized to extract various dynamical properties from multi-channel EEG signals derived from patients with dementia. The level of EEG complexity across brain areas was assessed statistically using analysis of variance (ANOVA) of the individual performance of estimated entropies. Afterwards, the nonlinear local tangent space alignment (LTSA) dimensionality reduction approach was utilized to enhance the automatic diagnosis of dementia patients' onset. Using $k - nearest$ $neighbors$ (kNN), support vector machine (SVM), and decision tree (DT) classifiers, the disabilities suffered by stroke survivors was finally identified. The comparative efficiency of the LTSA method for scaling down data dimensions with the kNN, SVM, and DT classifiers has been examined. LTSA with kNN achieved the highest classification accuracies for VD, $SMCI$, and NC, respectively.

According to the author's knowledge, this is the first time such an analysis has been performed for dementia-based discriminative processing of EEG information. The initial contribution of this research is the proposal of an novel EEG AICA-WT-$BubbEn$-LTSA mapping architecture to improve early dementia identification. The suggested framework uses the novel AICA-WT denoising method and bubble entropy to stabilize complexity parameters. The performance of the proposed framework with three class classification tasks was acquired utilizing three distinct machine learning models in order to provide dependable classification performance and demonstrate the robustness of our proposed mapping framework. The working memory methodology for capturing EEG signals from VD, $SMCI$, and NC subjects is the first to interpret graphical behavior from EEG-based background activity. Novel AICA-WT-$BubbEn$-LTSA could be a core for automated VD detection and a promising, highly efficient technique for identifying VD and $SMCI$ impaired effects on neuroelectrography alterations.

14.2 Related Works

Brain disorders like epilepsy, researchers have used EEG readings to diagnose both attention deficit hyperactivity disorder ($ADHD$) and AD. Using an EEG dataset with several channels spanning brain areas, it may be possible to evaluate a wide range of affective reactions. [4, 19–24]. Therefore, studies have demonstrated the potential for EEG signals to detect vascular dementia (VD) patients by examining working memory tasks and displaying brain alterations collected based on non-conscious EEG brainwave patterns in people with dementia [25, 26]. However, EEG data are typically polluted by motion, ocular, muscular, and cardiac activities [19, 27]. Greater magnitude artifacts distort the signal and mislead the analysis.

There is a growing body of research aimed at removing non-cerebral sources from EEG data, known as artifacts, which may imitate brain disease activity and so affect the analysis [19, 26]. Early techniques for detecting and removing artifacts included blind source separation (BSS) based on Independent Component Analysis (ICA) [28], wavelet denoising [29, 30] to enhance the performance [31]. However, wavelets are time-frequency spectrums that overlap, but ICA lacks redundancy in the number of signals relative to the number of sources. Al-Qazzaz [19, 32] have proposed the combination of ICA and wavelets approaches to solve these constraints.

In addition to being extremely informative on brain physiology, EEG signals may also serve as biomarkers of brain behavior [33–37]. The Hurst exponent (*Hur*) [32, 38] and fractal dimension (*FD*) [39, 40] nonlinear methods that have been used to represent and analyze cerebral cortex-generated complex dynamic data [41, 42]. Nonlinear parametric index of entropy can be used to quantify the uncertainty of dynamic systems like EEG signals that lack stability [43]. The field of cognitive neuroscience, sleep research, and the classification of emotional states have all profited from the use of entropy with EEG information [26, 40, 44, 45].

Entropy methods have been proposed throughout the previous three decades as a potent metric for quantifying the dynamic complexity of real-world systems such as EEG time series [43]. Entropies have been used to research cognitive thinking states, sleep states, and emotional level categorization techniques using the EEG signal [26, 40, 44, 45]. In addition, social emotion, personal identification, therapy uptake, clinical efficacy, and side effects are potential therapeutic uses of EEG-based biological gender recognition leveraging several entropies. [46]. Wang [47] employed *sample entropy* (*SampEn*), *approximate entropy* (*ApEn*), and *permutation entropy* (*PerEn*) to examine the human emotions in response to video clips due to the robustness of these entropies to noise and their ability to effectively assess the complexity of a time series [48, 49]. Researchers have proposed *fuzzy entropy* (*FuzzEn*) for EEG assessment. In addition, *Shannon entropy* (*ShEn*) and *conditional entropy* (*ConEn*) represent the amount of information and the rate at which new information is being made [50]. The widely-used *SampEn* is derived from *ConEn* [51], whereas *PerEn* and the newly developed *dispersion entropy* (*DispEn*) [52] are derived from *ShEn* [53]. *SampEn* gives unreliable or unknown entropy values for short time series and is inadequate for long signals [14, 15]. *PerEn* is intuitive and computationally efficient. However, it has a continuous distribution and is noise-sensitive. Fluctuation-based dispersion entropy (*FDispEn*) was proposed in [50] and Bubble entropy (*BubbEn*) was utilized in [54] to examine the dynamics of time series, specifically the distribution of symbol sequences, in order to address the inadequacies of *PerEn* and *SampEn*.

The advantage of this work is to find out how psychological EEG signals in different parts of the brain differ between *VD*, *SMCI*, and *NC* people by utilizing EEG markers to detect various dynamical features of dementia-based EEG background activity. Therefore, among the several empirical entropies, the *FuzzEn* [55], *FDispEn* [50] and *BubbEn* [54] entropies were chosen because they are noise-resistant and may provide important information for interpreting the time series complexity.

Methods like sequential feed-forward selection (*SFFS*), minimum redundancy maximum relevance (*mRMR*), genetic algorithm (*GA*), evolutionary computation (*EC*), and sparse discriminative ensemble learning (*SDEL*) algorithm, sparse linear discriminant analysis (LDA) and principle component analysis (*PCA*) have all been used to estimate the best features [56–61].

Xie [33] have utilized the *k*NN and *SVM* classifiers for seizure detection, whereas Subasi [62] have employed *PCA* as a dimensionality reduction technique and the *SVM* classifier with two outputs, either an epileptic seizure or not. In addition, for Brain Computer Interface (BCI) system applications, Vidaurre [63] examined brain-waves using a linear discriminant analysis (*LDA*) classifier, whereas Murugappan [64] classified discrete emotions using *k*NN and *LDA*. In addition, Lagun [65] cat-egorised the EEG datasets of AD, *SMCI*, and NC participants using logistic regres-sion (LR), naive Bayes (NB), and support vector machine (*SVM*). Chaovalitwongse [66] have presented a technique for classifying and detecting seizure precursors using *k*NN.

The majority of dementia detection investigations used EEG signals based on *AD*, and they concentrated on linear analysis employing spectral relative powers [67–69]. However, other studies [21, 70, 71] have employed nonlinear entropy char-acteristics to examine brain complexity behavior. To this goal, entropy features were computed to emphasize the diversity of dementia in affective-based EEG systems.

14.3   Methods and Materials

The recorded EEG requires several stages of signal processing and analysis in order to obtain relevant details from the EEG signal of *VD* and *SMCI* patients in order to enhance the accuracy of the diagnosis of degenerative changes. EEG may have a significant role in the diagnosis and severity categorization of dementia. Preprocessing, feature extraction, dimensionality reduction, and classification are the primary stages of EEG signal processing. Fig. 14.1 depicts the complexity of EEG processing algorithms.

14.3.1   Participants and EEG Recording

The *NicoletOne* (*V*32) system, developed and manufactured by *VIASYS* Healthcare Inc. in the United States, was used to gather the EEG data. The scalp was covered with 19 electrodes (including *ground* and system *reference* electrodes) in a cap elec-trode configuration. Here are the cutoff frequencies for the low-pass filter (*LPF*), high-pass filter (*HPF*), and notch hardware filters included in the EEG device: The 3 dB point for the LPF is at a frequency of 0.3 Hz, and the 70 Hz HPF upper cutoff frequency is adjustable. Typically, the notch filter is set at 50 Hz, and the frequency range is (0.3 to 70) Hz. The sampling frequency is determined by the application to be 256 Hz, etc., and a 12 *bit A/D* converter accurately digitizes the signal. 15 *NC* records, 15 *SMCI* patients, and 5 *VD* patients had their EEG data reviewed for this investigation. The participants serving as *NC* had no history of mental or neurologi-cal problems. The stroke patients were recruited from the *stroke ward* at *Pusat Perubatan Universiti Kebangsaan Malaysia* (*PPUKM*), the National University of

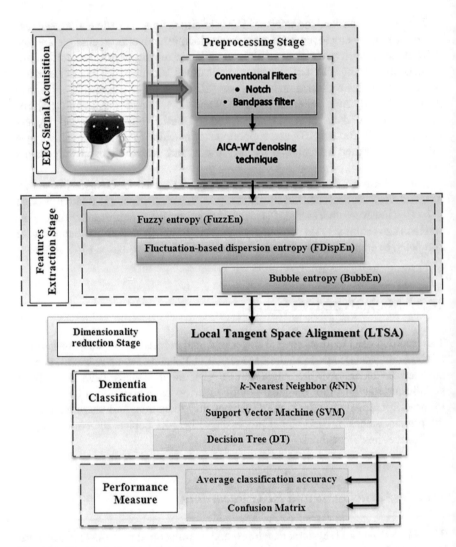

Fig. 14.1 The block diagram of current study

Malaysia's medical facility. Patients with *VD* were recruited through the *Neurology Clinic*. The stroke patient met the requirements of the *National Institutes of Health Stroke Scale (NIHSS)* [72]. All patients were diagnosed using magnetic resonance imaging (*MRI*) images of the brain, patient medical histories, and clinical and laboratory tests. The healthy *NC* group had no history of mental or neurological disorders. The *Mini − Mental State Examination (MMSE)* [73] and the *Montreal Cognitive Assessment (MoCA)* [74] were used to evaluate the cognitive abilities of both groups. In accordance with the 10–20 worldwide system, a total of 19 *electrodes* plus the *ground* and system reference electrode were placed (*Fp*1, *Fp*2, *F*7, *F*3, *Fz*, *F*4, *F*8, *T*3, *T*5, *T*4, *T*6, *P*3, *Pz*, *P*4, *C*3, *Cz*, *C*4, *O*1, *and O*2). Table 14.1

Table 14.1 Sociodemographic characteristics of the NC subjects and SMCI and VD patients.

Participant features	NC	SMCI	VD
Number	15	15	5
Age	60.06 ± 5.21	60.26 ± 7.77	64.6 ± 4.8
MMSE	29.6 ± 0.73	20.2 ± 5.63	14.8 ± 1.92
MoCA	29.06 ± 0.88	16.13 ± 5.97	13.2 ± 2.38
Gender	8 Females/7 Males	10 Females/5 Males	2 Females/3 Males

Age in years, MMSE Mini-Mental State Examination, MoCA Montreal Cognitive Assessment, SD meanstandard deviation

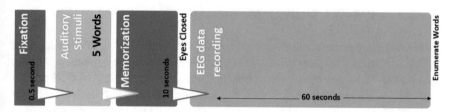

Fig. 14.2 The experimental model of working memory

displays the sociodemographic and cognitive characteristics of the *NC*, *SMCI* and *VD* patients.

The Human Ethics Committee of the *National University of Malaysia* authorized each protocol for an experiment. The participants also completed a consent form to receive information. In this EEG investigation, a session of auditory working memory (WM) test was done. Participants were given a 0.5 second fixation signal at the start of the session and asked to sit as still as possible for the duration of the test. Afterward, as a quick WM test, the participants were given five words to memorize for 10 seconds. Then, while EEG data was being recorded, participants were instructed to close their eyes and think about these words. The patients had to open their eyes once the allotted 60 seconds had passed and make a list of all the words and phrases they had remembered (Fig. 14.2) [3, 29].

14.3.2 Preprocessing Stage

EEG signal preprocessing is required to remove noise, due to the fact that EEG waves typically contain artifacts in the same frequency ranges, allowing for probable overlap with brain processes.

14.3.2.1 Conventional Filters

The *A/C* power interference noise was reduced by utilizing a *notch* filter with a 50 *Hz* cut-off frequency [4] and a band-pass filter (*BPF*) with a lower cutoff equating to 3 *dB* at 0.5 *Hz* and an upper cutoff frequency within the range of 64 *Hz*, as described in [69]. In a subsequent step of processing for the filtered EEG dataset, the data were split into 6 trials, with each trial including 10 seconds (6 *x* 10 second periods) and 15360 data points per ten seconds.

14.3.2.2 AICA–WT Technique Methodology

In this study, we present and describe the AICA-WT technique as a fully automatic hybrid approach. The purpose of this strategy is to address the limitations of both ICA and DWT by combining their benefits. To improve the quality of EEG recordings, AICA-WT is applied [75, 76]. ICA is a strong statistical approach for estimating a set of n unknown components, $s(t) = [s_1(t), \ldots, s_n(t)]$, that were linearly mixed by the ICA linear transform matrix A. The formula is as follows:

$$x(t) = As(t) \tag{14.1}$$

where the EEGs are denoted by x(t), and both x(t) and s(t) should average out to zero. The demixing matrix W, which is the inverse matrix of A used to represent the linearly ICs, is generated by the ICA from the higher-order statistics of x(t). The ICs can then be determined using Eq. (14.2) (based on the above assumptions) [75, 77, 78]:

$$y(t) = Wx(t) \tag{14.2}$$

where $y(t) = [y_1(t), \ldots, y_n(t)]$ is the vector that estimate the ICs

In this investigation, the FastICA algorithm described by Hyvärinen [79] was utilized to decompose EEG signals due to its simplicity, rapid convergence, and efficiency in decomposing the recorded EEG and extracting the new component matrix $\hat{s}$.

DWT, *symlet* mother wavelet (*MWT*) of *order* 9 'sym9', and the *SURE* threshold were chosen to denoise ICA-detected artifacts in a single or many channels [29]. A five-level decomposition of the EEG wave was performed (the sampling rate of the current work was 256 *Hz*). After applying the threshold for each level, the noise on the denoised ICs of the artificial sets was eliminated. Then coefficients were recreated utilizing the inverse *DWT* (*IDWT*). The denoised components have been restored to the initial set of ICs.

The calculated ICA of the original, artifact-free EEG data was then reconstructed as $\hat{x}$ from the corrected ICs using the following:

$$\hat{x}(t) = A\hat{s}(t) \qquad (14.3)$$

where $\hat{s}(t)$ is the new matrix of ICs.

14.3.3 Features Extraction

EEG signals are regarded as a non-invasive, effective diagnostic measure that can provide a more accurate description of emotional state variations across brain regions [21, 23, 80]. Consequently, it is crucial to detect dementia early using EEG signals. The complex dynamics structure of EEG signals can be assessed through the extraction of nonlinear dynamical attributes from the EEGs to identify the most significant features that improve the detection of dementia based on EEG brain mapping [25, 26, 80].

Nonlinear entropy approaches, such as *FuzzEn*, *FDispEn*, and *BubbEn*, have been used to quantify information regarding brain function based on dementia differences. $N = 15360$ samples and 6 windows of 10 second length (2560 samples) were taken from the EEGs for each of 19 channels over the course of 60 seconds.

14.3.3.1 Fuzzy Entropy (*FuzzEn*)

FuzzyEn has been used to characterize several biomedical data, including electromyograms [81], EEGs, or modulations in the heart rate [19, 20]. Moreover, new research [19] reveals that *FuzzEn* is a reliable entropy estimator for studying biological signals with incomplete data.

Given N data points from a time series $x(n) = x(1), x(2), \ldots, x(N)$, the following algorithm can be used to obtain *FuzzEn* [12]:

1. Create m-vectors $X_m(1), X_m(2), \ldots, X_m(N - m + 1)$, where $X_m(i) = [x(i), x(i + 1), \ldots, x(i + m - 1)] - x0(i)$ for all in the range $1 \leq i \leq N - m + 1$.
   These vectors are a sequence of m consecutive x values, starting at the ith point with the baseline $\left(x_0(i) = \dfrac{1}{m}\sum_{j=0}^{m-1} x(i+j) \right)$ eliminated.

2. Define the distance between vectors $X_m(i)$ and $X_m(j)$, $d_{ij, m}$, as the biggest absolute difference between their scalar components.

3. Using fuzzy function, determine the similarity degree $D_{ij, m}$ of the vectors $X_m(i)$ and $X_m(j)$ given n and r:

$$D_{ij,m} = \mu\left(d_{ij,m}, r\right) = \exp\left(\frac{-\left(d_{ij,m}\right)^n}{r} \right) \qquad (14.4)$$

4. Specify the function φ_m as follows

$$\varphi_m(n,r) = \frac{1}{N-m}\sum_{i=1}^{N-m}\frac{1}{N-m-1}\sum_{j=1,j\neq i}^{N-m}D_{ij,m} \tag{14.5}$$

5. We extend the dimension to $m + 1$, create vectors $X_{m+1}(i)$, and then derive the function φ_{m+1} by repeating steps 2 through 4.
6. $FuzzEn$ can be computed for time series with a finite number of samples N using the following Eq. [81]:

$$FuzEn(m,n,r,N) = \ln\varphi_m(n,r) - \ln\varphi_{m+1}(n,r) \tag{14.6}$$

14.3.3.2 Fluctuation-Based Dispersion Entropy (*FDispEn*)

The entropy metric *DispEn* was developed lately for measuring the randomness of time series. It's fast, and it's performed well in describing time series thus far. In this research, we looked at how different mapping approaches affected *DispEn*'s performance.

The D*ispEn* algorithm is as follows, given a unilabiate signal $x(n) = x(1), x(2), \ldots,$ $x(N)$ of length N:

At the outset, we map $x_j(j = 1, 2, \ldots, N)$ to c classes with indices from 1 to c. $u_j(j = 1, 2, \ldots, N)$ is the signal that has been categorized.

With an embedding dimension m and a time delay of d, we may generate a series of timestamps denoted by $u_i^{m,c}$: $u_i^{m,c} = \left\{u_i^c, u_{i+d}^c, \ldots, u_{i+(m-1)d}^c\right\}, i = 1, 2, \ldots, N - (m-1)d$ [52, 53]. Each dispersion pattern $\pi_{v_0 v_1 \ldots v_{m-1}}$ allocated to the m elements of the vector $u_i^{m,c}$, where $u_i^c = \left\{v_0, u_{i+d}^c = v_1, \ldots, u_{i+(m-1)d}^c = v_{m-1}\right\}$ has a corresponding integer value between 1 and c [52].

The relative frequency for the c^m possible dispersion patterns $\pi_{v_0 v_1 \ldots v_{m-1}}$, is calculated as follows:

$$p\left(\pi_{v_0 v_1 \ldots v_{m-1}}\right) = \frac{\#\left\{i|,i \leq N-1(m-1)d|, u_i^{m,c} \text{ has } \pi_{v_0 \ldots v_{m-1}}\right\}}{N-(m-1)d} \tag{14.7}$$

where # means cardinality. $p\left(\pi_{v_0 v_1 \ldots v_{m-1}}\right)$ illustrates the number of *dispersion* patterns of $\pi_{v_0 v_1 \ldots v_{m-1}}$ that is given as $u_i^{m,c}$ divided by the total number of *embedded* signals with *embedding* dimension m.

At last, the *DispEn* value is computed as follows, in accordance with Shannon's notion of entropy:

$$DispEn(x,m,c,d) = -\sum_{\pi=1}^{c^m}p\left(\pi_{v_0 v_1 \ldots v_{m-1}}\right) \cdot \ln p\left(\pi_{v_0 v_1 \ldots v_{m-1}}\right) \tag{14.8}$$

In fact, *FDispEn* accounts the variations in behaviour between neighboring elements in adjacent element dispersion patterns, which are based on fluctuation. Thus, we obtain vectors of length $m - 1$ in which every element is a different value between $-c + 1$ and $c - 1$. Thus, there are $(2c - 1)^{m-1}$ potential dispersion patterns based on random fluctuation. The only distinction between the *DispEn* and *FDispEn* algorithms is the potential patterns employed by each technique. Note that the normalized *FDispEn* is represented as [50]

$$\frac{FDispEn}{\ln\left((2c-1)^{m-1}\right)} \tag{14.9}$$

14.3.3.3   Bubble Entropy (*BubbEn*)

BubbEn is created by applying a metric to the permutation approach, which calculates a rough estimate of the work involved in the latter method. Similar vectors are grouped together to reduce the time and effort required to calculate the conditional R'enyi entropy. We limit the number of distinct potential states and generate a coarser distribution based on intrinsic correlations using this method. A sorting algorithm's number of steps is used as the unit of measurement. To determine how many iterations of bubble sort are necessary to sort the vector in ascending order, we count the number of insertions and deletions in the process. We'll call this entropy Bubble Entropy (*BubbEn*). Next, we count the number of swaps $\left(H^m_{swaps}\right)$ needed to arrange the vectors in ascending order, and use that information to calculate the conditional R'enyi entropy of this distribution.

$$BubbleEn = \left(H^{m+1}_{swaps} - H^m_{swaps}\right) / \log\left(m + 1 / m - 1\right) \tag{14.10}$$

For embedding dimensions m and $\log(1 + m(m + 1)/2)$, respectively, the maximum entropy is $\log(1 + m(m - 1)/2)$, and the normalization factor is the difference between these two values. In each case, it indicates how many possible states there are when bubble sort permits swaps between 0 to $m(m - 1)/2$. The state in which no swaps were performed was ignored in order to simplify the normalization factor because it was not relevant for non-zero values of m. The computation of *BubbEn* is shown in pseudo-code below:

1. We use a counting method to determine how many swaps n_i are required to arrange each vector X_i of m elements in in descending order.
2. The probabilities p_i (describing the likelihood of a given number of swaps) n_i are calculated by normalizing the histogram of n_i values by $N - m + 1$.
3. When $\alpha = 2$, the entropy H^m_{swaps} swaps is calculated from p_i using the following Equation:

$$H_2(X) = -\log \sum_{i=1}^{n} p_i^2 \qquad (14.11)$$

4. Iterating steps 1–3, we find H_{swaps}^{m+1} swaps for vectors with $m + 1$ elements.
5. Using Eq. 14.11, we determine *BubbEn*.

14.3.4   Statistical Analysis

To do ANOVA, the denoising findings, nonlinear entropy feature results of the 19 channels from the EEG datasets of 15 *NC*, 15 *SMCI*, and 5 *VD* patients were preliminarily classified into 5 recording regions that related to the *scalp* region of the cortex. Regionally averaged features aided in taking into account the differences between the scalp regions, which can directly demonstrate the effects of dementia following a stroke in terms of a reduction in brain complexity and a slowing of cognitive function. These regions include the frontal cortex (seven channels: *Fp*1, *Fp*2, *F*3, *F*4, *F*7, *F*8, *and Fz*), the temporal cortex (four channels: *T*3, *T*4, *T*5, *and T*6), the parietal cortex (three channels: *P*3, *P*4, *and Pz*), the occipital cortex (two channels: *O*1 *and O*2), and the central cortex (three channels: *C*3, *C*4, *and Cz*).

In order to assess the efficacy of the *FuzzEn*, *FDispEn*, and *BubbEn* entropies, three sessions of *two − way* analysis of variance (*ANOVA*) were statistically analyzed to determine the level of EEG complexity across brain areas. Version 22 of the SPSS program from IBM USA was selected for statistical analysis.

In each of the three sessions, the nonlinear (*FuzzEn, FDispEn, and BubbEn*) features were dependent variables, whereas the group factor and the five groups of the scalp areas were independent factors. The group factor included *NC* healthy participants, *SMCI* patients who had recently suffered a stroke, and *VD* patients. Then, *Levene's* test for homoscedasticity and the *Kolmogorov − Smirnov* evaluations for normality were applied. *Duncan's* test was used to determine the *post − hoc* contrast, and $p < 0.05$ was established as the significance level for each statistical evaluation.

14.3.5   Preliminary Feature Processing Prior Classification

In this work, each EEG channel was divided into 6 epochs, and each epoch was given three entropy features (*FuzzEn*, *FDispEn* and *BubbEn*).

Before being applied to the classifier, the extracted features from the preceding step must undergo additional analysis. The "curse of dimensionality," or difficulties caused by a large number of possible feature combinations, and the resulting increase in processing time can be avoided by employing dimensionality reduction techniques. In order to avoid classifier overload, improve classification model accuracy, and reduce overfitting concerns, this research made use of *dimensionality reduction* techniques. Thus, these solutions are necessary to reduce the dimension of feature vectors.

The dimension of the feature matrix for healthy *NC* and *SMCI* was (90 × 57), (15 *subjects* × 6 *epochs*) = 90 observations and (3 *features* × 19 *channels*) = 57 attributes, whereas for *VD* patients, the dimension was (30 × 57), where (5 *VD* ×6 *epochs*) = 30 observations and (3 *features* × 19 *channels*) = 57 attributes. Therefore, *VD* is an unbalanced set of data that may affect the performance of proposed model. Learning from unbalanced datasets is problematic because the imbalance hinders the performance of the learning algorithms. Given that the *majority* of learning models assume a balanced class distribution, their outcomes tend to favour the dominant *class* whose *class* predictions are inaccurate. Class imbalance in the dataset has a substantial effect on the classification model's precision. However, because the minority class cannot be readily distinguished, the classifier can simply classify each instance as a member of the majority class.

In this study, patients with *VD* serve as an example of the minority class. To rectify the data imbalance, *SMOTE* (Synthetic Oversampling Technique) was employed [82]. In order to reduce *overfitting* and bias in the classification analysis [83], the parameters of the classifier and the amount of oversampling were determined through 10 − *fold* cross-validation and grid search. The supplied dataset was divided into ten distinct subsets of equal size. One of these subsets was used as the test set, while the remaining nine were used to teach the classifier. This method was executed ten times with 10 successful outcomes. The arithmetic mean of these precisions represents the 10 − *fold* cross-validation precision of this dataset's learning algorithm [84].

Because *SMOTE* modifies the dataset, the %age of oversampling has been added to the parameters. Therefore, parameters discovered with various *SMOTE* percentages may not be identical. The *SMOTE* was utilized to balance the class frequency using only the training set [85, 86].

14.3.6   Local Tangent Space Alignment (LTSA)

With its speed and relative insensitivity to parameter choice, the local tangent space alignment (LTSA) method has found widespread application in dimension reduction across a variety of disciplines. In the LTSA method, the coordinates from the local tangent space are combined with the low-dimensional global coordinates using the local radiological transformation matrix. Using the surrounding area as a sample, a tangent space at the local level is constructed. Given the data $x(n) = x(1)$, $x(2), ..., x(M) \subset R^{M \times N}$, the, principle of LTSA can be described as following [87]:

1. Create a set X_i consisting of the k nearest neighbors of each sample x_i selected using the k nearest neighbors algorithm, and normalize the results $\hat{X}_i$. It can be written as

$$\hat{X}_i = \left[x_{i,1}, x_{i,2}, \ldots, x_{i,k} \right] \tag{14.12}$$

$$\hat{X}_i = X_i - \overline{x}_i l_k^T \tag{14.13}$$

where $\overline{x}_i = \dfrac{1}{k}\sum_j^k x_{i,j}$ and l_k is a unit vector of length k.

2. Perform singular value decomposition to determine the eigenvalues and eigenvectors of the matrix $\hat{X}_i$.

The tangent space H_i is the set of eigenvectors associated with the first d largest singular values.

$$\theta_{ij} = H_i^T \left(x_{ij} - \overline{x}_i \right) \tag{14.14}$$

3. In order to preserve as much data as possible during transformation, we must build the matrix $L_i = \theta_i^+$, where

$$min\mu(\gamma) = min \sum_{i=1}^{M} \left| \gamma_i \left(1 - \frac{1}{k} ll^T \right) - L_i \theta_i \right| \tag{14.15}$$

where θ_i^+ represents the generalized inverse matrix of θ_i, Y_i represents the set of nearest neighbors of Y after dimension reduction, that is, $Y_i = (y_{i1}, y_{i2}, \ldots, y_{ik})$.

4. Once the optimization problem in the previous equation has been solved by determining the matrix's eigenvalues and eigenvectors, the embedding matrix Y can be derived. The analogous Equations to (17) are

$$min\mu(\gamma) = min(YHW) = mintr\left(YHW^T H^T Y^T\right), \tag{14.16}$$

$$\left\{ \begin{array}{c} H = (H_1, H_2, \ldots, H_M) \\ W = diag(W_1, W_2, \ldots, W_M) \\ W_i = \left(I - \dfrac{1}{k} ll^T \right)(I - \theta_i^+ \theta_i) \\ I = YY^T \end{array} \right\}$$

The low-dimensional embedding matrix Y is obtained by computing the eigenvectors that correspond to the second through d^{th} smallest eigenvalues of the alignment matrix B.

$$B = HWW^T H^T \tag{14.17}$$

14.3.7   Dementia Classification Techniques

A thorough analysis of the EEG data was done to classify the individuals' cognitive and mental disability into three groups (NC, *SMCI*, and *VD*). The caliber of the generated features has a significant impact on classifier precision. As a result, the choice of *dimensionality reduction* techniques and the kind of classifier can both have an impact on how accurate the results of the classification are. Three popular methods for categorizing brain illnesses were used in this study: *k*NN, *SVM*, and *DT*.

The parameter *k* must be specified for the *k*NN classifier. The value of *k* was altered between 1 and 9 at 2-point intervals. The classifier was trained to determine the optimal value of *k*, and $k = 5$ was selected empirically. As a measure of similarity for classifying each trial using *k*NN, the Euclidean distance was computed.

Using ten-fold cross-validation to optimize the complexity parameter *C* with a range of $-4 \leq \log_{10}(C) \leq 4$ in *C* values $C \in \{0.0001, 0.001, 0.01, 0.1, 0, 10, 100, 1000, 10000\}$ on the training set produced optimal results for the *SVM* classifier. During testing, *C* equal to 10 yielded the best outcomes for *C* values. Based on the radial basis function (*RBF*) kernel, multi-class *SVM* classifiers were implemented. In addition, the training dataset was utilized to calculate the minimum mis-classification rate, which aided in obtaining the smoothing σ value for *SVM* training. The only way to determine the optimal value is by methodically varying during multiple training sessions. As a result, the σ value in this study was changed between 0.1 and 1 at intervals of 0.1. It was determined that a σ value of 0.5 corresponds to the lowest mis-classification rate [19, 22, 28, 32, 44, 88].

In addition, the *DT* classification tree model was utilized. It employs a recursive partitioning algorithm that generates nodes depending on certain criteria for splitting. The produced and divided nodes are then used to grow a tree. To use the split criteria, the optimal split point must be identified. The quality of the splitting criteria is measured by a function derived from the variance function. The optimal point for splitting is determined by a function that is applied to every split point beginning with binary splits and evaluating them based on an optimization criterion. Gini's diversity index has been used as an optimization criterion in this work. When the classification tree reaches the pure node, it stops partitioning the instance space; a node is pure if it contains only observations of one *class* [89]. 50 trees have been employed as the parameter for identifying *VD*, *SMCI*, and *NC* EEG signals using *DT*.

The *performance* of the suggested *framework* was assessed using the *average* classification accuracy reported as a percentage and the confusion matrix, which enabled to determination the effects of dementia recognition enhancement.

14.4 Results and Discussion

Utilizing the novel, 100% automatic AICA-WT denoising technique presented in [19], the EEG dataset was successfully denoised. In our previous investigations [19, 27, 28], we statistically analyzed the differences between the linear spectral distributions of EEG slowing in *VD* patients, *SMCI* patients, and healthy *NC* subjects. The training process is where the most important design decisions for the *k*NN, *SVM*, and *DT* classifiers are made, as they are based on the test set and training set sizes. However, the classifiers employed in this work were trained on the same training data set and assessed on the testing data set in order to compare the performance of the suggested classifiers.

14.4.1 Results of Preprocessing Stage

Compared to the original EEG recording, the artifactual components (red color) were successfully and adequately suppressed (blue color). As depicted in Fig. 14.3, the ocular artifacts were effectively inhibited in *Ch*2 (which represents F8 from the *frontal* region).

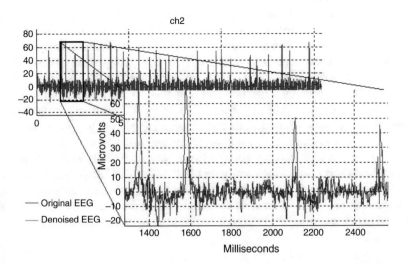

Fig. 14.3 The outcomes of applying the AICA–WT approach to EEG Ch2, which represents F8, to remove ocular artifact

14.4.2   Results of Dementia Recognition by Statistical Analysis

The brain states of *SMCI* patients with *VD* and *SMCI* were distinguished from those of healthy *NC* participants using *FuzzEn*, *FDispEn* and *BubbEn*. Table 14.2 presents a comparative average mean values of the three used entropies which are estimated over five scalp regions for the *VD* patients, *SMCI* patients, and healthy *NC* subjects.

The *VD*s exhibited lower complexity than the *SMCI*s and healthy *NC*s ($FuzzEn_{VaD}$ $< FuzzEn_{MCI} < FuzzEn_{NC}$) with significant differences were observed for the *NC* subjects ($p < 0.05$), ($FDispEn_{VaD} < FDispEn_{MCI} < FDispEn_{NC}$) and ($BubbEn_{VaD} < BubbEn_{MCI} < BubbEn_{NC}$) observable differences were identified between the *VD* patients and the *NC*. In line with expectations, the *complexity* of EEG signals decreases with increasing illness severity, especially in those with *SMCI* and *VD*.

The multiple comparisons have been looked at using the *Bonferroni post hoc* test. The *post − hoc* dementia multiple comparisons using *Bonferroni* corrections for the *FuzzEn*, *FDispEn*, and *BubbEn* characteristics are displayed in Table 14.3. The *NC* was statistically significant from *VD* ($p = 0.05$) and *SMCI* was statistically significant from *VD* ($p = 0.01$) for the *FuzzEn*, according to post hoc testing using the *Bonferroni* correction.

Additionally, the *SMCI* was statistically significant from *VD* for the *FDispEn* according to post hoc tests with the *Bonferroni* correction ($p = 0.023$).

Additionally, the *post hoc* analyses employing the *Bonferroni* correction for the BubbEn indicated statistically significant differences, especially for *VD*. The statistical difference between the *VD* and the *NC* was 0.05, while the statistical difference between the *VD* and the *SMCI* was 0.003.

Table 14.2 Lists the average values for *FuzzEn*, *FDispEn* and *BubbEn* across all five scalp regions for patients with *VD*, *SMCI*, and *NC* participants. An asterisk indicates differences between groups that are significant

Features	DSC	Frontal	Temporal	Parietal	Occipital	Central	*p*-value
FuzzEn	NC	1.147 ± 0.212	1.203 ± 0.171	1.03 ± 0.133	1.236 ± 0.197	1.09 ± 0.171	0.05*
	SMCI	1.08 ± 0.226	1.115 ± 0.264	1.015 ± 0.172	1.086 ± 0.196	1.038 ± 0.205	0.169
	VD	1.079 ± 0.204	1.056 ± 0.191	0.957 ± 0.151	1.073 ± 0.137	0.964 ± 0.254	0.653
FDispEn	NC	2.365 ± 0.388	2.514 ± 0.337	2.302 ± 0.243	2.276 ± 0.348	2.525 ± 0.329	0.114
	SMCI	2.333 ± 0.514	2.397 ± 0.524	2.249 ± 0.454	2.228 ± 0.506	2.352 ± 0.477	0.187
	VD	2.222 ± 0.398	2.29 ± 0.332	2.25 ± 0.33	2.111 ± 0.311	2.384 ± 0.302	0.163
BubbEn	NC	0.611 ± 0.033	0.609 ± 0.031	0.597 ± 0.027	0.601 ± 0.049	0.609 ± 0.037	0.011*
	SMCI	0.596 ± 0.039	0.592 ± 0.041	0.586 ± 0.046	0.576 ± 0.048	0.579 ± 0.04	0.921
	VD	0.592 ± 0.03	0.59 ± 0.035	0.59 ± 0.043	0.585 ± 0.032	0.593 ± 0.021	0.047*

Table 14.3 *VD*, *SMCI* patients and the *NC* subjects multiple comparison test using *Bonferroni* for *FuzzEn*, *FDispEn* and *BubbEn* entropy features

Dependent Variable	(I) DSC	(J) DSC	Mean Difference (I-J)	*p*-valuea
FuzzEn	NC	SMCI	−0.036	0.158
		VD	−0.113*	0.05
	SMCI	VD	−0.077*	0.01
FDispEn	NC	SMCI	0.06	0.344
		VD	−0.084	0.358
	SMCI	VD	−0.145*	0.023
BubbEn	NC	SMCI	−0.004	0.709
		VD	−0.020*	0.05
	SMCI	VD	−0.016*	0.003

*The mean difference is significant at the 0.05 level

14.4.3 Results of Dementia Recognition by Classification and Performance Measure

Figure 14.4 displays the *confusion matrix* for *VD*, *SMCI* patients and healthy *NC* subjects identification from EEGs using *FuzzEn* with *k*NN, *SVM* and *DT* classifiers, respectively, the correct recognition is observed on the diagonal whereas the off-diagonal represent the substitution errors.

The confusion matrix's two diagonal cells, as shown in Fig. 14.4 using *FuzzEn*, display the %age of correctly classified data from the *k*NN classifier. For instance, 93.33% of the time, *VD* and *SMCI* are correctly categorized. Likewise, all are accurately identified as *NC* subjects (100%) while 5.56% of *VD* are misclassified as *SMCI*, and 1.11% of *VD* and *SMCI* are misclassified as *NC* healthy patients.

Moreover, the *SVM* classifier results show that *VD* and *SMCI* are correctly classified with 64.44% and 97.78%, respectively. Like *NC* subjects, 100% are correctly classified, 28.89% of *VD* are incorrectly classified as *SMCI*, and 6.67% of *VD* and 2.22% of *SMCI* are incorrectly classified as *NC* healthy subjects, respectively.

Additionally, for the *DT* classifier, the confusion matrix shows that the *VD* and *SMCI* are correctly classified with 86.67% and 12.22%, respectively. Similarly, *NC* subjects are correctly classified, whereas 13.33% of *VD* and *SMCI* are incorrectly classified as *NC* healthy subjects. By contrast, 51.11% and 36.67% of *SMCI* are classified as *VD* and *NC* subjects, respectively.

The confusion matrix for *VD*, *SMCI* patients, and healthy *NC* subjects identification from EEG background signals using *DispEn* with *k*NN, *SVM*, and *DT* classifiers, respectively, are presented in Fig. 14.5.

Figure 14.5 illustrates the proportion of correct classification from the *k*NN classifier using *DispEn*. With 97.78% accuracy, *VD* and *SMCI*, whereas *NC* healthy patients are correctly classified with 100%. Similarly, 2.22% of *VD* are wrongly labeled as *SMCI* patients.

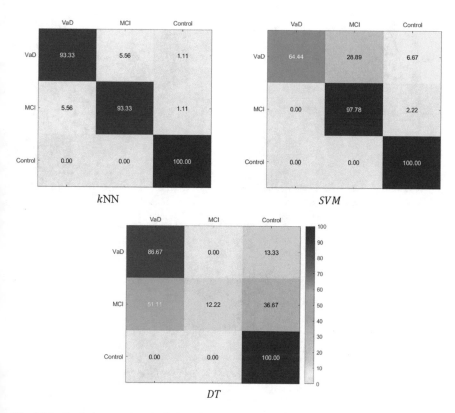

Fig. 14.4 *Confusion matrix* calculations for *VD, SMCI,* and *NC* from EEGs using *FuzzEn* and *k*NN, *SVM,* and *DT* classifiers

Furthermore, *VD, SMCI* and *NC* are appropriately diagnosed with 98.98%, 95.56% and 100%, respectively, according to the *SVM* classifier results. 1.11% of *VD* are incorrectly classified as *SMCI,* but 4.44% of *SMCI* are wrongly classified as *VD.*

VD are accurately categorized with 18.89%, whereas 81.11% of *VD* are mistakenly labeled as *SMCI* patients and healthy *NC* subjects. Similarly, *SMCI* are accurately classified with 86.67% and 13.33% wrongly labeled as *VD* patients and *NC* subjects, respectively.

NC participants are accurately classified with 91.11% but incorrectly classified as *SMCI* by 8.89%.

Figure 14.6 shows the confusion matrix for identifying *VD, SMCI* patients, and healthy *NC* participants from EEG background signals using *BubbEn* with *k*NN, *SVM,* and *DT* classifiers, respectively. On the diagonal, correct recognition is shown, whereas substitution errors are shown off-diagonal.

The proportion of correct classification from the *k*NN classifier utilizing *BubbEn* is shown in Fig. 14.6, *VD* and *SMCI* are correctly categorized with 96.67% accuracy, while *SMCI* and healthy individuals are correctly classified with 100%

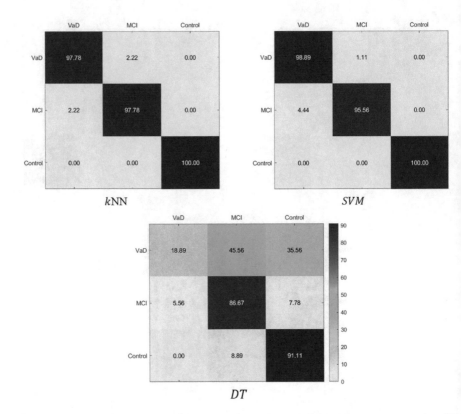

Fig. 14.5 *Confusion matrix* calculations for *VD*, *SMCI*, and *NC* from EEGs using *DispEn* and *k*NN, *SVM*, and *DT* classifiers

accuracy. Similarly, 1.11% and 2.22% of *VD* patients are mistakenly identified as *SMCI* patients and *NC* subjects, respectively.

Furthermore, according to the *SVM* classifier results, *VD*, *SMCI*, and *NC* are correctly diagnosed with 93.33% and 100%, respectively. *VD* is improperly diagnosed as *SMCI* in 1.11% and 5.56% as *NC*.

VD, *SMCI* and *NC* are correctly classified with 82.22%, 80% and 91.11%, respectively. Notably, 17.78% of *VD* are mislabeled as *SMCI* patients and healthy *NC* participants. Similarly, *SMCI* are incorrectly categorized, with only 20% mislabeled as *VD* patients and *NC* participants, respectively. With 8.89% accuracy, *NC* individuals are incorrectly classified as *VD* and *SMCI* patients.

To determine how well the LTSA *dimensionality reduction* technique works with the *k*NN, *SVM*, and *DT* classifiers, a comparative research has been done. The most accurate classifications of *VD*, *SMCI*, and *NC* patients were made using LTSA and *k*NN, in that order. Therefore, the effect of the *FuzzEn*, *FDispEn* and *BubbEn* entropies have been examine without applying the LTSA algorithm individually as shown in Fig. 14.7.

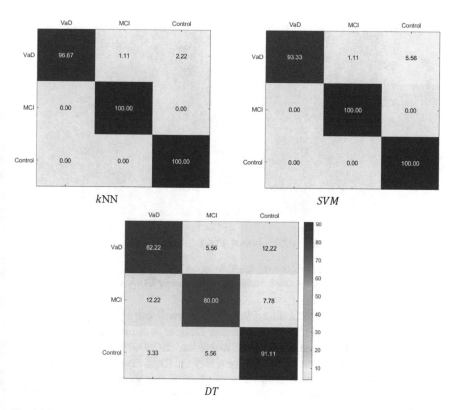

Fig. 14.6 *Confusion matrix* calculations for *VD*, *SMCI*, and *NC* from EEGs using *BubbEn* and *k*NN, *SVM*, and *DT* classifiers

The EEG-based dementia detection framework was evaluated in *MATLAB R*2021*a* on a laptop equipped with a 1.80 *GHz* and 1.99 *GHz* Intel *Core i*7 − 8550*U* processor, 16.0 *GB* of RAM, and a 64 − *bit* operating system.

The comparison of the proposed method with existing methodologies is shown in Table 14.4. Studies have used feature selection and dimensionality reduction techniques to estimate the optimal features. In order to improve the ability to identify *VD* and *SMCI* using EEGs, this study offers an automatic dementia recognition model employing the unique AICA-WT-*BubbEn*-LTSA dementia recognition framework. With the suggested strategy, the classification accuracy of *k*NN, *SVM*, and *DT* has improved somewhat. However, *VD* and *SMCI* recognition from *NC* subjects using the *BubbEn*-LTSA mapping process is the first to be taken into consideration in this study in order to maintain the best quality of features that enhanced the classification accuracy of *VD* and *SMCI* from *NC* subjects. These methods have also been used to study EEGs. Furthermore, the EEG dataset elicitation technique and the EEG estimate system have never been used for securing sensation information, which may make dementia contrasts more clear.

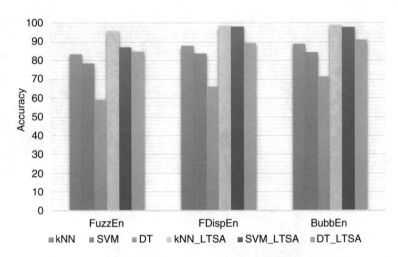

Fig. 14.7 Average accuracy (%) for the *k*NN, *SVM*, and *DT* classifiers as calculated from the *FuzzEn*, *FDispEn* and *BubbEn* entropies with and without using LTSA algorithm

This study has some limitations, including a small sample size and the need for a follow-up analysis with a larger database. Despite this, more research based on real-time online experiments is required to validate the results due to the differences between offline and online categorizations. Despite these caveats, the results of The findings of this study concur with those of other investigations showing that EEG signals can be used to distinguish between those with *VD*, *SMCI* and *NC* [3, 4, 30, 99, 100].

14.5   Conclusion

The pre-processing stage of the EEG datasets of 15 *SMCI* patients had mild cognitive *SMCI*, 15 *NC*, and 5 patients suffering *VD* involved the use of conventional filters and the novel AICA-WT method to denoise the data on WM task. Inh the next stage, the *complexity* and irregularity changes from EEGs have been investigated using the *FuzzEn*, *FDispEn*, and *BubbEn* characteristics. Additionally, the statistical analysis of the EEG complexity across the different brain regions has been done using ANOVA. Then, the nonlinear LTSA dimensionality reduction approach has utilized to enhance the automatic diagnosis of *VD* patients'. *k*-nearest neighbors (*k*NN), support vector machine (*SVM*), and decision tree (*DT*) classifiers have been performed in the final stage. The effectiveness of *FuzzEn*, *FDispEn*, and *BubbEn* have been compared, and the findings demonstrate that *BubbEn* is the technique that consistently separates *VD*, *SMCI* patients, and *NC* from the EEG signals. In order to create the innovative AICA-WT-*BubbEn*-LTSA dementia recognition framework, BubbEn has been chosen to construct a new BubbEn-LTSA mapping approach. The

Table 14.4 Comparative study of the suggested approach to the state-of-the-art

Study	EEG Dataset	Features types	Method	Classifiers	Best Accuracy (%)
Kortelainen et al. [56]	BPF	Frequency domain	SFFS	*kNN*	65
P. Ackermann et al. [61]	BPF	Statistical	mRMR	*SVM*, RF	*SVM* (55)
Al-Qazzaz et al. [45]	Conventional filtering, AICA-WT	*SpecEn, ApEn, PerEn*	IBGSA	*kNN*	90.52
Al-Qazzaz et al. [44]	SG	*RCMDE*	DEFS_Ch	*SVM*	95.24
H. Cai et al. [90]	BPF, Kalman	*Relative and Absolute* frequency, *Relative and absolute* power, CD, Entropy	*Correlation-*based method, *Wrapper* based method, *PCA*	*SVM* (RBF), RF, LR, *kNN, DT*	*DT* (76.4)
H. Cai et al. [91]	FIR, Kalman with DWT, Adaptive-Predictor Filter (APF)	Relative and absolute power, *Hjorth* parameters (*activity, mobility, complexity*), Shannon Entropy, SE, CD, Peak , Kurtosis, Skewness	Minimal-redundancy-maximal-relevance	*kNN, SVM, DT*	*kNN* (79.27)
Y. Li et al. [92]	Notch filter, LPF, HPF	AR model + max-power spectrum density, and Sum power, CD, Kolmogorov-Entropy (KE), Shannon Entropy, *PerEn*, LLE, Singular-Value Deposition Entropy (SVDE), Variance, Mean-square (*MS*), Mean of Peak-to-Peak (*P2P*)	Differential evolution	*kNN*	*kNN* (98.40)
H. Peng et al. [93]	BPF	Phase lag index (*PLI*), *alpha, beta, delta, and theta*	Kendall's tau coefficient	*SVM*, KNN, *DT*, NB	*SVM* (92.73)
S. Mahato et al. [94]	BPF	Asymmetry and paired asymmetry of *gamma*1, *gamma*2, *beta, alpha, theta, delta,* DFA, SE	ReliefF	Bagging, *SVM* (kernels such as polynomial,	*SVM* (96.02)

(continued)

Table 14.4 (continued)

Study	EEG Dataset	Features types	Method	Classifiers	Best Accuracy (%)
J. Zhu et al. [95]	LPF, HPF	AR model + Power-Spectrum Density (PSD), AR model + max-power spectrum density, and Sumpower, CD, Kolmogorov-Entropy (KE), Shannon Entropy, *PerEn*, Singular-Value Deposition Entropy (SVDE), Mean-square (MS), Mean of Peak-to-Peak (P2P)	Correlation Feature Selection	LR, *k*NN, RF, *SVM*, BayesNet, *NB*, J48	*k*NN (92.65)
R. A. Movahed et al. [96]	LPF, HPF	Synchronization likelihood (SL), Higuchi-Fractal Dimension (HFD), Detrended-Fluctuation Analysis (DFA), CD, Kolmogorov-Entropy (KE), Shannon Entropy, LLE, Kurtosis, Skewness, *DWT*, Relative-Wavelet Energy (*RWE*), Wavelet-Entropy (*WE*)	Sequential Backward Feature Selection (SBFS)	*SVM (RBF)*, LR, *DT*, *NB*, *RB*, *GB*, *RF*	*SVM* (99)
Narayan et al. [97]	BPF(8 to 30) Hz, notch filter, ICA	CSP	*PCA*	*SVM*, LDA	*SVM* (98.8)
Al-Qazzaz et al. [98]	Emotion	Entropy	*ESD*	*k*NN, *SVM*, RF	*SVM* (87.64)
Our Proposed Method (AICA-WT-*BubbEn*-LTSA)	Conventional filtering, AICA-WT	*FuzzEn*, *FDispEn* and *BubbEn*	LTSA	*k*NN	98.89
				SVM	91.11
				DT	98.89

unique AICA-WT-*BubbEn*-LTSA detection has improved automated *VD* dementia recognition, and it may be a potential framework for enhancing the distinction between *VD* and *SMCI* patients and *NC* participants.

References

1. C. Iadecola et al., Vascular cognitive impairment and dementia: JACC scientific expert panel. J. Am. Coll. Cardiol. **73**(25), 3326–3344 (2019)
2. N.K. Al-Qazzaz et al., Cognitive assessments for the early diagnosis of dementia after stroke. Neuropsychiatr. Dis. Treat. **10**, 1743 (2014)
3. N.K. Al-Qazzaz et al., Cognitive impairment and memory dysfunction after a stroke diagnosis: A post-stroke memory assessment. Neuropsychiatr. Dis. Treat. **10**, 1677 (2014)
4. N.K. Al-Qazzaz et al., Role of EEG as biomarker in the early detection and classification of dementia. Sci. World J. **2014**, 906038 (2014)
5. A.D. Korczyn, V. Vakhapova, L.T. Grinberg, Vascular dementia. J. Neurol. Sci. **322**(1–2), 2–10 (2012)
6. T.B. Cumming, R.S. Marshall, R.M. Lazar, Stroke, cognitive deficits, and rehabilitation: Still an incomplete picture. Int. J. Stroke **8**(1), 38–45 (2013)
7. S. Ankolekar et al., Clinical trials for preventing post stroke cognitive impairment. J. Neurol. Sci. **299**(1–2), 168–174 (2010)
8. A. Cedazo-Minguez, B. Winblad, Biomarkers for Alzheimer's disease and other forms of dementia: Clinical needs, limitations and future aspects. Exp. Gerontol. **45**(1), 5–14 (2010)
9. H. Hampel et al., Biomarkers for Alzheimer's disease: Academic, industry and regulatory perspectives. Nat. Rev. Drug Discov. **9**(7), 560–574 (2010)
10. S.T. DeKosky, K. Marek, Looking backward to move forward: Early detection of neurodegenerative disorders. Science **302**(5646), 830–834 (2003)
11. S.-S. Poil et al., Integrative EEG biomarkers predict progression to Alzheimer's disease at the MCI stage. Front. Aging Neurosci. **5**, 58 (2013)
12. J. Escudero et al., Assessment of classification improvement in patients with Alzheimer's disease based on magnetoencephalogram blind source separation. Artif. Intell. Med. **43**(1), 75–85 (2008)
13. C. Gómez, et al., Magnetoencephalogram background activity analysis in Alzheimer's disease patients using auto mutual information. in *Engineering in medicine and biology society, 2006. EMBS'06. 28th Annual International Conference of the IEEE.* (IEEE 2006)
14. R. Hornero et al., Nonlinear analysis of electroencephalogram and magnetoencephalogram recordings in patients with Alzheimer's disease. Philos. Trans. R. Soc. A Math. Phys. Eng. Sci. **2009**(367), 317–336 (1887)
15. R. Hornero et al., Spectral and nonlinear analyses of MEG background activity in patients with Alzheimer's disease. IEEE Trans. Biomed. Eng. **55**(6), 1658–1665 (2008)
16. P.R. Davidson, R.D. Jones, M.T. Peiris, EEG-based lapse detection with high temporal resolution. IEEE Trans. Biomed. Eng. **54**(5), 832–839 (2007)
17. F. Vecchio et al., Resting state cortical EEG rhythms in Alzheimer's disease: Toward EEG markers for clinical applications: A review. Suppl. Clin. Neurophysiol. **62**, 223–236 (2012)
18. J. Jeong, EEG dynamics in patients with Alzheimer's disease. Clin. Neurophysiol. **115**(7), 1490–1505 (2004)
19. N.K. Al-Qazzaz et al., Automatic artifact removal in EEG of normal and demented individuals using ICA–WT during working memory tasks. Sensors **17**(6), 1326 (2017)
20. P. Nguyen, et al. *Age and gender classification using EEG paralinguistic features.* in *2013 6th International IEEE/EMBS Conference on Neural Engineering (NER).* IEEE. (2013)
21. N.K. Al-Qazzaz et al., Electroencephalogram profiles for emotion identification over the brain regions using spectral, entropy and temporal biomarkers. Sensors **20**(1), 59 (2020)
22. N.K. Al-Qazzaz, M.K. Sabir, and K. Grammer. *Gender differences identification from brain regions using spectral relative powers of emotional EEG.* in *IWBBIO 2019* (2019)
23. N.K. Al-Qazzaz, M.K. Sabir, and K. Grammer. *Correlation indices of electroencephalogram-based relative powers during human emotion processing.* in *Proceedings of the 2019 9th international conference on biomedical engineering and technology.* (ACM 2019)

24. N.K. Al-Qazzaz, et al. *Effective EEG channels for emotion identification over the brain regions using differential evolution algorithm.* in *2019 41th annual international conference of the IEEE engineering in medicine and biology society (EMBC).* (IEEE 2019)

25. Al-Qazzaz, N.K., et al. *Stroke-related mild cognitive impairment detection during working memory tasks using EEG signal processing.* in *2017 fourth international conference on advances in biomedical engineering (ICABME).* (IEEE 2017)

26. Al-Qazzaz, N.K., et al. *Classification enhancement for post-stroke dementia using fuzzy neighborhood preserving analysis with QR-decomposition.* in *2017 39th annual international conference of the IEEE engineering in medicine and biology society (EMBC).* (IEEE 2017)

27. N.K. Al-Qazzaz et al., Discrimination of stroke-related mild cognitive impairment and vascular dementia using EEG signal analysis. Med. Biol. Eng. Comput. 56, 137–157 (2018)

28. N.K. Al-Qazzaz, S.H.M. Ali, and S.A. Ahmad. *Comparison of the effectiveness of AICA-WT technique in discriminating vascular dementia EEGs.* in *2018 2nd international conference on BioSignal analysis, processing and systems (ICBAPS).* (IEEE 2018)

29. N. Al-Qazzaz et al., Selection of mother wavelet functions for multi-channel EEG signal analysis during a working memory task. Sensors 15(11), 29015–29035 (2015)

30. N.K. Al-Qazzaz et al., Selection of mother wavelets thresholding methods in denoising multi-channel EEG signals during working memory task, in *Biomedical Engineering and Sciences (IECBES), 2014 IEEE Conference on,* (IEEE, 2014)

31. N. Bajaj et al., Automatic and tunable algorithm for EEG artifact removal using wavelet decomposition with applications in predictive modeling during auditory tasks. Biomed. Signal Proc. Control 55, 101624 (2020)

32. N.K. Al-Qazzaz et al., Discrimination of stroke-related mild cognitive impairment and vascular dementia using EEG signal analysis. Med. Biol. Eng. Comput. 56(1), 137–157 (2018)

33. S. Xie, S. Krishnan, Wavelet-based sparse functional linear model with applications to EEGs seizure detection and epilepsy diagnosis. Med. Biol. Eng. Comput. 51(1–2), 49–60 (2013)

34. D. Abásolo et al., Entropy analysis of the EEG background activity in Alzheimer's disease patients. Physiol. Meas. 27(3), 241 (2006)

35. N.K. Al-Qazzaz, et al. *EEG markers for early detection and characterization of vascular dementia during working memory tasks.* in *Biomedical engineering and sciences (IECBES), 2016 IEEE EMBS conference on.* 2016. (IEEE 2016)

36. N.K. Al-Qazzaz et al., EEG wavelet spectral analysis during a working memory tasks in stroke-related mild cognitive impairment patients, in *International Conference for Innovation in Biomedical Engineering and Life Sciences,* (Springer, 2016)

37. N.K. Al-Qazzaz et al., Entropy-based markers of EEG background activity of stroke-related mild cognitive impairment and vascular dementia patients, in *2nd International Conference on Sensors Engineering and Electronics Instrumental Advances (SEIA 2016),* (Barcelona, 2016)

38. J. Selvaraj et al., Classification of emotional states from electrocardiogram signals: A nonlinear approach based on Hurst. Biomed. Eng. Online 12(1), 44 (2013)

39. O. Sourina and Y. Liu. *A fractal-based algorithm of emotion recognition from EEG using arousal-valence model.* in *Biosignals* (2011)

40. N.K. Al-Qazzaz, et al. *EEG markers for early detection and characterization of vascular dementia during working memory tasks.* in *2016 IEEE EMBS Conference on Biomedical Engineering and Sciences (IECBES).* IEEE (2016)

41. B. García-Martínez et al., Application of entropy-based metrics to identify emotional distress from electroencephalographic recordings. Entropy 18(6), 221 (2016)

42. N. Thammasan et al., Continuous music-emotion recognition based on electroencephalogram. IEICE Trans. Inf. Syst. 99(4), 1234–1241 (2016)

43. W.-L. Zheng, J.-Y. Zhu, B.-L. Lu, Identifying stable patterns over time for emotion recognition from EEG. IEEE Trans. Affect. Comput. 10, 417–429 (2017)

44. N.K. Al-Qazzaz, S.H.M. Ali, and S.A. Ahmad. *Differential evolution based channel selection algorithm on eeg signal for early detection of vascular dementia among stroke survi-*

vors. in *2018 IEEE-EMBS conference on biomedical engineering and sciences (IECBES)*. (IEEE 2018)

45. N.K. Al-Qazzaz et al., Optimal EEG Channel selection for vascular dementia identification using improved binary gravitation search algorithm, in *International Conference for Innovation in Biomedical Engineering and Life Sciences*, (Springer, 2017)

46. A. Freeman et al., Inclusion of sex and gender in biomedical research: Survey of clinical research proposed at the University of Pennsylvania. Biol. Sex Differ. **8**(1), 22 (2017)

47. P. Wang, J. Hu, A hybrid model for EEG-based gender recognition. Cogn. Neurodyn. **13**(6), 541–554 (2019)

48. J. Tian, Z. Luo, Motor imagery EEG feature extraction based on fuzzy entropy. J. Huazhong Univ. Sci. Technol. **41**, 92–95 (2013)

49. Y. Cao et al., *Characterization of complexity in the electroencephalograph activity of Alzheimer's disease based on fuzzy entropy.* Chaos: An interdisciplinary. J. Nonlinear Sci. **25**(8), 083116 (2015)

50. H. Azami, J. Escudero, Amplitude-and fluctuation-based dispersion entropy. Entropy **20**(3), 210 (2018)

51. J.S. Richman, J.R. Moorman, Physiological time-series analysis using approximate entropy and sample entropy. Am. J. Physiol. Heart Circ. Physiol. **278**, H2039–H2049 (2000)

52. M. Rostaghi, H. Azami, Dispersion entropy: A measure for time-series analysis. IEEE Signal Proc. Letters **23**(5), 610–614 (2016)

53. C. Bandt, B. Pompe, Permutation entropy: A natural complexity measure for time series. Phys. Rev. Lett. **88**(17), 174102 (2002)

54. G. Manis, M. Aktaruzzaman, R. Sassi, Bubble entropy: An entropy almost free of parameters. IEEE Trans. Biomed. Eng. **64**(11), 2711–2718 (2017)

55. W. Chen et al., Measuring complexity using fuzzyen, apen, and sampen. Med. Eng. Phys. **31**(1), 61–68 (2009)

56. J. Kortelainen and T. Seppänen. *EEG-based recognition of video-induced emotions: Selecting subject-independent feature set.* in *2013 35th annual international conference of the IEEE engineering in medicine and biology society (EMBC).* (IEEE 2013)

57. Z. Wang, Z. Zhang, W. Wang, Emotion recognition based on framework of badeba-svm. Math. Probl. Eng. **2019**, 1–9 (2019)

58. H. Ullah et al., Internal emotion classification using EEG signal with sparse discriminative ensemble. IEEE Access **7**, 40144–40153 (2019)

59. B. Nakisa et al., Evolutionary computation algorithms for feature selection of EEG-based emotion recognition using mobile sensors. Expert Syst. Appl. **93**, 143–155 (2018)

60. J. Atkinson, D. Campos, Improving BCI-based emotion recognition by combining EEG feature selection and kernel classifiers. Expert Syst. Appl. **47**, 35–41 (2016)

61. P. Ackermann, et al. *EEG-based automatic emotion recognition: Feature extraction, selection and classification methods.* in *2016 IEEE 18th international conference on e-health networking, applications and services (Healthcom).* (IEEE 2016)

62. A. Subasi, M. Ismail Gursoy, EEG signal classification using PCA, ICA, LDA and support vector machines. Expert Syst. Appl. **37**(12), 8659–8666 (2010)

63. C. Vidaurre et al., Time domain parameters as a feature for EEG-based brain–computer interfaces. Neural Netw. **22**(9), 1313–1319 (2009)

64. M. Murugappan, N. Ramachandran, Y. Sazali, Classification of human emotion from EEG using discrete wavelet transform. J. Biomed. Sci. Eng. **3**(04), 390 (2010)

65. D. Lagun et al., Detecting cognitive impairment by eye movement analysis using automatic classification algorithms. J. Neurosci. Methods **201**(1), 196–203 (2011)

66. W.A. Chaovalitwongse, Y.-J. Fan, R.C. Sachdeo, On the time series k-nearest neighbor classification of abnormal brain activity. IEEE Trans. Syst. Man Cybern. Part A Syst. Hum. **37**(6), 1005–1016 (2007)

67. D. Abásolo, et al. *Approximate entropy and mutual information analysis of the electroencephalogram in Alzheimer's disease patients.* in *Advances in medical, signal and information processing, 2006. MEDSIP 2006. IET 3rd international conference on* (IET 2006)

68. J. Escudero et al., Analysis of electroencephalograms in Alzheimer's disease patients with multiscale entropy. Physiol. Meas. **27**(11), 1091 (2006)

69. D. Abásolo et al., Approximate entropy and auto mutual information analysis of the electroencephalogram in Alzheimer's disease patients. Med. Biol. Eng. Comput. **46**(10), 1019–1028 (2008)

70. E. Bullmore, O. Sporns, Complex brain networks: Graph theoretical analysis of structural and functional systems. Nat. Rev. Neurosci. **10**(3), 186–198 (2009)

71. X. Jie, R. Cao, L. Li, Emotion recognition based on the sample entropy of EEG. Biomed. Mater. Eng. **24**(1), 1185–1192 (2014)

72. T. Brott et al., Measurements of acute cerebral infarction: A clinical examination scale. Stroke **20**(7), 864–870 (1989)

73. M.F. Folstein, L.N. Robins, J.E. Helzer, The mini-mental state examination. Arch Gen Psychiatry **40**, 812 (1983)

74. T. Smith, N. Gildeh, C. Holmes, The Montreal cognitive assessment: Validity and utility in a memory clinic setting. Can. J. Psychiatr. **52**(5), 329 (2007)

75. J. Escudero, et al., Blind source separation to enhance spectral and non-linear features of magnetoencephalogram recordings. Application to Alzheimer's disease. Med. Eng. Phys., 2009. 31(7): p. 872–879

76. G. Barbati et al., Optimization of an independent component analysis approach for artifact identification and removal in magnetoencephalographic signals. Clin. Neurophysiol. **115**(5), 1220–1232 (2004)

77. C.J. James, C.W. Hesse, Independent component analysis for biomedical signals. Physiol. Meas. **26**(1), R15 (2005)

78. J. Escudero et al., Artifact removal in magnetoencephalogram background activity with independent component analysis. Biomed. Eng. IEEE Trans. **54**(11), 1965–1973 (2007)

79. A. Hyvarinen, Fast and robust fixed-point algorithms for independent component analysis. IEEE Trans. Neural Networks **10**(3), 626–634 (1999)

80. N.K. Al-Qazzaz, et al., *Entropy-Based Markers of EEG Background Activity of Stroke-Related Mild Cognitive Impairment and Vascular Dementia Patients*, in *2nd International Conference on Sensors Engineering and Electronics Instrumental Advances (SEIA' 2016)* 2016: Barcelona, Spain. p. 92-94

81. W. Chen et al., Characterization of surface EMG signal based on fuzzy entropy. IEEE Trans. Neural Syst. Rehabil. Eng. **15**(2), 266–272 (2007)

82. N.V. Chawla et al., SMOTE: Synthetic minority over-sampling technique. J. Artif. Intell. Res. **16**, 321–357 (2002)

83. R. Kohavi. *A study of cross-validation and bootstrap for accuracy estimation and model selection.* in *Ijcai.* (1995)

84. Y. Song, J. Zhang, Discriminating preictal and interictal brain states in intracranial EEG by sample entropy and extreme learning machine. J. Neurosci. Methods **257**, 45–54 (2016)

85. I.H. Witten, E. Frank, *Data Mining: Practical Machine Learning Tools and Techniques* (Morgan Kaufmann, 2005)

86. M. Hall et al., The WEKA data mining software: An update. ACM SIGKDD Explorations Newsletter **11**(1), 10–18 (2009)

87. H. Esmaiel et al., Multi-stage feature extraction and classification for ship-radiated noise. Sensors **22**(1), 112 (2021)

88. N.K. Al-Qazzaz, et al. *The role of spectral power ratio in characterizing emotional EEG for gender identification.* In *2020 IEEE-EMBS conference on biomedical engineering and sciences (IECBES).* (IEEE 2021)

89. S.E. Sánchez-Hernández et al., Evaluation of feature selection methods for classification of epileptic seizure EEG signals. Sensors **22**(8), 3066 (2022)

90. H. Cai et al., Study on feature selection methods for depression detection using three-electrode EEG data. Interdiscip. Sci. Comput. Life Sci. **10**(3), 558–565 (2018)
91. H. Cai et al., A pervasive approach to EEG-based depression detection. Complexity **2018**, 1–3 (2018)
92. Y. Li et al., EEG-based mild depressive detection using differential evolution. IEEE Access **7**, 7814–7822 (2018)
93. H. Peng et al., Multivariate pattern analysis of EEG-based functional connectivity: A study on the identification of depression. IEEE Access **7**, 92630–92641 (2019)
94. S. Mahato et al., Detection of depression and scaling of severity using six channel EEG data. J. Med. Syst. **44**(7), 1–12 (2020)
95. J. Zhu et al., An improved classification model for depression detection using EEG and eye tracking data. IEEE Trans. Nanobioscience **19**(3), 527–537 (2020)
96. R.A. Movahed et al., A major depressive disorder classification framework based on EEG signals using statistical, spectral, wavelet, functional connectivity, and nonlinear analysis. J. Neurosci. Methods **358**, 109209 (2021)
97. Y. Narayan, Motor-imagery EEG signals Classificationusing SVM, MLP and LDA classifiers. TURCOMAT **12**(2), 3339–3344 (2021)
98. N.K. Al-Qazzaz et al., An integrated entropy-spatial framework for automatic gender recognition enhancement of emotion-based EEGs. Med. Biol. Eng. Comput. **60**, 531–550 (2022)
99. N.K. Al-Qazzaz et al., EEG wavelet spectral analysis during a working memory tasks in stroke-related mild cognitive impairment patients, in *International Conference for Innovation in Biomedical Engineering and Life Sciences*, (Springer, 2015)
100. N.K. Al-Qazzaz, et al. *Entropy-based markers of EEG background activity of stroke-related mild cognitive impairment and vascular dementia patients. in Sensors and electronic instrumentation advances: proceedings of the 2nd international conference on sensors and electronic instrumentation advances* (2016)

Printed in the United States
by Baker & Taylor Publisher Services